T0137488

Assessment of Population Health Risks of Policies

Gabriel Guliš • Odile Mekel
Balázs Ádám • Liliana Cori
Editors

Assessment of Population Health Risks of Policies

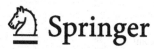
Springer

Editors
Gabriel Guliš
Unit for Health Promotion Research
University of Southern Denmark
Esbjerg, Denmark

Balázs Ádám
University of Southern Denmark
Esbjerg, Denmark

University of Debrecen
Debrecen, Hungary

Odile Mekel
Unit Innovation in Health
NRW Centre for Health
Bielefeld, Germany

Liliana Cori
Institute of Clinical Physiology
National Research Council
Rome, Italy

ISBN 978-1-4939-4629-7   ISBN 978-1-4614-8597-1 (eBook)
DOI 10.1007/978-1-4614-8597-1
Springer New York Heidelberg Dordrecht London

Foreword

Health impact assessment claims to be applicable to policies, programmes and projects but relatively little work on policy has been reported. The appearance of a book on assessing the health consequences of national policies in several countries is to be warmly welcomed. The contrasting of a top-down approach (assessing the health consequences of a proposed or an existing policy) and a bottom-up approach (starting with a health problem and working back to policy solutions for that problem) is a useful addition to our thinking on this subject. The bottom-up approach chimes with the suggestions made elsewhere that impact analysis should not be a final step, which is only undertaken when a policy has been finalised, but should be an integral part of the whole policy-making process. Throughout the book emphasises how causal diagrams and full-chain thinking help to unpick the consequences of policy. The approach in RAPID relies very heavily on epidemiological thinking and pays little attention to the stakeholder participation, which is emphasised in other approaches.

The analysis of health consequences of policy becomes even more informative if it is possible to quantify the impacts. A chapter in this book explores how far this is the case for the impacts described in the top-down and bottom-up case studies. It demonstrates both how far quantification is possible and the knowledge gaps which limit quantification.

While most of the book is concerned with national policy one chapter looks at international policy taking the example of the European Union Health Strategy. This demonstrates how the approaches developed in RAPID can add to our understanding and should be adopted by European policy makers.

However in order to improve policy it is necessary both that policy advisers explore and assess the health consequences and that policy makers take notice of those assessments. It is encouraging that EU policy makers in DG SANCO chose to support and commission this RAPID project but its success will depend on the degree to which policy makers take note of the work described. In some of the cases described in this book the analysis of health consequences was requested by the relevant policy-making body in the country concerned. In other cases it appears that the consequences of a policy were examined but it is not clear whether the relevant policy makers requested or took notice of the work.

The RAPID team recognised the key role played by policy makers and another chapter describes the series of workshops involving health experts and crucially policy makers which explored the findings of RAPID. We are told that the policy makers were favourably impressed by the progress made but it will be fascinating to know if the policy-making process in these countries changes to pay more attention to health consequences.

The work described in this book is far too important to gather dust on the book-shelf. It could make a valuable contribution to making Health in All Policies a reality. Policy advisers need to take notice of it even if they sometimes need help to understand the more technical aspects of some chapters. Equally policy makers need to be aware that they can be helped to a clearer knowledge of the likely health consequences of policy options and so make better trade-offs between the various policy goals, thus improving the health of the populations they serve.

In summary the writing team are to be congratulated on producing a fascinating book and substantially moving forward our thinking on assessing the health consequences of national and international policy.

John Kemm

Introduction

Human activities are mostly guided with the intention to improve well-being and lives of people, increase security and improve conditions of living environment. Yet, history provides us with many cases where a good intention proved to have harmful impact on environment and human health. A well-known example is the case of introduction of pesticides, a group of chemicals to protect agricultural production, increase harvest and provide necessary nutrition to people. Time has shown that this good intention has serious negative impact on environment and human health. A methodology to assess potential risks of different chemicals has been developed and widely introduced to minimise such risks; risk assessment as a scientific discipline began to influence human lives and minimise potential negative impacts. While concerned with, e.g., individual chemicals or even a mix of them, risk assessment fulfils the expectations and contributes significantly to extended lifespan.

The end of the twentieth century presented a new challenge to risk assessment and public health. Interaction of different determinants of health such as social and environmental, economic and behavioural has been described and a call for a methodology to assess potential impacts of policies on health has been raised. Health impact assessment responded to this need, mostly focusing on projects and programmes rather than policies. The assessment of economic, social and environmental effects of policies have acquired in the last decade an increasing relevance, especially in the European Union context, where the harmonisation of different cultures and legislative background requires an effort toward common standards and understanding.

The present book, based on products of a European Commission, Directorate for Health and Consumers (DG SANCO) via Executive Agency for Health and Consumers (EAHC)-funded project called "Risk Assessment from Policies to Impact Dimension (RAPID)", aims to provide readers with a developed guidance to assess population health risks of policies.

Major development in public health operations, risk assessment, health impact assessment and the Health in All Policies approach is described in first two chapters guiding the reader to get acquainted to the "full-chain reasoning". In the context of the work presented in this book a link from a policy via main determinants of health and risk factors to concrete health outcomes is understood under the term "full chain."

Following, in two chapters the development of the guidance is described. First, the classical impact assessment angle is employed and a top-down (from policy to health effect) path is followed in a set of national case studies as well as in the summarised guidance document. Responding to the fact that public health practice is often in the opposite position, e.g. based on existing health problems public health practitioners need to argue on the role of other than health sectors on health, a separate set of case studies presents the development of the guidance on bottom-up direction (from health outcome to policy/policies).

In both directions while conducting the case studies quantification of effects on different levels of the full chain proved to be the most important cross-cutting issue. Reflecting on this a full chapter is devoted to discuss quantification and reviews the "state of the art" in this field.

In the current globalised world applicability of any method, tool or guidance on international level is a key issue. The RAPID guidance based on agreement with EAHC and DG SANCO has been tested on the Health Strategy of the European Commission and Chap. 6 provides the summary of findings.

Any tool, method or guidance has little value if there is no user to use it in everyday life. A set of consultations with experts coming from different sectors and expertise areas conducted in the format of workshops in ten countries of Europe provided valuable insights into the practical use of the RAPID guidance. Moreover, the workshops provided an excellent setting for recognition of how important the national context is. Language is a key issue even in a globalised world. Risk assessment, similar to public health, has different meaning in different languages and cultures. As a consequence, an instrument developed, discussed and implemented by a multinational and multidisciplinary group of researchers can bear an added value.

The present book highly acknowledges not only the financial support provided by EC via DG SANCO and EAHC but also most importantly the willingness and openness of all colleagues in ten countries who were doing their best to overcome the language and context barrier and provide significant input to international readers and users of policy risk assessment methodology.

Acknowledgements

Editors and authors of chapters of this book acknowledge a research grant from the European Commission Health and Consumer Protection Directorate-General via Executive Agency for Health and Consumers grant agreement no. 20081105 which made the presented work possible.

Contents

1 **Public Health, Policy Analysis, Risk Assessment,
 and Impact Assessment**.. 1
 Gabriel Guliš, Joanna Kobza, Jana Kollárová, Ingrida Zurlyte,
 Mariusz Geremek, Ágnes Molnár, and Fabrizio Bianchi

2 **Risk Assessment, Impact Assessment, and Evaluation**.......................... 13
 Piedad Martin-Olmedo and Odile Mekel

3 **Top-Down Policy Risk Assessment** 37
 Balázs Ádám, Ágnes Molnár, Gabriel Guliš, Peter Otorepec,
 Razvan Chereches, Joanna Kobza, Jana Kollárová, Nunzia Linzalone,
 Marek Majdán, Sarah Sierig, Odile Mekel, Peter Mochungong,
 Jozef Pastuszka, Ingrida Zurlyte, and Rainer Fehr

4 **Bottom-Up Policy Risk Assessment**.. 131
 Peter Otorepec, Piedad Martin-Olmedo, Julia Bolivar, Odile Mekel,
 Jutta Grohmann, Daniela Kállayova, Mária Kvaková, Jana Kollárová,
 Ágnes Molnár, Balázs Ádám, Stella R.J. Kræmer, Mariusz Geremek,
 Joanna Kobza, and Rainer Fehr

5 **Quantification of Health Risks**.. 199
 Odile Mekel, Piedad Martin-Olmedo, Balázs Ádám, and Rainer Fehr

6 **Application of RAPID Guidance on an International Policy**............... 233
 Gabriel Guliš, Liliana Cori, Sarah Sierig, and Odile Mekel

7 **Use of Policy Risk Assessment Results
 in Political Decision Making**... 249
 Liliana Cori, Gabriel Guliš, Joanna Kobza, Ágnes Molnár,
 and Jana Kollárová

Index.. 263

Contributors

Balázs Ádám University of Southern Denmark, Esbjerg, Denmark
University of Debrecen, Debrecen, Hungary

Fabrizio Bianchi Institute of Clinical Physiology, National Research Council, Pisa, Italy

Julia Bolivar Escuela Andaluza de Salud Pública, Granada, Spain

Razvan Chereches Babes-Bolyai University, Cluj-Napoca, Romania

Liliana Cori Institute of Clinical Physiology, National Research Council, Rome, Italy

Rainer Fehr University of Bielefeld, Bielefeld, Germany

Mariusz Geremek Medical University of Silesia, Katowice, Poland

Jutta Grohmann NRW Centre for Health (LZG.NRW), Bielefeld, Germany

Gabriel Guliš University of Southern Denmark, Esbjerg, Denmark

Daniela Kállayova Trnava University, Trnava, Slovakia

Joanna Kobza Medical University of Silesia, Katowice, Poland

Jana Kollárová Regional Public Health Authority, Kosice, Slovakia

Stella R.J. Kræmer University of Southern Denmark, Esbjerg, Denmark

Mária Kvaková Trnava University, Trnava, Slovakia

Nunzia Linzalone Institute of Clinical Physiology, National Research Council, Pisa, Italy

Marek Majdán Trnava University, Trnava, Slovakia

Piedad Martin-Olmedo Escuela Andaluza de Salud Pública, Granada, Spain

Odile Mekel NRW Centre for Health (LZG.NRW), Bielefeld, Germany

Peter Mochungong Environmental Health Centre Health Canada, Ottawa, ON, Canada

Ágnes Molnár Centre for Research on Inner City Health, Li Ka Shing Knowledge Institute, St. Michael's Hospital, Toronto, ON, Canada

University of Debrecen, Debrecen, Hungary

Peter Otorepec National Institute of Public Health, Ljubljana, Slovenia

Jozef Pastuszka Silesian University of Technology, Gliwice, Poland

Sarah Sierig NRW Centre for Health (LZG.NRW), Bielefeld, Germany

Ingrida Zurlyte Health Education and Disease Prevention Center, Vilnius, Lithuania

Chapter 1
Public Health, Policy Analysis, Risk Assessment, and Impact Assessment

Gabriel Guliš, Joanna Kobza, Jana Kollárová, Ingrida Zurlyte, Mariusz Geremek, Ágnes Molnár, and Fabrizio Bianchi

Introduction

Public health has been defined as "the science and art of preventing disease, prolonging life and promoting health through the organized efforts and informed choices of society, organizations, public and private, communities and individuals" (Winslow 1920) or as "the art of applying science in the context of politics so as to reduce inequalities in health while ensuring the best health for the greatest number" (WHO 1998). As the challenges of public health have evolved, from sanitary

G. Guliš (✉)
Unit for Health Promotion Research, University of Southern Denmark, Niels Bohrsvej 9-10, 6700 Esbjerg, Denmark
e-mail: ggulis@health.sdu.dk

J. Kobza • M. Geremek
Medical University of Silesia, 18 Medykow Street, 40-752 Katowice, Poland
e-mail: koga1@poczta.onet.pl; m.geremek@poczta.onet.pl

J. Kollárová
Regional Public Health Authority, Ipelska 1, 04011 Kosice, Slovakia
e-mail: kollarova@ruvzke.sk

I. Zurlyte
Health Education and Disease Prevention Center, Kalvariju Street 153, LY-08221 Vilnius, Lithuania
e-mail: Ingrida@post.omnitel.net

Á. Molnár
Centre for Research on Inner City Health, Li Ka Shing Knowledge Institute,
St. Michaels's Hospital, 209 Victoria St., Rm. 3-26.22, Toronto, ON M5B 1C6, Canada
e-mail: MolnarAg@smh.ca

F. Bianchi
Institute of Clinical Physiology, National Research Council, Regione Toscana,
Pisa Area di Ricerca di San Cataldo, Via Moruzzi,1-56127, Pisa, Italy
e-mail: fabrizio.bianchi@ifc.cnr.it

G. Guliš et al. (eds.), *Assessment of Population Health Risks of Policies*,
DOI 10.1007/978-1-4614-8597-1_1, © Springer Science+Business Media New York 2014

surveillance and infectious diseases in the past, to chronic diseases, lifestyle factors, socioeconomic conditions, occupational and environmental health determinants, health reforms and others, so have the methods of assessment advanced by research technologies development. The new health threats and epidemics, such as AIDS, SARS (Severe Acute Respiratory Syndrome), influenza H5N1, or emergencies like natural disasters or bioterrorism, effects of globalization and migration present new tasks to public health governance requiring new working methods.

There is no common consensus on the meaning of public health (Kaiser and Mackenbach 2008) and its future goals (Weil and McKee 1998) and there are different understandings among states about objectives and how public health services are organized (Allin et al. 2004). The new public health can be generally defined as an integrative approach to protect and promote the health status of the individuals and population. New public health focuses especially on disease prevention, health promotion, education and cross-sectoral action, including decisions and activities beyond the health system, well-being and health of society, communities, and individuals (Baum 2007).

The policy of new public health is based on responsibility of national, regional, and local governments, with significant international engagement (e.g., World Health Organization—WHO, European Commission—EC) for the well-being and health of society and self-care by the community and the individual. From European perspective, the new public health policy no longer concentrates on a series of separate or specific condition-oriented programs as it had over the past several years. Currently, the focus has been switched to health status, health determinants and health systems. This is also reflected by the key European health documents such as the EC health strategy (EC 2007).

Terms used to define public health functions are also numerous and develop over time. The most mentioned in core global health policy documents are: monitoring health status of population; identification of main health problems and hazards in the communities; health education; enforcement of laws to protect health; developing policies and plans which support individual and community health; ensuring of professional medical and public health workforce; evaluation of accessibility, quality and effectiveness of health services for individuals and population; supporting research for implementation of best practices and innovative solutions to health problems; and developing community partnerships to protect population health and promote health improvement. The newest public health action must adapt to an ever changing environment, taking into consideration a conjunction of financial, demographic and technological pressures and barriers. Yach highlighted that governments should respect and ensure the structure and sustainable delivery of essential public health functions, because they represent public goods (Yach 1996).

The intersectoral nature of contemporary public health leads to necessity to develop the relations between partners from many sectors. Among them are policy makers, public health experts and practitioners, business representatives, community leaders, media, NGOs, volunteer committees.

The Institute of Medicine in its report highlighted assessment as one of the three key functions of public health as important as policy development and service assurances (IOM 2002). It stated that health data monitoring involves regular assessment of community health status and identification of main health risks.

The assessment process must be conducted on both national and community level. The key aim is to identify potential health hazards and benefits and consider their importance for society.

Although numerous political documents express the inclusion of health considerations into decision making process and policy, e.g., the Amsterdam Treaty of the European Union, article 152 (in Lisbon treaty article 168), mentions protection of human health in all Community policies and activities as a main task, only few impact assessment guidelines give detailed information how to assess health impacts of policies and how to include health experts in decision making processes. The possibility to influence policy making process in other sectors by public health professionals is often limited and the capacity of research institutions to support public health goals and programs is still very weak. The technical capacity to conduct risk assessment is also not adequately developed across Europe (WHO 2012) especially with regard policies.

Essential Public Health Functions (Operations) and Place of Policy Analysis and Impact Assessment

There are different views and understanding of the term "public health" by different countries and cultures. There are countries where public health is equal to health protection and the need to enter the field of policy analysis and impact analysis of policies is not that strongly perceived. The essential public health functions defined first by CDC (http://www.cdc.gov/nphpsp/essentialservices.html) and later adopted by WHO (Bettcher et al. 1998) served as a unifying element around the globe on content of public health. Recently WHO Europe modified the terminology to Essential public health operations (http://www.euro.who.int/en/what-we-do/health-topics/Health-systems/public-health-services/policy/the-10-essential-public-health-operations) and updated the list. The ten Essential public health operations are as presented in Table 1.1.

The first five operations are considered as core operations and the second five as supportive ones. The issue of policy analysis and impact analysis is clearly linked to operation No. 4 "health promotion including action to address social determinants and health inequity" and also No. 6 "assuring governance for health and well-being." Both these operations require knowledge of policy cycles, policy making processes, policy analysis, and impact assessment.

Health promotion including action to address social determinants of health and health inequity simply must include policy development and impact assessment parts. Health inequities are related to inequities in social determinants of health. Low income, low educated people living in poor neighborhoods have less opportunities to pursue healthy lifestyles. Income redistribution policies, social policies, neighborhood planning policies, transportation policies, employment and education policies are all contributing to development of inequities. Health promotion by enhancing responsibility for one's health and determinants of health includes not

Table 1.1 Essential public health operations

1. Surveillance of population health and well-being
2. Monitoring and response to health hazards and emergencies
3. Health protection including environmental, occupational, food safety, and others
4. Health promotion including action to address social determinants and health inequity
5. Disease prevention, including early detection of illness
6. Assuring governance for health and well-being
7. Assuring a sufficient and competent public health workforce
8. Assuring sustainable organizational structures and financing
9. Advocacy, communication, and social mobilization for health
10. Advancing public health research to inform policy and practice

only the level of individual behavior and community action but also the structural policy level becoming a natural place for policy impact assessment processes.

To ensure governance for health and well-being policies need to be developed and implemented on the way which minimizes any hazard on health status of the population and on the other hand allows for maximum positive health impacts. Mechanisms, guidance's and tools, preferable standardized tools are needed to ensure development of policies to promote health and being able to assess their impact on health.

Largely, but not exclusively these two essential public health operations are to identify policies relevant to be assessed for their health impacts. The task of policy impact assessment is not a new issue. The Ottawa charter (WHO 1986) is often credited with bringing this issue into public health by introducing the term "healthy public policy."

Healthy Public Policies

Health promotion by its principles goes beyond health care. It aims to put health on the agenda of policy makers in all sectors and at all levels, directing them to be aware of the health consequences of their decisions and to accept their responsibilities for health. This approach builds up the principle of healthy public policies. It is believed that coordinated action on legislation, fiscal measures, taxation and organizational change leads to better health, income and social policies that foster greater equity. The aim must be to make the healthier choice the easier choice for policy makers as well.

Health in All Policies

The principle of building healthy public policies was revised at beginning of twenty-first century and presented by Finland as the "health in all policies" approach. Health in All Policies (HiAP) is the approach of including, integrating or internalizing health in other policies that shape or influence the determinants of health. These determinants include transport, housing, education, social, tax, and agricultural policies for example. Health in All Policies is more concerned with the structural issues on any level of governance (local, regional, national, and international) and less with individual programs or projects. Relevant issues could also be dispersed in multilevel governance systems. Health considerations should, according to HiAP, be included in the development, implementation and evaluation of policies. This approach requires a new form of governance where there is joined-up leadership within governments, across all sectors and between levels of government (Adelaide Statement 2010).

To implement the HiAP principle in addition to personal capacities, tools and methods to recognize potential hazards of a developed policy on health and conduct an assessment of hazards are necessary. In optimal situation this can be done by public health experts; however in real life scenario it is hard to expect that each sector will have own trained public health experts who are involved in development of new policies. The importance of availability of standardized tools and methods is therefore increasing.

A key question which needs to be answered is at which stage or moment of policy development should the assessment of potential impacts on health be completed. Knowledge of policy development process theories is therefore necessary to estimate the proper timing.

Policy Making Models and Public Health

In most cases the policy cycle is described by needs assessment, policy development, implementation and evaluation. Often, impact assessment procedures are considered best when prospective, so at the stage of policy approval or adoption in between development and implementation. To apply fully the HiAP principle the best choice however is inclusion of policy impact assessment into developmental phase of a policy.

According to the literature, policymaking can take place in several different ways, some more rational than others. There are many different categorizations of the policy making process. The models presented in the following should not be construed as exhaustive but have been selected on the basis of their previously identified relevance in studies of evidence use (Hanney et al. 2003).

It is an ongoing discussion, whether policy is being developed on a rational basis. The rational model for policy making is characterized by the idea of a direct, linear relationship between means and ends. Evidence should be used as a means to achieve a defined goal. The rational model has formed the basis for several modified models of both normative character (The Satisfying Model, The Limited Rational Model, The Extended Rational Model) and positive character (Muddling Through, Mixed Scanning, Garbage Can, Appropriateness Model). These models describe either how policy processes should proceed (normative), or how this is really happening (positive).

Normative Models

A modification of the rational model can be found in the idea of *bounded rationality*. Humans' ability to process information is perceived to be limited, and it is also limited how much information can be taken into account when a decision must be made. The cost of searching for information and exploring alternatives and consequences may outweigh the benefits. In addition, time is a limiting factor since policy processes often runs within a limited time frame (Pedersen 2006; Hanney et al 2003; Nutley and Davis 2007).

Studies show that people frequently act from experience and new knowledge is understood from what is already known. Knowledge that contradicts current assumptions can be rejected, while knowledge that confirms these assumptions are chosen. Moreover, a satisfying solution is many times chosen over an optimal solution. This leads to the concept of *the administrative man*, who is not rational, but limited rational. Limited rationality can be characterized by (Pedersen 2006; Hanney et al 2003; Nutley and Davis 2007; Jacobsen and Thorsvik 2002):

- Goals are unclear and changeable
- Only selected solutions and their impact is assessed
- Solutions are evaluated sequentially, as there is capacity to assess them
- The first satisfying solution is chosen

Positive Models

It has long been recognized that policymaking is a complex process. The process may involve evidence as well as a series of other factors such as different interests, values, personal ambitions of policy makers etc. In the policy process, evidence must also "compete" with other sources of knowledge derived from common sense, general knowledge, empirical data etc. Incremental models of policy making allow different stakeholders a role in the policy debate and use many sources of information that may influence policymakers (Hanney et al 2003; Nutley and Davis 2007).

Incrementalism is a part of the decision-making model called "Muddling Through." According to this model, the order of the policy making process is not necessarily that of the perfect rational model. In the analysis of alternative solutions and their consequences new targets can be discovered. For this reason, it is not possible to formulate policies in a straightforward manner. Furthermore, analysis of alternatives and consequences is incomplete and thus incremental decisions are taken. This process is in contrast with the rationality assumption, since policy makers do not necessarily have clear goals, and they can return to goal formulation later in the policy process (Jacobsen and Thorsvik 2002).

Another model of the positive nature of policy making is "garbage can" model. This model suggests that solutions not previously used still are present in the policy-making system. When other problems occur later, these solutions can be used. Kingdon (Kingdon 1984, 1995) has developed a model for the policy process inspired by the garbage can model. He envisions three independent streams: a problem stream, an alternative stream, and a political stream. At various times these streams are brought together. A problem becomes urgent, and then a solution from alternative stream is chosen, which then is fed into the policy stream. The probability that the three streams meet depends on whether there is an opening, a so-called window of opportunities. This calls for specific solutions when one suddenly sees an opportunity and exploits it (Pedersen 2006; Hanney et al 2003; Nutley and Davis 2007). Models such as the garbage can model highlight the way in which policy making can be seen as a "sloppy" process more than a process that systematically follows several relevant processes (Hanney et al 2003; Nutley and Davis 2007).

These models for policy making are all important for different policy processes within public health (Nutley and Davis 2007) and public policy making.

Do any of the presented policy making models favor the use of impact assessment? Is there a higher chance to employ policy risk assessment by any of the presented models? Answers to these questions are not yet known.

Principles of Risk Assessment and Application of Them for Policies

Risk assessment is a scientific method to establish information about the hazards usually related to a single concrete chemical, biological or physical substance or mixture of substances. It consists of well-defined steps and usually leads to establishment of numerical, quantitative information about a hazard. The standard steps of risk assessment are described more in depth in following Chap. 2.

The application of principles of risk assessment to policies is not a simple task. The reasons are highly variable;

- Standard risk assessment deals with concrete subject (usually a chemical substance), e.g., in public health language a concrete risk factor.
- Although cumulative risk assessment deals with mixtures of substances it still rather rarely considers social risk factors in assessment.
- Policies mostly influence the distribution of such risk factors. An example could be given on air pollution. Risk assessment allows us to establish limit values for PM_{10}, SO_2, NO_x, and other chemicals in air, but an energy policy of a country is influencing via selection of power generation means which of these pollutants and at what extent are expected to be present in ambient air over coming years.
- Projects and programs can be banned based on established limit values; policies however are rather rarely banned. They might be modified or updated but in most of cases they are applied. An example can be given based on DDT use. DDT as single substance is banned from use due to its long-term toxic effect. But by policy of WHO this substance is still allowed to be used under specific circumstances if there is no other chemical available to prevent against mosquitoes and malaria. Another example can be on traffic injuries, the risk of fatal traffic injuries

is usually expressed in number of fatalities compared to overall volume of traffic. But humans are not banning traffic; we modify policies to decrease the risk, but do not ban traffic.

Due to these differences in case of policy related risk assessment it seems to be more appropriate to speak about policy health impact assessment as direct risk assessment.

These examples lead to the need to apply the full chain principle while doing policy risk assessment. In contrary to a single or mixed substance hazards policies usually influence a set of determinants of health which are leading to changes in distribution and prevalence of risk factors (the "single substances") and they in turn influence prevalence and distribution of health outcomes. This approach we call further in book the "full chain approach." In scientific literature as well as in practice risk assessment (including cumulative risk assessment) deals with relation of a concrete hazard (or mix of hazards) and health effect; the full chain approach aims to analyze also factors influencing presence and distribution of hazards. In public health literature the "causes of causes" approach (CSDH 2008) or causal diagrams (Joffe and Mindell 2006) are described mostly in relation to either the social determinants of health or to health impact assessment. When constructing the full impact chain the hardest issue is to distinguish between determinants of health and risk factors. This is a general issue within public health and there are several explanations description including terminology. The Commission on social determinants of health of WHO following work of Rose (Rose 1992) introduced the term "causes of the causes" (CSDH 2008), Keleher is using the term proximal and distal determinants of health (Keleher and Murphy 2004) and the term "wider determinants of health" is also used in public health literature (Bambra et al 2010). For Risk Assessment from Policy to Impact Dimension (RAPID) project which provides background for this book and for the RAPID guidance we understand determinants of health those structural determinants which are directly linked to policies and represent the two upper levels of the Dahlgren & Whitehead model of health (Dahlgren and Whitehead 1991). Risk factors are on other hand directly linked to concrete population at risk and are direct outcome of changes in determinants of health.

Does policy risk assessment differ from policy evaluation? Yes, it does! Policy evaluation can be better defined as a process by which general judgments about quality, goal attainment, program effectiveness, impact, and costs can be determined. In essence, policy evaluation is the process used to determine what the consequences of public policy are and what has and has not been achieved (Theodoulou and Kofinis 2003). Policy evaluation consists of process, outcome, impact, and cost–benefit evaluation and it is mostly done retrospective, e.g., after a policy is implemented.

Impact Assessment of Policies

Impact assessment (IA) is a process aimed at structuring and supporting the development of policies. It identifies and assesses the problem at stake and the objectives pursued. It identifies the main options for achieving the objective and

Table 1.2 Review of impact assessments

Impact assessment	Determinants of health targeted	Differences
Environmental impact assessment (Barker and Wood 1999)	Environment	Focus on environmental determinants of health, mostly on physical environment on local, regional, or national level
Strategic environmental impact assessment (WHO 2005)	Environment on international and strategic level	Focus on environmental determinants of health, mostly on physical environment on international, trans-boundary level
Social impact assessment (WHO 2005)	Social	Focus on social determinants of health
Economic impact assessment (Rushton et al. 1999)	Economic	Focus on economic determinants of health, cost–benefit, and other types of economic analysis
Health technology assessment (Douma et al. 2007)	Health technologies	Focus on health care technologies used within health sector
Health system impact assessment	Health system	Focus on impact of policies, plans, projects on health system of a country
Health impact assessment	All	Includes all determinants and focuses on impact on health of the population

analyzes their likely impacts in the economic, environmental, and social fields. It outlines advantages and disadvantages of each option and examines possible synergies and trade-offs (http://ec.europa.eu/governance/impact/index_en.htm accessed 19/04/2013).

There are several impact assessment methods; Table 1.2. summarizes different impact assessments and describes differences compared to Health Impact Assessment (HIA) and target areas in terms of the determinants of health.

All mentioned impact assessment aims to assess impacts of policies, plans, projects on usually a single determinant of health or group of determinants of health. Health impact assessment (HIA) as defined by Gothenburg consensus paper (WHO 1999), aims to assess future impacts of recent plans, policies, projects, and programs on health and determinants of health. As HIA aims to inform and influence decision making process it is preferably used *prospectively* (before the decision is made), but it could be applied also as concurrent (during implementation of a decision) or retrospective (after a decision is implemented; in this case it helps to develop capacities and prepare for future updates of a decision). As given by Kemm (Kemm et al. 2004) it targets decision making both in non-health and within health sectors. Health impact assessment picks up the information from all sectors and aims to assess their impact on determinants of health and if possible directly on health. By doing so, it provides information to decision makers both in non-health and health sectors to make decision which have a potential to harm human health.

Not all of mentioned impact assessments are dealing with impacts of policies.

Conclusion

Risk assessment, impact assessment, and understanding policy making are crucial issues of contemporary public health. The following chapter is going to discuss more in depth the principles of risk assessment and health impact assessment and their application specifically on policies.

References

Adelaide Statement on Health in All Policies. (2010). Moving towards a shared governance for health and well-being. Report from the International Meeting on Health in All Policies, World Health Organization (WHO), Adelaide.

Allin, S., Mossialos, E., Mc, K. M., & Holland, W. (2004). *Making decisions on public health: A review of eight countries.* Brussels: WHO, European Observatory on Health Systems and Policies.

Bambra, C., Gibson, M., Sowden, A., Wright, K., Whitehead, M., & Petticrew, M. (2010). Tackling the wider social determinants of health and health inequalities: Evidence from systematic reviews. *Journal of Epidemiology and Community Health, 64*(4), 284–291.

Barker, A., & Wood, C. H. (1999). An evaluation of EIA system performance in eight EU countries. *Environmental Impact Assessment Review, 19*, 387–404.

Baum, F. (2007). *The new public health.* Melbourne: Oxford University Press.

Bettcher, D. W., Sapirie, S., & Goon, E. H. (1998). Essential public health functions: Results of the international DELPHI study. *World Health Statistics Quarterly, 51*(1), 44–54.

CSDH (WHO Commission on Social Determinants of Health). (2008). *Closing the gap in a generation: Health equity through action on the social determinants of health. Final Report of the Commission on Social Determinants of Health.* Geneva: World Health Organization.

Dahlgren, G., & Whitehead, M. (1991). *Policies and strategies to promote social equity in health.* Stockholm, Sweden: Institute for Future Studies.

Douma, K. F. L., Karsenberg, K., Hummel, M. J. M., Bueno-de-Mesquita, J., & van Harten, W. H. (2007). Methodology of constructive technology assessment in health care. *International Journal of Technology Assessment in Health Care, 2*, 162–168.

Hanney, S. R., Gonzalez-Block, M. A., Buxton, M. J., & Kogan, M. (2003). The utilisation of health research in policy-making: Concepts, examples and methods of assessment. *Health Research Policy and Systems, 1*(1), 2.

Health impact assessment toolkit for cities; Document 1; From vision to action, WHO Copenhagen. (2005). Retrieved on 18 Apr, 2013, from http://www.euro.who.int/en/what-we-do/health-topics/environment-and-health/urban-health/publications/2005/health-impact-assessment-from-vision-to-action

Health impact assessment; Main concepts and suggested approach. (1999). WHO. Retrieved on 27 Jun, 2007, from http://www.euro.who.int/document/PAE/Gothenburgpaper.pdf

Health Report. (1998). *Life in the 21st century, a vision for all.* Geneva: World Health Organization.

Jacobsen, D. I., & Thorsvik, J. (2002). *Hvordan organisationer fungerer. Indføring i organisation og ledelse.* København: Hans Reitzels Forlag.

Joffe, M., & Mindell, J. (2006). Complex causal process diagrams for analyzing the health impacts of policy interventions. *American Journal of Public Health, 96*, 473–479.

Kaiser, S., & Mackenbach, J. P. (2008). Public health in eight European countries: An international comparison of terminology. *Public Health, 122*(2), 211–216.

Keleher, H., & Murphy, B. (2004). *Understanding health: A determinants approach.* London: Oxford University Press.

Kemm, J., Parry, J., & Palmer, S. (2004). *Health impact assessment*. Oxford: Oxford University Press.

Kingdon, J. D. (1984, 1995). *Agendas, alternatives and public policies*. Boston, MA: Little Brown and Company.

Nutley, S. W., & Davis, T. O. (2007). *Using evidence, how research can inform public services*. Bristol: The Policy Press.

Pedersen, K. M. (2006). *Sundhedspolitik, Beslutningsgrundlag, beslutningstangen og be-slutninger i sundhedsvæsnet*. Odense: Syddansk Universitetsforlag.

Preliminary review of institutional models for delivering essential public health operations in Europe, WHO. (2012). Accessed 18 Apr, 2013, from http://www.euro.who.int/en/what-we-do/health-topics/Health-systems/public-health-services/publications2/2012/preliminary-review-of-institutional-models-for-delivering-essential-public-health-operations-in-europe

Rose, G. A. (1992). *The strategy of preventive medicine*. Oxford, NY: Oxford University Press.

Rushton, J., Thornton, P. K., & Otte, M. J. (1999). Methods of economic impact assessment, Rev. sci.tech. Off. int. Epiz., *18*(2), 315–342.

The EU Health Strategy, White paper. Together for health: A strategic approach for the EU 2008–2013. European Commission (2007). Retrieved on 14 Jan, 2013, from http://ec.europa.eu/health-eu/doc/whitepaper_en

The Future of the Public's Health in the 21st Century, 2002, Committee on Assuring the Health of the Public in the 21st Century, Board on Health Promotion and Disease Prevention, Institute of Medicine, The National Academies Press, Washington, DC. (2002). Retrieved on 27 Jan, 2013, from   http://www.iom.edu/Reports/2012/For-the-Publics-Health-Investing-in-a-Healthier-Future.aspx

Theodoulou, S. Z., & Kofinis, C. (2003). The Art of the Game: Understanding Public Policy, Wadsworth Publishing, USA.

Weil, O., & McKee, M. (1998). Setting priorities for health in Europe: Are we speaking the same language? *European Journal of Public Health, 8*, 256–258.

WHO. (1986). *The Ottawa charter on health promotion*. Geneva: World Health Organization.

Winslow CEA. (1920). The untitled fields of public health, *Science 51*(*1306*), 23–33, DOI: 10.1126/science.51.1306.23

Yach, D. (1996). Redefining the scope of public health beyond the year 2000. *Current Issues in Public Health, 2*, 247–252.

Chapter 2
Risk Assessment, Impact Assessment, and Evaluation

Piedad Martin-Olmedo and Odile Mekel

Introduction

Public health evolution has experienced some relevant hits throughout history. One was the improvement of sanitary conditions and the control of infectious diseases. The second focused on the contribution of individual behaviors to non-communicable diseases and premature death. The most recent one conceptualizes health as a key dimension of quality of life (Kickbusch 2003).

The World Health Organization (WHO) has shown in subsequent reports that global health can extensively be improved both by a systematic identification and assessment of more relevant underlying causes of diseases and injury, and by taking actions for preventing or reducing those risk factors. Behavioral risks including alcohol, tobacco and drugs consumption, unsafe sex or eating habits (leading in some countries to high rates of overweight, obesity and high levels of blood pressure and cholesterol), together with environmental factors such as poor water sanitation or indoor and ambient air pollution have proved to be responsible for about one-third of the total global burden of disease throughout the world. Tackling causal risk factors effectively offers the prospect of millions of premature deaths being prevented, and a great improvement on quality of life for populations in all countries (WHO 2002, 2004, 2009). Health services, although very relevant in defining the course of the illness process, are less important in determining population's health (Kemm 2001; WHO 2004, 2009). In this way health protection and health promotion, averting and diminishing major risk factors, have been set up as core priorities worldwide for the last decades.

P. Martin-Olmedo (✉)
Escuela Andaluza de Salud Pública, Cuesta del Observatorio 4, 18080 Granada, Spain
e-mail: piedad.martin.easp@juntadeandalucia.es

O. Mekel
Unit Innovation in Health, NRW Centre for Health (LZG.NRW), Bielefeld 33611, Germany
e-mail: odile.mekel@lzg.gc.nrw.de

G. Guliš et al. (eds.), *Assessment of Population Health Risks of Policies*,
DOI 10.1007/978-1-4614-8597-1_2, © Springer Science+Business Media New York 2014

An early model developed to get a better understanding of what contribute to sickness and health was the one proposed by Lalonde (Lalonde 1974), which grouped risk factors into four levels: human biology, lifestyles, environment and health organization. Under this framework it was considered that the greatest efforts to improve population's health status should be done in the field of individual behavior changes, using a narrow approach of epidemiological association between individual risk factors and health outcomes.

However, it is now widely accepted that the causal pathway leading to an adverse health outcome does not depend on isolate risk factors but on the intricate relation of those elements with broader socioeconomic, cultural, environmental, and political conditions (WHO 2002; Dahlgren and Whitehead 2007; Kemm 2007; Metcalfe and Higgins 2009). This approach was already acknowledged in the preamble of the constitution of WHO when referring to the concept of "health" (WHO 1948), and in the Ottawa Charter (WHO 1986). The so-called social view of health generated under this new framework focused its attention not on individual behaviors and communities at risk but in the whole population within a setting. Public health targets moved towards building healthy communities, healthy workplaces, strengthening the wide range of social networks for health, and increasing people's capacity to lead healthy lives (Kickbusch 2003).

From late 1980s, this approach was widening by considering not only the models and determinants explaining the health status of the population, but also how certain factors (unemployment, unsafe workplaces, housing deprivation, etc.) contribute to health disparities within a population both at group and individual level (Wilkinson and Marmot 2003; Sen 2004; Gehlert et al. 2008; Harris-Roxas and Harris 2011). Analyzing social, environmental, and working conditions as upstream factors in multilevel models can improve the design and implementation of interventions targeted at levels downstream from those conditions (Gehlert et al. 2008). WHO has placed significant emphasis on this perspective by establishing the Commission on Social Determinants of Health (Solar and Irwin 2010).

The design and implementation of healthy public policies that, directly or indirectly, address health determinants was proposed by the Ottawa Charter (WHO 1986) as a valuable promoting action to achieve a substantial improvement in quality of life, conceptualizing health as a "resource for living" (Kickbusch 2003). In this way, the Charter urged health to be included on the agenda of policy makers in all sectors that might affect the every-day life of people at all levels. Healthy public policies has been defined as a policy that takes accountability of all possible health impacts, acknowledging the causal pathways resulting from the modification of upstream health determinants (mostly environmental conditions, living and working conditions, and community influences), and related risk factors downstream (WHO 1986; Kemm 2001; Joffe and Mindell 2004; Metcalfe and Higgins 2009; Kearns and Pursell 2011). This approach was strengthened by subsequent revisions and strategies such as *Health for All in the Twenty-first century* (WHO 1999) which underlined that the majority of health determinants reside outside the health sector, and highlighted the need for a complex intersectoral political and social collaboration.

To this respect, the European Union, first at the Treaty of Maastricht and more explicitly at the Amsterdam Treaty, declared that "a high level of health protection shall be ensured at the definition and implementation of all Community policies activities" (European Communities 1997). The strategy of "Health in All Policies" (HiAP), adopted at the Finnish European Union (EU) Council Presidency in 2006 (Ståhl et al. 2006), has become increasingly important in Europe as governments realize that reducing inequalities and improving health are fundamental enablers for economic development (Solar and Irwin 2010; Lin et al. 2012). The second programme of Community action in the field of health (2008–2013) of the European Parliament and Council also calls "to support the mainstreaming of health objectives in all Community policies and activities" (European Commission 2007).

The increasing call for a better protection of citizen's health demands a better understanding of the existing forms for characterizing health impacts of policies, and the purposes for which they are undertaken. Differences in concepts, frameworks and procedures among various approaches (risk assessment, health impacts assessment, etc.) have arisen in relation to specific issue of concern (i.e., waste disposal; electromagnetic fields, biotechnology, social disparities, urban planning, etc.), or due to perceived weakness in practice (i.e., the food safety crisis that took place in late 1980s and 1990s as the occurrence of BSE (mad-cow)). The present chapter intends to provide an overview of some of those approaches, especially risk assessment for health and health impact assessment, considering them in the political context they appeared, and the purpose they have been applied for. Finally some attention will be paid to the process called "policy evaluation," as a different tool used in the improvement of healthy policy formulation and practice.

Risk Assessment

Every aspect of life involves risk, and how we deal with it depends largely on our understanding of the concept and its assessment. Although there are many possible definitions about "risk," from a public health perspective it is broadly conceived as "the probability of an adverse health outcome, or a factor that raises this probability" (WHO 2002, pp. 9). The introduction of this concept establishes quite an advantageous step forward by contrast with the idea of "hazard," which refers to any agent (biological, chemical or physical) or situation having the potential to cause harmful effects when a person or population is exposed to that agent or situation (IPCS 2004; FAO/WHO 2006). In this way, hazard refers only to a qualitative perspective related to the inherent characteristics of the agent (i.e., intrinsic toxicity of a chemical, or pathogenicity and virulence of a microorganism). However, the use of risk implies the possibility to quantify how probable is that a person or a population might get in contact with an hazardous agent or a risk factor (this means to become exposed to), and at the same time allows to quantify the severity of the possible consequences of that exposure, mainly in terms of health outcomes but also as socioeconomic impact.

So, in summary risk assessment methods consist of models that describe and predict how potential sequences of events, resulting from human actions or natural failures, can lead to exposure, while accounting for the magnitude and severity of the consequences (Ricci 2006).

This terminology and approach has been widely used in the fields of chemical or food safety when, as an example, we refers to the human exposure to toxic substances present in the environment or in foodstuff. It can however also be applied to other hazardous situations or risk factors related to behavioral options or to the socioeconomic environment where people live (WHO 2002, 2009). In this way, and assuming the framework of the social determinants of health mentioned before, the causal pathway leading to a particular health outcome can be displayed as complex diagrams where public interventions (policies and programs) are key upstream health determinants, which implementation would generate different exposure scenarios by modifying downstream the distribution of certain risk factors in the population (Joffe and Mindell 2002, 2006; Dahlgren and Whitehead 2007; Solar and Irwin 2010). In the *World Health report 2002* by WHO focused on "Reducing Risk, Promoting Healthy life," a different terminology is used, referring to upstream health determinants as distal risk factors, and downstream health determinants as proximal risk factors (WHO 2002). Whatsoever, it is essential to consider the whole causal chain when addressing the potential impacts of a policy on health. This broader analysis of the potential impacts of a policy on the population health is the main objective of the present book, being discussed in several chapters.

Early Framework and Procedure for Risk Assessment

The different aspects of the physical environment that can influence human health have been the focus of many studies in the last decades, and build the roots of the risk assessment approach. A wide range of human and natural activities from protecting air and water to ensuring the safety of food, drugs, and consumer products such as toys, have made of risk assessment an important public-policy tool for informing regulatory and technologic decisions, setting priorities among research needs, and developing approaches for considering the costs and benefits of regulatory policies. Today, national and international legislation dealing with environmental and health protection require from risk assessment to rank and guide the selection of optimal management choices (Ricci 2006; NRC 2009).

The National Environmental Policy Act (NEPA 1969), adopted in 1969 set up the foundation for the environmental policy in the United States (USA), including as a major objective the protection of human health and welfare. This far-reaching legislation is a reference in the early development of the risk assessment procedure as a tool to understand and address a wide variety of hazards and situations that pose chronic health risks. This process was instrumental for the U.S. Environmental Protection Agency (EPA) and other federal and state agencies, industry, the academic community and others for several years, although, it is not till 1983 that a harmonized definition and uniform guideline was proposed by the U.S. National Research Council (NRC) in the *Risk Assessment in the Federal Government: Managing the Process* (NRC 1983). In this document also known as the Red Book, risk assessment was defined as "the characterization of the potential adverse health effects of human exposures to environmental hazards," including both, quantitative and qualitative expressions of risk. Excluded from this concept were the analysis of perceived risks, comparisons of risks associated with different regulatory strategies, and the analysis of the economic and social implications of regulatory decisions (functions assigned to risk management) (NRC 1983, pp. 18).

In this initial model, risk assessment procedure was divided into four major steps:

(a) *Hazard identification* involving the identification of all situations or agents capable of causing adverse health effects in a particular exposure scenario, characterizing the nature and strength of causation based on data from epidemiological studies, animal-bioassays, in vitro effects studies, and comparison of molecular structures. Key information to be considered under this stage refers also to toxicokinetics (how the body absorbs, distributes, metabolizes, and eliminates chemicals) and toxicodynamics (effects that chemicals have on the body) as well as potential mode of actions (or toxicity pathways) related to the health effects identified (NRC 1983; EPA 2012).

(b) *Dose–response assessment* describing the relationship between the amount and condition of exposure to an agent (the dose provided), and the probability and severity of an adverse health effect (the responses) in the exposed population. The response assessed may be the incidence of some endpoint or health outcome (i.e., cancer incidence, incidence of a critical effect, etc.), or it may describe the magnitude of response (i.e., magnitude of IQ loss). Traditionally different mechanisms were proposed for carcinogenic (non-threshold) and other health effects (threshold), although this is currently under revision (NRC 2009). The information is obtained by reviewing the scientific evidence generated in epidemiological and toxicological studies, which implies the use of extrapolating methods and assumptions (i.e., from high to low dose or from animal bioassay to humans). Those statements introduce quite an important source of biological uncertainty that need to be properly described and justified (NRC 1983; EPA 2012).

(c) *Exposure assessment*, as a process of measuring the intensity, frequency, and duration of human exposures to an agent currently present in the environment, or hypothetically released as result of future human actions. The information gathered at this stage refers normally to the distribution and concentration of a hazard in the environment allowing the characterization of the exposure pathways (contaminant source or release, environmental fate and transport, exposure point or area, exposure route, and potentially exposed population), as well as data on behavioral and physiological characteristics of the actually or potentially exposed population (NRC 1983). Modeling is often used to estimate the environmental concentration of hazards that people are exposed to in relation to a source of emission (NRC 1994). Biomonitoring (measuring concentrations of the chemicals, their metabolites, or their adducts in human specimens) is another approach used for exposure assessment (Calafat et al. 2006).

(d) *Risk characterization* is the final step where the exposure and dose–response assessments are combined in estimating the nature and the magnitude of human risk according to the different exposure scenarios identified. As a fundamental step in supporting decision making, all key findings and important considerations about risk need to be clearly reported at this stage, including factors such as the nature and weight of evidence for each step of the process, the estimated uncertainty of the component parts, the distribution of risk across various sectors of the population, and the assumptions contained within the estimates (NRC 1983, 1994; EPA 1984, 2000, 2012).

The risk assessment process was proposed to be objective, transparent, systematic, science-based, well-planned, fully documented, subjected to peer review, and updated as new evidence become available (NRC 1983). Those attributes and values are currently shared by any field and context where risk assessment is being applied (IPCS 2004; FAO/OMS 2006; NRC 2009; EPA 2012).

Each step of the risk assessment process is subject to scientific judgments and policy options such as how to deal with uncertainty, type of inferences and assumptions applied when data availability is inconsistent (also known as defaults), or those choices affecting the utility of the assessment's results for decision making. The expression "risk assessment policy" is used to refer to all those considerations which should be explicitly distinguished from the political, economic, and technical concerns inherent to the design and choice of regulatory strategies (risk management) (NRC 1983, 2009; FAO/WHO 2006). Default values should be scientifically justified, and be based on existing data and representative of the missing parameter. The different agencies and international organizations involved in risk assessment have established and published a set of defaults values used in their evaluations (i.e., EFSA 2012; EPA 2011a, b). Documentation of all assumptions contributes to the consistency and transparency of risk assessment.

Under this framework, risk assessment was proposed to be undertaken independently from risk management to ensure the impartiality of the outcomes, although a fluid communication and interaction in both directions was strongly encouraged (NRC 1983). However, this independency has been taken sometimes to the extreme of making of the risk assessment a tool with no clear purpose within the policy-decision process, generating a gap between science and policy action (Montage 2004).

Some Application of Risk Assessment in the Formulation of Policies and Strategies

A wide variety of guidelines and methodological guidance have been produced worldwide on the bases of this procedure, especially to support the regulation of chemical substances and to assess the health risk of human exposure to environmental hazards. It is worth mentioning the extensive work done by EPA applying risk assessment to inform a broad range of regulatory decisions such as: restriction of pesticide usage, setting remediation goals to hazardous waste site, usage of hazardous materials, establishing standards for ambient air quality, or standards to control the emissions of hazardous air pollutants. EPA's 2012 report, *Framework for Human health Risk Assessment to Inform Decision Making*, provides a detailed list of guidance and manuals that EPA has developed for different topics, and for the performance of each one of the four steps of the risk assessment process. A comprehensive set of links to key EPA tools and guidelines can also be accessed at EPA's Risk Assessment Portal (http://www.epa.gov/risk/). The general output of the process applied by EPA, especially as part of site remedial investigations, refers to numeric estimate of theoretical risk, focusing on current and potential future exposures and considering all contaminated media regardless if exposures are occurring or are likely to occur. By design, it generally uses standard (default) protective exposure assumptions when evaluating site risk (EPA 2000, 2011b, 2012).

The ATSDR (U.S. Agency for Toxic Substances and Disease Registry) also developed a procedure called *Public Health Assessment* (PHA) that incorporates the same four steps of the risk assessment process, but differing from EPA approach by focusing more closely on site-specific exposure conditions regarding past, present or future polluting activities affecting particular communities. In addition to environmental and exposure data, PHA also incorporates specific community health concerns, and any available health effects data (toxicological, epidemiological, medical, and health outcome data) to provide a site-specific evaluation, and identify appropriate public health actions (ATSDR 2005).

The International Programme on Chemical Safety (IPCS) set up by WHO intends to provide governments as well as international and national organizations with consistent procedures and tools to ensure the safety of human health and the environment regarding all activities involving chemicals. It covers a full range of exposure situations from the natural presence of chemicals in the environment to their extraction or synthesis, industrial production, transport, use, and disposal. So it comprises aspects related to environmental health, occupational health or food safety, among others.

In last decades, IPCS has produced harmonized risk assessment methods, as well as risk assessments reports on specific chemicals based on the Red Book's four steps-procedure. These products include Concise International Chemical Risk Assessment Documents, International Chemical Safety Cards, Pesticide Data Sheets, Poisons Information Monograph, Standards for drinking water quality, or Monographs and evaluations of contaminants and additives in foodstuff. IPCS also plays a very important role in the implementation of international agreements such as the *Globally Harmonized System of Classification and Labelling of Chemicals* or the *Global Environment Monitoring System—Food Contamination Monitoring and Assessment Programme (GEMS/Food)*. An exhaustive list of publications, tools and links referring to IPCS activities can be obtained from the IPCS Web site (http://www.who.int/ipcs/en/).

Risk assessment has also been an important element in improving the formulation of policies in the domain of food safety. The increasing complexity of the food chain, the rapid globalization with greater movement of people and goods, the drastic changes in dietary patterns and food preparation preferences, the emergence of new pathogens, or the introduction of new technology in food processing and manufacturing operations are just some of the challenges that modern food safety systems must confront. The food safety crises in the 1990s, particularly the one related to the bovine spongiform encephalitis, generated a significant controversy regarding existing monitoring and control measurements, and highlighted the need to assume a more systematic, scientific and interactive approach to respond to food safety problems. To this respect, and in order to meet the new demands of modern food safety, FAO and WHO proposed from 1995 that governmental bodies would adopt a new structured decision-making process called "*Risk analysis.*" Under this framework the formulation of new food safety policies should be done following an iterative, ongoing and highly interactive process involving a systematic and transparent collection, analysis, and evaluation of all relevant scientific and nonscientific information about food hazards, so the best option to manage the associated risks could be selected (FAO/WHO 1995, 2003). Risk analysis can be used for example to characterize the level of risk associated to the presence of a certain chemical in a foodstuff helping governments to decide which, if any, actions should be taken in response (i.e., setting or revising a maximum limit for that contaminant, review of labeling requirements, etc.). This process also enables authorities to identify the various points of control along the food chain at which measures could be applied, to weigh up the costs and benefits of different options, and to determine the most effective one(s) (FAO/WHO 2006). In Europe, this framework was adopted in 2002 by the General Food Law Regulation (Article 6 of Regulation 178/2002) as the basis for the future development of all EU food safety legislation.

Risk analysis includes three independent but closely interrelated components: risk management, risk assessment and risk communication (FAO/WHO 2003, 2006). As stated in the Red Book, risk analysis framework also emphasis the need for a quite distinctive separation between risk assessment and risk management though keeping a frequent and continuous dialogue between the two components. At international level, risk management defining food safety standards is undertaken by different Codex Committees (Committees on Food Hygiene, Meat Hygiene, Food Additives, Contaminants, Pesticide Residues, and Residues of Veterinary Drugs in Foods), while risk assessment providing the science-based support for those standards is assumed by the three Joint FAO/WHO Expert Bodies: the Joint Expert Committee on Food Additives (JECFA); the Joint Meeting on Pesticide Residues (JMPR); and the Joint Expert Meeting on Microbiological Risk Assessment (JEMRA). Additional risk assessments may be provided, on occasion, by ad hoc expert consultations, and by member governments that have conducted their own assessments (FAO/WHO 2006). In Europe, the European Commission, European Parliament and EU Member States are the key risk managers in the EU system. They are responsible for making European policies and taking decisions to manage risks. The European Food Safety Authority (EFSA), based in Parma (Italy), is the responsible for food related risk assessment in the EU, producing scientific opinions and advice to support the Commission and other risk managers in the policy-making processes. Other EU agencies who apply risk assessment are: European Centre for Disease Prevention and Control (ECDC), the European Medicines Agency (EMA), the European Chemicals Agency (ECHA), and the European Environment Agency (EEA). In addition three non-food Scientific Committees managed by DG SANCO (SCCS, SCHER, SCENIHR) and the Scientific Committee on Occupational Exposure Limits (SCOEL), managed by DG Employment complete the EU risk assessment system.

The process to conduct risk assessment within the risk analysis framework consists of the same four steps proposed in the Red Book's procedure, with the exception that the "dose–response assessment" step is here designated as "hazard characterization" (FAO/WHO 2003, 2006), but keeping a similar approach. An additional phase to the procedure in this field is the so-called "*risk profile*," a frame that contextualizes the food safety problem, defines public health objectives, and identifies priorities before starting the risk assessment itself. Information gathered for a risk profile helps in deciding about the feasibility, depth and length of the risk assessment to be conducted according to available resources, legal and political considerations. A risk profile is similar to the scoping and screening stages used under other forms of impact assessment. Typically the risk profile includes a brief description of: the situation, foodstuff or commodity involved; information on pathways by which consumers are exposed to the hazard; potential risks associated with that exposure; consumer perceptions of the risks; the distribution of possible risks among different population groups; and current control measures. The risk profile is considered to be a responsibility of risk managers but in practical terms is primarily developed by risk assessors or others with specific technical expertise, and finally discusses and agreed by managers (FAO/WHO 2006).

In the field of food safety (and other fields of public health), specific differences in the procedure to conduct a risk assessment are mainly related to the type of hazard (i.e., chemical, biological, or physical hazard), the exposure scenario (i.e., known hazards versus emerging hazards, technological issues, complex hazard pathways such as for antimicrobial resistance) and the time and resources available. One of the most relevant issues refers to the different nature between chemical and biological hazards. The first ones are considered to enter in the food chain as part of row ingredients or through very concrete processing steps (i.e., additives or packaging migrants), remaining stable after the point of introduction, and causing mainly chronic health effects with some exceptions as potential acute health effects related to pesticide exposure. On the contrary, biological hazards are extremely ubiquitous and can radically change over time, growing, declining, or dying before a food is consumed. They cause normally acute health problems from a single edible portion of food, and generate a wide variability in health response (FAO/WHO 2006).

Risk Assessment Outputs

Results from risk assessment can be expressed in qualitative or quantitative terms with various intermediate formats.

Qualitative risk assessments outputs are the quickest to be obtained, but their value could be controversial for being rather subjective. Nonetheless, this approach could be quite useful depending on the context. They can be obtained by creating matrix that assigns risk ratings (low, moderate or high) to each one of the parameters affecting risk (likelihood of exposure, severity of the associated health outcomes, vulnerability or susceptibility of the population). A basic problem is that the three descriptors (high, medium, low) are often inadequate, and it is necessary to introduce some kind of numerical ranking for each category. The qualitative assessment outputs require even do of an extensive understanding of all the parameters affecting risk, reliable and accurate data about each factor, as well as a predefinition of the criteria used for assigning weight to each parameter (FAO/WHO 2006). An example of how to apply this approach is proposed by Fletcher (Fletcher 2005) for the field of fishery management. Traditional methods to incorporate expert knowledge in these circumstances and improve the quality and transparency of final qualitative outputs, include the Delphi method, the nominal group approach, focus groups, scenario analysis, rational consensus, self-scoring, collective scoring, surveys and questionnaires, interviews and case studies, among others.

In quantitative risk assessments, the outputs are expressed numerically, either in deterministic or probabilistic terms. The former used numerical point values (generally the mean or the 95th percentile value) for each parameter contributing to the risk (i.e., concentration of a chemical in a specific environmental media; the average daily consumption of drinking water, average body weight of the affected population, etc.), to generate a single risk estimate. Usually choices are the values that represent the most likely value, or alternatively values that capture the so called worst case situation or "worst case scenario" (i.e., the highest environmental concentration of a pollutant that population might be exposed to, or dietary exposures for frequent consumers). Using most likely values may be sufficient if the variability affecting most of the parameters is low, and the problem is well characterized. The use of a worst case scenario is more protective but could also lead to an unrealistically overly conservative output, of difficult applicability in adopting risk management options according to available resources. Deterministic techniques have been for years the approach most widely applied in risk assessment involving chemical hazards.

In the probabilistic approach the input values are distributions, and the final output is a range of possible scenarios of risk (characterized by a probabilistic distribution too), informing also about the variability and uncertainty associated with the calculated risk estimate. These two terms are often interchanged but they are not equivalent in the risk assessment process. According to the NRC, *uncertainty is the lack of precise knowledge as what the truth is, whether qualitative or quantitative* (NRC 1994 cited by Ricci 2006), for example because inadequate data exist, or because the biological phenomena involved are not well understood (FAO/WHO 2006; IPCS 2008). Risk assessors should provide an explicit description of uncertainties in the risk estimate and their origins, including a description of how assumptions may have influenced the final outputs. *Variability* describes the *range of possible values for any measurable characteristic inherent of a population, inasmuch as people vary substantially in their exposures and their susceptibility to potentially harmful effects of the exposure* (NRC 2009). Variability cannot be reduced, but it can be better characterized with improved information.

The probabilistic modeling is considered to address more effectively and realistically the characterization of risk, but it demands larger resources and data, being more difficult and complex to be applied. It is increasingly used for the risk assessment of biological hazards.

A more exhaustive description of methods available for quantitative health risk assessment is described in Chap. 5 of this book.

Epidemiological Approach for Health Risk Assessment

A slightly different approach used in public health for risk assessment considers this process as the *systematic evaluation of changes in the population health resulting from modifying the distribution of population exposure to a risk factor or a group of risk factors* (Murray et al. 2003; WHO 2004). The major difference with previously reported procedures refers to the risk estimates which are not presented in terms of absolute risk (yes/no), excess risk (i.e., 3–4 times higher risk), or added risk. The so called *comparative quantification of health risk assessment* involves calculating the *population attributable risk*, or where multilevel data are available, *potential impact fraction (PIF)*, defined as the proportion of future burden of disease or injury that could be avoidable if current or future exposure levels to a risk factor or group of risk factors are reduced to hypothetical scenarios. Maldonado and Greenland (2002) and Murray et al. (2003) refer to those scenarios as *counterfactual*, and they imply a reduction in the distribution of a risk factor in the population to a theoretical minimum level (zero or as low as possible), or to a better achievable level (i.e., by 5, 10, 20, or 30 %). The counterfactual approach is considered more useful for policy-makers than the binary categorization into "exposed" and "non-exposed" which can substantially underestimate the importance of the continuous risk factor–disease relationship. The final avoidable burden of disease would be obtained by multiplying the total disease burden for the population (in deaths, hospital admissions or other metrics) by the PIF (Murray et al. 2003; WHO 2002, 2004). Those results could also be combined with cost-benefit analysis techniques to present results both in terms of health impacts and economic terms, of greater utility for policy-makers.

In summary the key methodological steps required are:

(a) Choice of most relevant health endpoint in terms of consistent definition, impact, strength of evidence of relationship with studied risk factors, and availability of baseline occurrence rates
(b) Identifying the population at risk (overall and/or susceptible groups)
(c) Selection of exposure indicators and study area for exposure assessment

(d) Definition of exposure scenarios
(e) Choice of the most suitable exposure–response function (i.e., relative risk for a given change in exposure) obtained from a systematic revision of the scientific literature that best fit to the studied population and exposure scenarios

The epidemiological health risk assessment approach has been a main focus of WHO early work on environmental health risk assessment and comparative burden of diseases (WHO 2000, 2002, 2004, 2009). This procedure has also been applied in several projects focused on the assessment of the health impacts related to a group of risk factors such as certain ambient air pollutants (Hurley et al. 2005; Pascal et al. 2013) or other environmental stressors (Prüss-Üstün et al. 2003; Hänninen and Knol 2011) or lifestyle risk factors (Soerjomataram et al. 2010; Lim et al. 2012).

The use of the terminology "health impact assessment" to refer to this methodology has created some misunderstanding and confusion with a much broader concept of the assessment of potential health impacts of a policy, programs or project on the health of a defined population, which will be described later in this chapter.

Improving Risk Assessment Procedure

The application of risk assessment has been increasingly extended to new issues and far-reaching public health and environmental questions as the scientific evidence and analytical techniques improved through time. However, its credibility is being challenged. Risk assessment findings have been accused of being unnecessarily complex sometimes, and not well connected to the needs and demands of the decision-making process. Furthermore, the lack of adequate procedure for involving all stakeholders at appropriate point in the risk assessment process has been identified as a pitfall that reduces reliability and transparency to the outputs (Montage 2004; Schreider et al. 2010).

The NRC's *Science and decisions: Advancing Risk assessment* (NRC 2009) provides recommendations for the improvement of the technical aspects and utility of risk assessment. Some of the most relevant suggestions, from a decision-support perspective, refer to:

- Better engagement in formative stages to the questions formulated by decision-makers, planning and designing risk assessment to evaluate the merits of different risk management options, rather than making of the risk assessment an end in itself. In this way, it is suggested to enclose the Red Book's paradigm (NRC 1983) into a new framework with enhanced problem formulation and scoping, and detailed definition of the required depth of the scientific analysis.
- The need to move from a narrow scope involving a single cause–effect pathway (i.e., a single chemical and a single adverse effect) to a more holistic assessment addressing risk posed by multiple stressors throughout multiple pathways.

- The level of detail for characterizing uncertainty and variability within the risk assessment process should be planned from the beginning, adjusting its complexity to the decision-making needs.
- It is also suggested to establish a formal process for stakeholder involvement throughout all stages but with time constraints to ensure that decision making schedules are met.

Similar developments can be observed in Europe: the European Commission is aware of the need for a new conceptual framework in risk assessment which should be an *"exposure-driven, flexible, tiered approach, drawing continually on advances in technology and scientific understanding of biology, which meets the needs of stakeholders"* (EU 2012, pp. 76). Currently, a public consultation on the discussion paper addressing the new challenges for risk assessment is under way.

Many of the proposed changes match with the evolution of the concept of health previously described.

Health Impact Assessment

The Gothenburg consensus paper defined Health Impact Assessment (HIA) as "a combination of procedures, methods and tools by which a policy, program or project may be judged as to its potential effects on the health of a population, and the distribution of those effects within the population" (WHO Europe 1999). HIA intends to assist decision makers by providing a set of evidence-based recommendations on the causal pathways that link the different possible scenarios related to the implementation of a policy to potential health outcomes through a set of upstream health determinants and downstream risk factors (Kemm 2001, 2007; Joffe and Mindell 2002, 2006; Metcalfe and Higgins 2009). Its ultimate goal is to support the development of healthy policies by adjusting the design or adding new components to original proposals that maximize health gains, and minimize negative outcomes and health inequalities (Joffe and Mindell 2005; Mindell et al. 2008; Harris-Roxas and Harris 2011).

The most widely current practice of HIA takes as a reference the social view of health and equity, which as described above, gives a great importance to health determinants linked to interventions from non-health sectors (i.e., economy, agriculture, housing, occupation, transport), and to major equity indicators (gender, ethnicity and social class) (Metcalfe and Higgins 2009; Solar and Irwin 2010). In this way, HIA has been considered as a promising tool for promoting an effective implementation of the HiAP strategy, as well as for addressing potential health inequalities that might arise from a proposal (European Commission 2007; Wismar et al. 2007; WHO-Government of South Australia 2010; Harris-Roxas and Harris 2011; McQueen et al. 2012; Kemm 2013). Furthermore, HIA intends to promote coordinated cross-governmental actions, and a better understanding of the decision making process, adding transparency and democracy by involving other stakeholders (Kemm 2007; Salay and Lincoln 2008).

HIA Categorization and Forms

There is a broad variety of forms in which HIA is undertaken in practice. To categorize these forms, different criteria have been used (see Table 2.1). Some of those conditions refer somehow to technical aspects such as kind of intervention, its extension or complexity, the spatial scale to which it is applied, timing for conducting the HIA, or the methodology used. One of the critical points discussed for long refers to the appropriateness and utility to conduct concurrent or retrospective HIA. Those approaches although interesting from a scientific point of view, allowing gathering evidence for improving future HIAs, are late in providing useful information to the decision-making process. Therefore, there is a broad consensus that HIA should be performed preferably prospectively (Kemm 2001, 2013).

Cole et al. (2005), and Harris-Roxas and Harris (2011) proposed two different ways for categorizing HIA, the former based on the diverse origin of HIA, and the second on the purposes for which HIA is been conducted. Both proposals, complementary to a certain extent, allow a better understanding of the existing forms of HIA, and also identify major challenges to build capacity for a larger HIA implementation in the future.

Table 2.1 HIA characterization according to different criteria

Criteria	Type of HIA[a]
Type of proposal	Policies/programs
	Projects
Level of application	Supranational
	National
	Local
Extent	Desk-top
	Rapid
	Comprehensive
Health's model	Broad
	Tight
Timing	Prospective
	Concurrent
	Retrospective
Origin	Quantitative/analytic approach
	Participatory approach
	Procedural approach
Purpose	Mandated
	Decision-support
	Advocacy
	Community-led

[a]Cole et al. 2005; Joffe and Mindell 2005; Davenport et al. 2006; Mahoney et al. 2007; Kemm 2000, 2007; Veerman et al. 2005; Mindell et al. 2008; Bhatia and Werham 2008; Bhatia and Seto 2011; Harris-Roxas and Harris 2011

According to Cole et al. (2005), variations in HIA practice is very much related to the different fields from which they were promoted, detailed as follows:

- The "quantitative/analytic approach" strongly linked to the risk assessment framework applied mostly in the field of environmental health, but also in toxicology, epidemiology, engineering, economics and food safety. As described previously, this approach used for a long time a biomedical health model involving a single cause–effect pathway, although more recently HIA practitioners from those fields are considering multiple stressors and health outcomes, including some equity analysis. The functionalities of this approach from the decision-makers' perspective are: (1) the possibility to compare management alternatives (see previous description for *counterfactual scenarios*), and (2) its apparent objectivity in spite of the fact that it incorporates numerous assumptions. However, not all important health determinants and health outcomes can be measured, so the final picture in terms of health impacts provided by this approach is frequently quite partial, and responds to very specific purposes (i.e., alternatives for water treatment; defining maximum exposure values for air pollutants). Other limitations of this approach are quite similar to the ones already reported for risk assessment; basically its high cost, high demand of time and data, and its little stress on public participation procedures. Some examples of this approach were reported by Cole et al. (2005), Veerman et al. (2005), and Bhatia and Seto (2011).
- The "participatory approach" grounded on the Ottawa Charter's principles (WHO 1986), incorporates a more holistic health model, where all major causal pathways linking policy options, upstream health determinants, and health outcomes are tried to be identified in the assessment process. Under this framework the key input for analysis is the information provided through stakeholder participation, using mostly qualitative methodologies. This approach is considered to bring greater democratization and transparency to the decision-making process. However, the qualitative nature of the information generated makes more difficult the comparison among policy options, and also, depending on the context, is given less legitimacy for claiming changes in formulating a policy. Examples can be found in the USA (Dannenberg et al. 2008) as well as the extensive practice developed in European countries (Cole et al. 2005; Metcalfe and Higgins 2009; Kemm 2013).
- The "procedural approach" is coupled to the Environmental Impact assessment (EIA), a process legally binding for many countries worldwide that intends to ensure that environmental considerations (including social and health effects) are explicitly addressed and incorporated into the development of certain large projects, such as a dam, a motorway, or the construction of a factory (Salay and Lincoln 2008). The potential barriers and opportunities for integrating HIA within EIA process are still challenging tasks (Bhatia and Werham 2008). The existence of methods broadly disseminated and understood is proposed to ensure a relatively easy, transparent and reproducible manner to conduct HIA. On the contrary, some authors claimed that health considerations in this context have received only isolated attention, and that its emphasis on bureaucratic expediency

are at the root of many of its limitations (Cole et al. 2005; Lock and McKee 2005; Martin-Olmedo 2013).

According to Harris-Roxas and Harris (2011), the use alone of the possible HIA's origin as criteria to classify HIA practice, only leads to futile disagreements and conflicts among practitioners from different fields who claim the primacy of their approach, under-evaluating other disciplines. These authors proposed a typology of four different forms of HIA (see Table 2.1) based primarily on the purpose for which HIA might be undertaken, and also on its origin, the values underpinning the assessment, who should be conducting the assessment and, very important, on the learning that takes place through the process of conducting an HIA (technical, conceptual, and social learning). Those different forms are not totally exclusive from each other, existing in practice some overlaps between different categories (i.e., between advocacy and community-led HIA).

Procedure for HIA

There is no a single correct procedure of HIA as it can be applied to different types of decisions (from international policy to local projects), and a wide range of topics. The appropriate procedure varies depending on the framework and the purpose for which HIA is undertaken (Kemm 2007; Mindell et al. 2008; Harris-Roxas and Harris 2011). Different methodologies are proposed for characterizing the impacts, ideally combining multidisciplinary approaches which involve quantitative and qualitative techniques from a broad variety of academic domains (Joffe and Mindell 2005, 2006; Kemm 2007). Even so most of the different approaches share a five stage procedure with some variations in the terminology. Those phases are generally described (Cole et al. 2005; Joffe and Mindell 2005; Kemm 2007) as:

- *Screening*: a judgment on the added value and feasibility for conducting an HIA on view of the preliminary assessment of potential health impacts of an intervention. It main purpose therefore is to filter out proposals that do not need of a HIA because the impacts on health are either too obvious or not relevant. Screening implies a systematic process using a set of criteria usually listed in a checklist or algorithm, a rapid systematic review of the literature, and if necessary, the consultation to experts and affected stakeholders.
- *Scoping*: it sets the boundaries or term of reference for the HIA; this means a detailed roadmap of the analysis to follow, specifying the concerns of the decision makers and possible policy scenarios under evaluation, the causal pathways to be addressed (from policy to upstream health determinants, risk factors, and health outcomes), methodological aspects (depth of the assessment, geographical and time boundaries, availability of data, methods with equal recognition to qualitative and quantitative approaches), resources, and timetable. A steering committee is established in the scoping part, and the involvement of stakeholders as well as public is clarified.

- *Assessment of impacts*: also known as appraisal or risk assessment is the main stage which clarifies the nature and size of the health impacts likely to result from the scenarios related to a proposed policy. Differential distribution assessment of those impacts in the community is also an important task, although data required for this evaluation is not always readily available, and results are frequently controversial. As described before, this stage is being used wrongly in some context as synonymous of "health impact assessment" by itself. More detailed information on methodological aspects related to this stage, especially about quantification approaches, is developed in Chap. 5 of this book.
- *Reporting to decision-makers*: about the results of the assessment, and suggesting possible actions (including the no action option) for improving the intervention if necessary. The main content of the report should also be presented to all stakeholders who have participated in the process. It is very important that the timeframe for submitting this report meets the schedules of the decision making process. Communication skills are crucial at this stage, being necessary to adjust the language and format of the report to the audience needs.
- *Monitoring and evaluation*: depending on the approach it might include the following aspects: (1) evaluation of the HIA process (a mechanism of quality assurance in terms of planned outputs, cost and equity, and a source of learning for improving future practice); (2) monitoring the acceptance of recommendations (a way to analyze the effectiveness of the HIA process in improving the formulation of healthy policies); and (3) the outcome evaluation, monitoring the predicted impacts once the proposal has been implemented. This last aspect is considered by some authors as a complete different discipline called "policy evaluation".

A set of links to get access to a variety of HIA methodological guidelines, and practical experiences are listed in Table 2.2.

HIA Outputs

The evidence of impacts obtained from different sources at different stages of the HIA process can be both qualitative and quantitative, and include published literature, local data, and stakeholder's experiences (Joffe and Mindell 2005).

This evidence can be presented in different formats. Matrices are visual tools very extensively used for summarizing and structuring the evidence of potential health impacts in a qualitative way. In those matrices, the information gathered refers to:

a. Main health determinants and health outcomes affected;
b. The direction of change (+ if it is a health gain; or − if the impacts means a loss);
c. The severity of the impact (more or less signals of positive or negative depending on the scale of the impact) (Abrahams et al. 2004)

Table 2.2 HIA resources: methodological guidelines, and practical experiences

Name (URL)
WHO HIA Portal (http://www.who.int/hia/en/)
The HIA Gateway (part of Public Health England from 1 April 2013) (http://www.apho.org.uk/default.aspx?QN=P_HIA)
Centers for Disease Control and Prevention (CDC), Atlanta, USA—HIA resources (http://www.cdc.gov/healthyplaces/hiaresources.htm)
Institute of Public Health in Ireland (http://www.publichealth.ie/hia)
New Zealand Ministry of Health (http://www.health.govt.nz/our-work/health-impact-assessment)
Scottish Health Impact Assessment (HIA) Network (http://www.healthscotland.com/resources/networks/HIAresources.aspx)
Wales Health Impact Assessment Support Unit (WHIASU) Web site (http://www.wales.nhs.uk/sites3/home.cfm?orgid=522)
UCLA HIA-Clearing House—HIA-CLIC (USA) (http://www.hiaguide.org/)
CREIS (HIA portal in Spanish), Escuela Andaluza de Salud Pública (Spain) (http://www.creis.es/)
Austrian HIA Web site (HIA portal in German) Gesundheit Österreich (GÖG) (http:// www. goeg.at/)
Swiss HIA Portal (in French and German language), EIS association/GFA Verein (http://www.impactsante.ch/)

Causal pathways diagrams are also a visual way of presenting the multicausal relationships between an intervention and health effects. Each political option, through separate causal pathways, can be considered as different exposure scenario affecting a variety of health outcomes. Some of these causal relationships can be characterized by a function, and its combination may result in some modeling and quantitative outputs. However, very rarely it is possible to quantify the entire model (Joffe and Mindell 2002, 2006; Abrahams et al. 2004; Metcalfe and Higgins 2009)

A number of different quantitative approaches can be used to estimate the changes of the health status of the population due to an intervention. This topic is more extensively developed in Chap. 5 of this book.

Policy Evaluation

Policy evaluation is conceived as a discipline aiming to characterize the results of a policy or any other intervention during or following its implementation rather than predicting in advance potential impacts. This is the most critical difference from the tools previously described, risk assessment and HIA, both focusing mostly in improving policy formulation prior its implementation.

As reference guidance we highlight the H.M. Treasure' 2011 report *The Magenta Book. Guidance for evaluation,* which provides standards of good practice in conducting evaluations, and seeks to meet the specific and practical needs of policy makers and analysts working in public policy at all levels (local and national). According to this guidance a deep understanding of how and why policies work is essential in developing more effective and efficient policies in the future, allowing reinvestment or resource savings.

Policy evaluation is an objective process based on quantitative and qualitative techniques which encompasses three dimensions: (1) "process evaluation" accounting for all aspects related to whether a policy is implemented as intended; (2) "impact evaluation" referring to whether an intervention is effective in meeting its objectives, and (3) "economic evaluation," which compares the benefits of a policy and its cost.

Conclusions

The overview provided in the present chapter has shown that risk assessment and HIA are both valuable tools in supporting the decision-making process, sharing principles and approaches, but with important differences and particularities derived mainly from their origins and evolution through time.

Both frameworks are meant to be objective and systematic processes that intend to provide a set of evidence-based recommendations for the improvement of populations' health in the design of polices and interventions. Other attributes such as being transparent, science-based, well-planned, fully documented, open to participation or independent to the decision making process itself are also common values to both processes under current practice.

Risk assessment, having its roots on environmental health, used for long a biomedical health model involving a single cause–effect pathway which focuses on the relationship of single proximal risk factor and health outcomes, using mainly quantitative techniques for characterizing the impacts. Through time we have seen how the process has been reformulated, incorporating a more holistic approach, considering qualitative techniques, placing more emphasis on the early stage of planning and designing (scoping) to better adapt to questions formulated by risk managers, and improving the involvement of stakeholders.

HIA, linked from its origin to the strategy of HiAP, gives a great importance to health determinants linked to interventions from non-health sectors, adopting as a reference the social view of health and equity. The multidisciplinary approach needed for its compliance has not always been a reality, with confrontations from practitioners from different disciplines who claimed that the emphasis should be placed in one or other methodology (quantitative versus qualitative), when in fact all of them are necessary and/or complementary. Some misunderstanding have arisen regarding the appraisal stage of the process, also named risk assessment, and considered as "health impact assessment" in itself in some contexts.

A current debate is focusing on the convenience for integrating HIA into other forms of impacts assessment (i.e., environmental impact assessment). Enthusiasts of HIA claim that other forms of impact have paid only isolated attention to health considerations so far, and consider that HIA needs to be undertaken independently.

Still, application of risk assessment principles to policies and conduct of health impact assessment of policies is a rather complex and time consuming task. The following two chapters review experience from 10 top-down (policy to health effect direction) and 7 bottom-up (from health effect to policies direction) policy risk assessment case studies coming from ten countries with the aim to develop a methodological guidance for policy risk assessment within or outside HIA.

References

Abrahams, D., Pennington, A., Scott-Samuel, A., Doyle, C., Metcalfe, O., den Broeder, L., et al. (2004). *European Policy Health Impact Assessment (EPHIA) – A guide. IMPACT*. Liverpool: University of Liverpool.

ATSDR (U.S. Agency for Toxic Substances and Diseases Registry). (2005). *Public health assessment: Guidance manual (update)*. Atlanta, GA: U.S. Department of Health and Human Services-Agency for Toxic Substances and Disease Registry.

Bhatia, R., & Seto, E. (2011). Quantitative estimation in health impact assessment: Opportunities and challenges. *Environmental Impact Assessment Review, 31*(3), 301–309.

Bhatia, R., & Werham, A. (2008). Integrating human health into Environmental Impact Assessment: An unrealized opportunity for the environmental health and justice. *Environmental Health Perspectives, 116*(8), 991–1000.

Calafat, A. M., Ye, X., Silva, M. J., Kuklenyik, Z., & Needham, L. L. (2006). Human exposure assessment to environmental chemicals using biomonitoring. *International Journal of Andrology, 29*(1), 166–171.

Cole, B. L., Shimkhada, R., Fielding, J., Kominski, G., & Morgenstern, H. (2005). Methodologies for realizing the potential of health impact assessment. *American Journal of Preventive Medicine, 28*(4), 382–389.

Dahlgren, G., & Whitehead, M. (2007). *European strategies for tackling social inequities in health: Levelling up, Part 2*. Copenhagen: WHO Regional Office for Europe.

Dannenberg, A. L., Bhatia, R., Cole, B. L., Heaton, S. K., Feldman, J. D., & Rutt, C. D. (2008). Use of health impact assessment in the U.S.: 27 case studies, 1999-2007. *American Journal of Preventive Medicine, 34*(3), 241–256.

Davenport, C., Mathers, J., & Parry, J. (2006). Use of health impact assessment in incorporating health considerations in decision making. *Journal of Epidemiology and Community Health, 60*, 196–201.

EFSA (European Food Safety Authority). (2012). Guidance on selected default values to be used by the EFSA Scientific Committee, Scientific Panels and Units in the absence of actual measured data. *EFSA Journal, 10*(3), 2579.

EPA (U.S. Environmental Protection Agency). 1984. *Risk assessment and management: Framework for decision-making*. EPA/600/985/002. Washington, DC: Office of Policy, Planning and Evaluation, U.S. Environmental Protection Agency.

EPA (U.S. Environmental Protection Agency). 2000. *Science policy council handbook: Risk characterization*. EPA/100/B-00/002. Washington, DC: Science Policy Council, U.S. Environmental Protection Agency.

EPA (U.S. Environmental Protection Agency). 2011. *Recommended use of body weights the default method in derivation of the oral reference dose*. EPA/100/R11/0001. Washington, DC: Office of the Science Advisor Risk Assessment Forum, U.S. Environmental Protection.

EPA (U.S. Environmental Protection Agency). 2011b. *Exposure handbook-2011 edition*. EPA/600/R-09/052F. Washington, DC: Office of Research and Development, U.S. Environmental Protection Agency.

EPA (U.S. Environmental Protection Agency). 2012. *Framework for human health risk assessment to inform decision making: EPA risk assessment forum external review draft*. EPA/601/D12/001. Washington, DC: Office of the Science Advisor Risk Assessment Forum, U.S. Environmental Protection Agency.

EU (European Union). (2012). *Addressing the new challenges for risk assessment.* Brussels: European Union.

European Commission. 2007. Decision No 1350/2007/EC of the European Parliament and of the Council of 23 October 2007 establishing a second programme of Community action in the field of health (2008–13). Official Journal L 301, 20/11/2007. Luxembourg.

European Communities. (1997). *Article 152, Treaty of Amsterdam amending the Treaty on European Union, the Treaties establishing the European Communities and certain related acts.* Luxembourg: Office for Official Publications of the European Communities.

FAO (Food and Agriculture Organization) and WHO (World Health organization). (1995). *Application of risk analysis to food standards issues.* Geneva: Joint FAO/WHO Expert Consultation.

FAO (Food and Agriculture Organization) and WHO (World Health organization). (2003). *Codex alimentarius commission. Procedural manual* (13th ed.). Rome: Joint FAO/WHO Food Standards Programme.

FAO (Food and Agriculture Organization) and WHO (World Health organization). (2006). *Food safety risk analysis: A guide for national food safety authorities.* Rome: FAO and WHO.

Fletcher, W. J. (2005). The application of qualitative risk assessment methodology to prioritize issues for fisheries management. *ICES Journal of Marine Science, 62*, 1576–1587.

Gehlert, S., Sohmer, D., Sacks, T., Mininger, C., McClintock, M., & Olopade, O. (2008). Targeting health disparities: A model linking upstream determinants to downstream interventions. *Health Affairs, 27*(2), 339–349.

Hänninen, O., & Knol, A. (Eds.). (2011). *European perspectives on environmental burden of disease. Estimates for nine stressors in six countries.* Helsinki: National Institute for Health and Welfare (THL).

Harris-Roxas, B., & Harris, E. (2011). Differing forms, differing purposes: A typology of health impact assessment. *Environmental Impact Assessment Review, 31*, 396–403.

Hurley, F., Hunt, A., Cowie, H., Holland, M., Miller, B., Pye, S., et al. (2005). *Methodology for the cost-benefit analysis for CAFE Volume 2: Health impact assessment.* Oxon: AEA Technology Environment.

IPCS (International Programme on Chemical Safety). (2008). *Guidance document on characterizing and communicating uncertainty in exposure assessment. In: IPCS Harmonization Project Document. IPCS. Uncertainty and Data Quality in Exposure Assessment No. 6.* Geneva: World Health Organization.

IPCS (International Programme on Chemical Safety)-World Health Organization. (2004). *IPCS risk assessment terminology Harmonization project document no. 1.* Geneva: World Health Organization.

Joffe, M., & Mindell, J. (2002). A framework for the evidence base to support Health Impact Assessment. *Journal of Epidemiology and Community Health, 56*, 132–138.

Joffe, M., & Mindell, J. (2004). A tentative step towards healthy public policy. *Journal of Epidemiology and Community Health, 58*, 966–968.

Joffe, M., & Mindell, J. (2005). Health impact assessment. *Occupational and Environmental Medicine, 62*, 907–912.

Joffe, M., & Mindell, J. (2006). Complex causal process diagrams for analyzing the health impacts of policy interventions. *American Journal of Public Health, 96*, 473–479.

Kearns, N., & Pursell, L. (2011). Time for a paradigm change? Tracing the institutionalisation of health impact assessment in the Republic of Ireland across health and environmental sectors. *Health Policy, 99*, 91–96.

Kemm, J. (2000). Can health impact assessment fulfil the expectations it raises? *Public Health, 114*, 431–433.

Kemm, J. (2001). Health impact assessment: A tool for healthy public policy. *Health Promotion International, 16*(1), 79–85.

Kemm, J. (2007). What is HIA and why might be useful? In M. Wismar, J. Blau, K. Ernst, & J. Figueras (Eds.), *The effectiveness of health impact assessment: Scope and limitations of supporting decision-making in Europe* (pp. 3–13). Copenhagen: WHO, European Observatory on Health Systems and Policies.

Kemm, J. (Ed.). (2013). *Health impact assessment: Past achievement, current understanding, and future progress*. Oxford: Oxford University Press.

Kickbusch, I. (2003). The contribution of the World Health Organization to a new public health and health promotion. *American Journal of Public Health, 93*, 383–388.

Lalonde, M. (1974). *A new perspective on the health of Canadians*. Ottawa, NJ: Ministry of National Health and Welfare, Government of Canada.

Lim, S. S., Vos, T., Flaxman, A. D., Danaei, G., Shibuya, K., et al. (2012). A comparative risk assessment of burden of disease and injury attributable to 67 risk factors and risk factor clusters in 21 regions, 1990-2010: A systematic analysis for the Global Burden of Disease Study 2010. *The Lancet, 380*(9859), 2224–2260.

Lin, V., Jone, C. M., Synnot, A., & Wismar, M. (2012). Synthesizing the evidence: How governance structures can trigger governance actions to support Health in all policies. In D. V. MacQeen, M. Wismar, V. Lin, C. M. Jones, & M. Davies (Eds.), *Intersectoral governance for health in all policies. Structures, actions and experiences* (pp. 23–55). Copenhagen: World Health Organization, European Observatory on Health Systems and Policies.

Lock, K., & McKee, M. (2005). Health impact assessment: Assessing opportunities and barriers to intersectoral health improvement in an expanded European Union. *Journal of Epidemiology and Community Health, 59*, 356–360.

Mahoney, M., Potter, J. L., & Marsh, R. (2007). Community participation in HIA: Discods in teleology and terminology. *Critical Public Health, 17*, 229–241.

Maldonado, G., & Greenland, S. (2002). Estimating causal effects. *International Journal of Epidemiology, 31*, 422–429.

Martin-Olmedo, P. (2013). Implementing and institutionalizing health impact assessment in Spain: Challenges and opportunities. In M. O'Mullane (Ed.), *Integrating health impact assessment into the policy process: Lessons and experiences from around the world*. Oxford: Oxford University Press.

McQueen, D. V., Wismar, M., Lin, V., & Jones, C. M. (2012). Introduction Health in all policies, the social determinants of health and governance. In D. V. MacQeen, M. Wismar, V. Lin, C. M. Jones, & M. Davies (Eds.), *Intersectoral Governance for Health in all policies: Structures, actions and experiences* (pp. 3–22). Copenhagen: World Health Organization, European Observatory on Health Systems and Policies.

Metcalfe, O., & Higgins, C. (2009). Healthy public policy – is health impact assessment the cornerstone? *Public Health, 123*, 296–301.

Mindell, J. S., Boltong, A., & Forde, I. (2008). A review of health impact assessment frameworks. *Public Health, 122*, 177–187.

Montage, P. (2004). Reducing the harms associated with risk assessments. *Environmental Impact Assessment Review, 24*, 733–748.

Murray, C. J., Ezzati, M., Lopez, A. D., Rodgers, A., & Vander Hoorn, S. (2003). Comparative quantification of health risk: Conceptual framework and methodological issues. *Population Health Metrics, 1*, 1–20.

NEPA (National Environmental Policy Act of 1969). 1969. *Public Law 91-190, 42* U.S.C. 4321–4347.

NRC (National Research Council). (1983). *Risk assessment in the federal government: Managing the process*. Washington, DC: National Academy Press.

NRC (National Research Council). (1994). *Science and judgement in risk assessment*. Washington, DC: National Academy Press.

NRC (National Research Council). (2009). *Science and decisions: Advancing risk assessment*. Washington, DC: National Academy Press.

Pascal, M., Corso, M., Chanel, O., Declercq, C., Badaloni, C., Cesaroni, G., et al. (2013). Assessing the public health impacts of urban air pollution in 25 European cities: Results of the APHEKOM project. *Science of the Total Environment, 449*, 390–400.

Prüss-Üstün, A., Mathers, C., Corvalan, C., & Woodward, A. (2003). *Introduction and methods: Assessing the environmental burden of disease at national and local levels. WHO Environmental Burden of Disease Series 1.* Geneva: World Health Organization.

Ricci, P. (2006). *Environmental and health risk assessment and management: Principles and practices.* Dordrecht, The Netherlands: Springer.

Salay, R., & Lincoln, P. (2008). *The European Union and health impact assessments: Are they an unrecognised statutory obligation?* London: National Heart Forum.

Schreider, J., Barrow, C., Birchfield, N., Dearfield, K., Devlin, D., Henry, S., et al. (2010). Enhancing the credibility of decisions based on scientific conclusions: Transparency is imperative. *Toxicological Sciences, 116*(1), 5–7.

Sen, A. (2004). Why health equity? In S. Anand, F. Peter, & A. Sen (Eds.), *Public health, ethics and equity* (pp. 21–34). New York: Oxford University Press.

Soerjomataram, I., de Vries, E., Engholm, G., Paludan-Müller, G., Brønnum-Hansen, H., Storm, H. H., et al. (2010). Search. Impact of a smoking and alcohol intervention programme on lung and breast cancer incidence in Denmark: An example of dynamic modelling with Prevent. *European Journal of Cancer, 46*(14), 2617–2624. doi:10.1016/j.ejca.2010.07.051.

Solar, O., & Irwin, A. (2010). *A conceptual framework for action on the social determinants of health. Social determinants of health discussion. Paper 2 (Policy and Practice).* Geneva: World Health Organization.

Ståhl, T., Wismar, M., Ollila, E., Lahtinen, E., & Leppo, K. (Eds.). (2006). *Health in all policies. Prospects and potentials.* Finland: Ministry of Social Affairs and Health.

Treasury, H. M. (2011). *The magenta book: Guidance for evaluation.* London: H.M. Treasury.

Veerman, J. L., Barendregt, J. J., & Mackenbach, J. P. (2005). Quantitative health impact assessment: Current practice and future directions. *Journal of Epidemiology and Community Health, 59*, 361–370.

WHO. (1948). *Preamble to the constitution of the World Health Organization.* Geneva: World Health Organization.

WHO. (1986). *The Ottawa Charter on health promotion.* Geneva: World Health Organization.

WHO. (1999). *Health 21—Health for all in the 21st century.* Copenhagen: World Health Organization.

WHO. (2000). *Evaluation and use of epidemiological evidence in environmental health risk assessment. A WHO guideline document.* Copenhagen: World Health Organization.

WHO. (2002). *The world health report 2002: Reducing risks, promoting healthy life.* Geneva: World Health Organization.

WHO. (2004). *Comparative quantification of health risks: Global and regional burden of disease attributable to selected major risk factors.* Geneva: World Health Organization.

WHO. (2009). *Global health risks: Mortality and burden of disease attributable to selected major risks.* Geneva: World Health Organization.

WHO and Government of South Australia. (2010). *Adelaide statement on health in all policies: Moving towards a shared governance for health and well-being.* Adelaide: World Health Organization and Government of South Australia.

WHOEurope. (1999). *Gothenburg consensus paper on health impact assessment: Main concepts and suggested approaches.* Brussels: European Centre for Health Policy.

Wilkinson, R., & Marmot, M. (2003). *The solid facts: Social determinants of health* (2nd ed.). Geneva: World Health Organization.

Wismar, M., Blau, J., & Ernst, K. (2007). Is HIA effective? A synthesis of concepts, methodologies and results. In M. Wismar, J. Blau, K. Ernst, & J. Figueras (Eds.), *The effectiveness of health impact assessment: Scope and limitations of supporting decision-making in Europe* (pp. 15–33). Copenhagen: WHO, European Observatory on Health Systems and Policies.

Chapter 3
Top-Down Policy Risk Assessment

**Balázs Ádám, Ágnes Molnár, Gabriel Guliš, Peter Otorepec,
Razvan Chereches, Joanna Kobza, Jana Kollárová, Nunzia Linzalone,
Marek Majdán, Sarah Sierig, Odile Mekel, Peter Mochungong,
Jozef Pastuszka, Ingrida Zurlyte, and Rainer Fehr**

Introduction

Several factors can influence human health and the wide range of these factors relate
to virtually all sectors of life. Since the Lalonde report was published in the 1970s
it has been realized that besides the traditionally accepted role of genetics, health care,
and physical environment, socioeconomic determinants have a crucial contribution

B. Ádám (✉)
University of Southern Denmark, Niels Bohrsvej 9-10, 6700 Esbjerg, Denmark

University of Debrecen, Kassai 26, 4028 Debrecen, Hungary
e-mail: badam@health.sdu.dk; adam.balazs@sph.unideb.hu

Á. Molnár
Centre for Research on Inner City Health, Li Ka Shing Knowledge Institute, St. Michael's
Hospital, 209 Victoria St., Rm. 3-26.22, Toronto, ON M5B 1C6, Canada M5B 1C6
e-mail: MolnarAg@smh.ca

G. Guliš
Unit for Health Promotion Research, University of Southern Denmark, Niels Bohrsvej 9-10,
6700 Esbjerg, Denmark
e-mail: ggulis@health.sdu.dk

P. Otorepec
National Institute of Public Health, Trubarjeva 2, SI 1000 Ljubljana, Slovenia
e-mail: peter.otorepec@ivz-rs.si

R. Chereches
Babes-Bolyai University, Strada Mihail Kogalniceanu 1, Cluj-Napoca 3400, Romania
e-mail: razvan.chereches@publichealth.ro

J. Kobza
Medical University of Silesia, 18 Medykow Street, 40-752 Katowice, Poland
e-mail: koga1@poczta.onet.pl

J. Kollárová
Regional Public Health Authority, Ipelska 1, 04011 Kosice, Slovakia
e-mail: kollarova@ruvzke.sk

G. Guliš et al. (eds.), *Assessment of Population Health Risks of Policies*,   37
DOI 10.1007/978-1-4614-8597-1_3, © Springer Science+Business Media New York 2014

to the health status of the individual and population alike (Lalonde 1974). Because health is largely determined by factors which lie outside of the health sector, not only health policy but any sectoral policy making has the potency to affect health. Conducting healthy public policy appears as the first of the five action areas in the Ottawa Charter for Health Promotion (WHO 1986). As concluded, the task requires political commitment and needs to be based on coordinated efforts in legislation, fiscal, and organizational measures aiming at providing a physical and social environment supportive for health. The formulation of public policy with a strong focus on health is discussed in the Adelaide Recommendations on Healthy Public Policy that emphasizes human health and well-being as one of the main principles of policy development in all sectors (WHO 1988). One step further is the recognition that not only public but any policy can have an effect on health, which leads to the concept of Health in All Policies (HiAP). The Finnish Presidency of the European Union first introduced the consideration of health as a fundamental issue in policy making and made it a major health theme on European level in 2006 (Ståhl et al. 2006). The Adelaide Statement on Health in All Policies has recently formulated HiAP into a global issue stating that although many sectors already contribute to better health, significant gaps still exist (WHO, Government of South Australia 2010).

Making policies that promote health to the largest possible extent is best achievable if the consideration of human health is integrated into the policy making process in a structured way. The assessment of health risks related to policy options is indispensable in this regard because it allows policy decisions to be based on absolute

N. Linzalone
Institute of Clinical Physiology, National Research Council, Regione, Via Moruzzi 1,
56127 Pisa, Italy
e-mail: linunzia@ifc.cnr.it

M. Majdán
Trnava University, Univerzitne namestie 1, 91701 Trnava, Slovakia
e-mail: mmajdan@truni.sk

S. Sierig • O. Mekel
Unit Innovation in Health, NRW Centre for Health (LZG.NRW), Westerfeldstraße 35–37,
Bielefeld 33611, Germany
e-mail: sarah.sierig@gmx.de; odile.mekel@lzg.gc.nrw.de

P. Mochungong
Environmental Health Centre Health Canada, 50 Colombine Driveway, Tunney's Pasture,
Ottawa, ON, Canada K1A 0K9
e-mail: peter.mochungong@hc-sc.gc.ca

J. Pastuszka
Silesian University of Technology, Akademicka 2A, 44-100 Gliwice, Poland
e-mail: jozef.pastuszka@polsl.pl

I. Zurlyte
Health Education and Disease Prevention Center, Kalvariju Street 153, LY-08221 Vilnius, Lithuania
e-mail: Ingrida@post.omnitel.net

R. Fehr
University of Bielefeld, Universitätsstraße 25, 33615 Bielefeld, Germany
e-mail: rainer.fehr@uni-bielefeld.de

measures of risk (Rose 1992). However, a generic, detailed mechanism that could fulfill all the requirements of such an ambitious goal is still under development. Evidence-based handling of health issues is not readily accommodated in the decision-making process of sectoral policies, even in areas closely related to health, that calls for appropriate methodology.

Health impact assessment (HIA) provides a powerful tool to make predictions on the health impacts of policies, programs, and projects (WHO European Centre for Health Policy 1999). Its primary aim is to assist policy makers so as to make as health friendly decisions as possible. While experience with the use of HIA has accumulated in the last decade, demand for the assessment of health effects of various initiatives has grown substantially (Veerman et al. 2005; Dannenberg et al. 2006, 2008). Several guidelines have been developed that unify methodology and aid users to predict health impacts (Scott-Samuel et al. 2001; Taylor and Blair-Stevens 2002; Health Canada 2004; Abrahams et al. 2004; Quigley et al. 2006; Harris et al. 2007; Metcalfe et al. 2009; Bhatia 2010a; Bhatia et al. 2010b; Human Impact Partners 2011).

HIA collects information from various sources and processes them in the risk appraisal phase. This central step is responsible for the assessment of health risks related to policy options; therefore it has a crucial role in determining the quality and usability of the output. Traditional risk assessment procedures work well for the characterization of health effects related to environmental exposures, especially in case of a one risk factor—one health outcome scenario (Basham 2001; McCarthy et al. 2002; Veerman et al. 2005; Steenland and Armstrong 2006; Lhachimi et al. 2010). Guidance used in environmental health impact assessments to integrate quantitative assessment of health effects has recently been developed (Briggs 2008). But traditional tools fail to be effective when the complex impact scheme of a policy ought to be assessed. In a comprehensive HIA of a policy proposal, the impact scheme always includes social determinants of health and related risk factors the quantitative assessment of which cannot be based on toxicological principles but needs exposure-effect functions best provided by epidemiological studies. Even then quantification of several causal pathways may often remain unfeasible. In practice, qualitative predictions of health impacts are still dominant. If quantification is carried out for some impact pathways, qualitative and quantitative estimates exist side by side in a comprehensive assessment. In addition, the several causal chains of an impact scheme can interact with each other on different levels that pose further difficulties to the complex evaluation of the health impact.

The above-mentioned methodological problems make the practice of considering health risks of policies in the political decision-making process challenging (Davenport et al. 2006; Mannheimer et al. 2007; Ádám 2012). Another barrier is that the scientific results of impact assessments often cannot be readily translated to the practice of policy development, being the perspectives and understanding of scientists and policy makers so different. Decision makers can find the interpretation of qualitative estimates too subjective, therefore difficult to work with, especially if there is a need for comparison. Quantitative estimates may work more effectively in the policy-making process, provided that they rely on robust and rigorous models (Mindell et al. 2001; Milner et al. 2003; O'Connell and Hurley 2009). Numerical predictions can better describe the size of effects that helps to prioritize and summarize positive and negative impacts. It gives possibility to balance the pros and cons of a policy option in health terms, especially if estimates are provided in unified measures. One favored possibility is to monetize health impacts which can prove to be particularly useful in assisting the bargaining process.

Few studies exist that provide a comprehensive analysis of health risks related to policy proposals, just like those that apply quantitative methods of assessment. Although health impact assessments are designed to be able to characterize policy impact, experience of the Health Impact Assessment in New Member States Accession and Pre-Accession Countries (HIA—NMAC) 2006–2008 EU project pointed out a lack of adequate methodology and guidelines for the appraisal phase of policy level HIAs. Certain need has been recognized for the development of a concise, applicable guide that can effectively aid the assessment of the complex causal web of policies that includes, among others, social determinants of health. The primary aim of the Risk Assessment from Policy to Impact Dimension (RAPID) 2009–2012 EU project was to develop such a methodological guidance. The main idea was that the systematic analysis of complex impact schemes requires the description of the "full chain" of causal pathways considering all levels of causality in an integrated manner. The analysis should proceed from the top to the bottom of the causal chain, i.e. from the cause, that is the policy, through health determinants and risk factors to the effect that are health outcomes. The top-down risk assessment approach follows a logical structure that can be readily applied in the risk appraisal phase of policy health impact assessments.

Lessons learned from case studies were used in the RAPID project to achieve the goal of developing a methodological model, formulate recommendations, and finally to prepare a unified guidance on top-down full chain assessment of health risks of policies, that can be then pilot tested as applied for the assessment of an international policy. Project partners worked on separate case studies representing diverse topics. They enjoyed a high level of freedom to decide on topics, information sources, and tools used in the assessment process. Only the main steps of the assessment were determined in advance. The work started with the selection and detailed description of a specific policy. Following this step, each partner identified and characterized the wider determinants of health influenced by the policy and risk factors linked to these determinants. As the final step, health outcomes related to the selected risk factors were assessed. A significant aim of the project was to harmonize the methodology of classical risk assessment with that of health impact assessment and apply quantitative risk assessment techniques in the assessment of health impacts of policies. The experiences of case studies allowed for making recommendations on various practical aspects, such as information need and feasibility, integration of quantitative and qualitative assessment elements in specified pathways and characterization of uncertainty.

In the next section short summaries of the case studies are presented. They discuss different topics except the two studies on road safety. However, the policy context is essentially different even for them, as one assesses a new legislation but the other a completed program. The elaboration of the assessment, the understanding of the elements of the causal chain, as well as the use of quantitative methods shows high diversity among the studies. Nevertheless, all case studies provided opportunities to draw valuable conclusions that could be applied in the formulation of a unified guidance.

Case Studies

The New Hungarian Anti-smoking Policy

Introduction

Tobacco use is one of the leading preventable causes of morbidity and mortality worldwide. Tobacco smoke exposure has been related to a wide range of health effects. Notwithstanding, smoking as a lifestyle factor affects not only smokers, but, via environmental tobacco smoke (ETS) exposure, anybody in the vicinity, especially in indoor environments (U.S. DHHS 2006).

In the last decade, several countries implemented comprehensive anti-smoking policies for the protection of nonsmokers. Among the possible actions, ban of smoking in public places is one of the most effective measures (WHO 2008a).

Since 2006, Hungarian political decision-makers have also got to realize the need for amending the existing anti-smoking legislation by further restricting smoking in indoor public places. Changes were urged by the extensive scientific information and experiences accumulated in the topic during the last decade, as well as by the county's international obligations. Moreover, the prevalence of smoking is high and the burden of smoking-related health outcomes is especially severe in Hungary. In 2009, a proposal for the tightening of the existing Hungarian anti-smoking legislation was prepared. The Ministry of Health deemed a comprehensive prospective health impact assessment (HIA) of the proposal necessary and entrusted the HIA workgroup of the Faculty of Public Health, University of Debrecen with the preparation. The assessment carried out in 2009–2010 and completed with quantitative assessment in the RAPID project was the first comprehensive prospective HIA of a policy proposal in Hungary.

Policy Description

The public health importance of smoking is well established. Several preventive measures have been developed and initiatives launched by various institutions on international, national, and local level to decrease the disease burden related to tobacco smoke exposure. The European Strategy for Tobacco Control prepared by the WHO provides guidelines for governments to work out national level anti-smoking policies, regulations, and action plans. A separate section of the document discusses passive smoking with the conclusion that considering existing scientific evidence, rigorous actions are needed to prevent environmental tobacco smoke exposure (WHO Regional Office for Europe 2002). The WHO Framework Convention on Tobacco Control (FCTC) that was ratified by Hungary has the goal to decrease smoking to a minimal level by global intervention, to put a stop to the smoking epidemic, to mitigate health effects, and to reduce smoking-related burden on societies to an acceptable level (WHO 2003). One of the main issues of the framework convention is the protection of nonsmokers from passive smoking and the only effective strategy to prevent environmental ETS exposure indoor is the provision of fully smoke-free environment.

In the last decades the European Union issued several nonobligatory legal instruments as means of tackling second-hand smoke exposure so as to urge member states to formulate adequate national legislations: Council Resolution 89/C 189/01 of 1989 and Recommendation 2003/54/EC, Directives 89/391/EEC, 89/654/EEC, 2004/37/EC, 83/477EGK, 92/85/EEC on occupational health and safety. In order to launch a broad public consultation on the best way to promote smoke-free environments in the EU, the Commission adopted a Green Paper "Towards a Europe free from tobacco smoke: policy options at EU level" in 2007 followed by a Council Recommendation on smoke-free environments in 2009 (European Commission 2007; Council of the European Union 2009).

In recent years the tightening of anti-smoking policies took place in the majority of the European countries. In line with the EU policies, prohibition of smoking was introduced first in public places—in hospitals, schools, offices, theaters, cinemas— then in public transport vehicles. The restrictions were later adopted in workplaces then in hospitality and leisure venues. The first significant step in this direction was made by Ireland when banning smoking in pubs, restaurants, and workplaces in 2004. The Irish example was soon followed by Norway (2004), Malta (2004), Italy, Sweden (2005), Scotland (2006), England (2007), and other countries.

The professional background for the provision of tobacco smoke-free environment was offered in Hungary by the National Public Health Program announced by the Resolution No. 46/2003. (IV. 16) of the National Assembly. As a contracting party to the FCTC of the WHO, Hungary had the legal obligation to take measures to provide tobacco smoke-free public places. The FCTC proclaimed by the Act No III of 2005 meant an international covenant for the introduction of restrictions of smoking in public places. Relating to the Green Paper of the European Commission, the Hungarian Government has stated that the provision of the right for health and the reduction of smoking are among its highest priorities. The prohibition of smoking in closed public places as a final goal was an acknowledged and targeted commitment of both the EU and the Hungarian Government.

The majority of measures protecting individuals from ETS exposure in Hungary used to be included in the Act No XLII of 1999 on the protection of nonsmokers and on certain rules of consumption and trade of tobacco products (referred to as Act in the case study). By that it is forbidden to smoke in several public venues except in designated smoking places but is allowed without restrictions in institutions of the catering industry where hot meal for local consumption is not served (pubs). The need for the tightening of the Hungarian anti-smoking policy has emerged several times among policy makers and the first proposal for the amendment of the Act was presented in 2009 with the basic concept that all indoor public places become nonsmoking establishments. It also placed a restriction on smoking in some open public areas, such as playgrounds, underpasses, and stations of public transport. In addition, the proposal called for changes in the regulation of selling and promotion of tobacco products.

The policy analysis found clear drivers and actors of the policy as discussed above. Since the policy was formulated as a national Act, the whole population of Hungary could be regarded as the target group. Examples from other countries for the introduction of similar regulations supported the judgment about the feasibility of its implementation. The public support of anti-smoking policies and law-respecting behavior is essential for any long-term success and study findings show that public support typically increases before their introduction and after implementation (Fong et al. 2006). The 2009 Eurobarometer survey found that 87 % of the Hungarian supported the introduction of banning smoking in workplaces, 81 % in restaurants and 62 %—lagging behind the EU average—in pubs.

Determinants of Health and Risk Factors

Restriction of smoking in public places influences several health determinants and risk factors in direct or indirect ways.

Tobacco Smoking

There are several thousand chemicals identified in tobacco and in tobacco smoke. Cigarette smoke consists of a vapor and a particulate phase. The vapor-phase components, such as carbon dioxide and monoxide, acetaldehyde, formaldehyde, and nitrogen oxides contribute to 95 % of the mass of smoke. Particulate matter (tar) constitutes the rest of the mixture with nicotine being distributed between the two phases. Tobacco smoke contains several probable and 17 proven carcinogens (IARC 2004). Since carcinogens act in a stochastic dose–response manner, the threshold of safety can be determined neither for them nor for tobacco smoke. During the combustion of tobacco free radicals are formed. These highly reactive molecules can enter into contact with and damage the macromolecules of the body.

A smoking ban in public places and workplaces decreases the prevalence of active smoking and consumption volumes, as well. The effect is attributed to the reduction of opportunities for smoking and to the nuisances, such as the inconvenience of smoking outdoor or in isolated boxes (Eriksen and Chaloupka 2007). Anti-smoking policies increase people's awareness about the health effects of active and passive smoking and contribute to the decreasing acceptance of smoking by the society (Fong et al. 2006; Gorini et al. 2007). In Italy smoking prevalence dropped from 2004 to 2006 of about 7.3 % (Gorini et al. 2007), and an even larger decrease was observed in other countries. The fear that smoking would be relocated from public places to homes was not verified.

Smoking prevalence is high in Hungary. A study of the School of Public Health, University of Debrecen, corresponding well with the findings of the 2003 National Health Survey, found 27.4 % and 40.7 % prevalence of active smoking among females and males in 2006, respectively. Taking into consideration cultural similarities between societies and the precaution to rather underestimate the effect of the policy on exposure, 7 % reduction in the prevalence of active smoking was used in the study for exposure assessment.

Air Quality (Environmental Tobacco Smoke Exposure)

Environmental tobacco smoke is a mixture of side stream smoke and residual mainstream smoke exhaled by the smoker and diluted in the atmosphere. In the mixture the proportion of mainstream smoke varies between 1 and 43 % depending on conditions. Due to quick dilution the physicochemical properties of ETS alter, the concentration of components usually decreases and additional free radicals are formed. Some components, among them CO and several carcinogens (e.g. benzo[a]pyrene, formaldehyde, cadmium, arsenic) have a higher level in side stream than in mainstream smoke (IARC 2004).

Experiences from countries introducing full restriction of smoking in indoor public places indicate significant reduction in ETS exposure. The air concentration of nicotine and particulate matter as well as the carbon monoxide level of exhaled air and the cotinine content of saliva of potentially exposed individuals were decreased. The first comprehensive national workplace smoke-free law in Ireland led to dramatic declines in reported smoking in workplaces (77.4 %), restaurants (96.5 %) and bars/pubs (by 94.9 %). There was a significant decrease (5.9 %) in the proportion of Irish homes where smoking was allowed, too (Fong et al. 2006). Employee's exposure to ETS at the workplace was reported to drop by 66.7–76.5 % in Finland. Using the above observations, 95 % decrease in the prevalence of ETS exposure in the hospitality sector, 70 % in the workplace, and 5.9 % in the households were used to estimate the policy effect on the high Hungarian ETS exposure rates.

Economic Impact: Costs, Income, and Employment

Smoking poses heavy burden on the society. Costs include loss of productivity related to smoking breaks, direct expenses of increased health care costs of smoking-related diseases, as well as indirect expenses deriving from the decreased productivity of the victims of active and passive smoking resulting in loss of income tax and social insurance tax (European Commission 2007). The total costs of smoking in the EU/EFTA countries reached 1–1.4 % of the region's GDP in 2000, similar to the 0.8 % found in the USA. 1.5–2 % loss of GDP due to smoking was estimated in Hungary in 2004.

The introduction of anti-smoking policies faced strong opposition from the catering and hospitality industry and from the tobacco lobby in most of the countries.

According to the arguments, anti-smoking regulations entail negative economic effects that are reduced income, closed down businesses, and increasing unemployment in the catering sector (Eriksen and Chaloupka 2007). In contrast, studies investigating objective indicators of tax income or employment did not find long-term negative economic effects of anti-smoking policies (U.S. DHHS 2006). An evaluation of the 1999 anti-smoking Act in Hungary found no negative economic squeal in the catering sector, too.

Anti-smoking policies cause income loss to the tobacco industry and to the government due to the reduced consumption of tobacco products. The latter can be compensated by increasing the tax content. The ASPECT Consortium reported negligible impact of anti-smoking policies on the overall employment of the European tobacco industry.

Social Contacts and Recreation

Some studies estimate smoking ban having negative effect on social contacts due to the physical separation of smoker and nonsmoker acquaintances and friends (Gorini et al. 2007). Other authors consider increasing stigmatization and exclusion of smokers, sometimes by creating inhuman environments, alarming.

The conditions of recreation improve due to the provision of smoke-free environments for nonsmokers.

Built Environment and Land Use, Housing, and Working Conditions

Tobacco smoke-free environment has an increasing esthetic and financial value. 55 % of the US and 90 % of the Canadian population live in smoke-free houses that have steadily increasing value on the real estate market (WHO 2008a). Despite of the misgivings prior the smoking ban in Ireland, 90 % found smoke-free bars more pleasant and comfortable according to a public surveys after the introduction.

Banning smoking in public places and workplaces results in a perceptible reduction of ETS exposure level not just in the restricted places but elsewhere, even in homes (Eriksen and Chaloupka 2007), that contributes to the improvement of various built environments, housing, and work conditions, as well.

Summary

The proposed restrictions result in a substantial decrease of the level of ETS exposure and prevalence of smoking in closed public places, workplaces, and public transport vehicles contributing positively to air quality, built environment, housing, and workplace conditions, as well (Table 3.1).

Table 3.1 Health determinants and risk factors predicted to be influenced by the tightening of the Hungarian anti-smoking regulations

Health determinant	Effect on risk factors
Lifestyle Substance use (smoking)	Moderate decrease of the frequency and quantity of smoking
Physical environment Air	Significant decrease of ETS exposure in public places, workplaces, and public transport vehicles
Built environment and land use	Increased value of the built environment as becoming tobacco smoke-free
Working environment and housing conditions	Significant decrease of ETS exposure in workplaces and homes
Socioeconomic environment Income and social status	Favorable restructuring of family expenses due to decreased purchase of tobacco products Decreased income of the tobacco industry and the government due to reduced consumption Savings in the health care and private sector
Employment and working conditions (job safety)	Insignificant effect on the employment and turnover of the catering industry
Social contacts	Exclusion of smokers
Culture	Decreased smoking prevalence and consumption quantities
Recreation	Improved conditions for recreation in tobacco smoke-free environments

Health Outcomes

Smoking harms not only smokers´ health but also those exposed to environmental tobacco smoke in the vicinity. Beside the several health damages, the few possibly positive effects are negligible (IARC 2004).

Health Effects of Active Smoking

Tobacco smoke is classified as a proven human carcinogen (IARC 2004). Lung cancer is the most frequent malignant cause of death related to smoking. In a meta-analysis on the correlation of smoking and cancer Gandini et al. (2008) found that smoking increases the risk for developing lung cancer 8.96-fold. There is also causal relationship between smoking and the development of oral cavity, nasal and para-nasal cancers, pharyngeal, laryngeal, esophagus, stomach, pancreas, liver, renal, urinary tract, and cervical cancer, as well as of myeloid leukemia. The level of risk is mainly determined by the length of smoking history and by the number of cigarettes smoked daily. There are data but insufficient to prove that smoking can cause colon cancer and there is no established relationship between smoking and breast, endometrial, and prostate cancer (IARC 2004; U.S. DHHS 2004).

Tobacco smoke irritates mucus membranes of the respiratory tract causing coughing, increased mucus production, wheezing, and dyspnea. Smoking induces the development of chronic obstructive respiratory diseases, increases the risk for airway infections and aggravates the symptoms of asthma. Tobacco smoke exposure of the fetus, children, and youth hinders the normal development of the lung (Thun et al. 2000; U.S. DHHS 2004).

Smoking induces atherosclerosis of blood vessels; therefore, it is a strong independent risk factor of coronary heart diseases and stroke. The effect shows dose–response relationship with consumption volume, years of smoking, extent of smoke inhalation, and with early onset. Smoking can contribute to the development of heart failure and peripheral arterial diseases (Thun et al. 2000; U.S. DHHS 2004).

Smoking is proven to increase the risk for developing peptic ulcer. It promotes the development of Crohn's disease and the formation of gallstones. Smoking reduces female fertility; maternal smoking may contribute to preterm delivery, low birth weight, and sudden infant death. Smoking induces osteoporosis, periodontitis, and cataract and impairs the effectiveness of several immune functions (U.S. DHHS 2004).

Among the health outcomes, the prioritization process found four diseases of public health importance: lung cancer, chronic obstructive respiratory diseases, coronary heart diseases, and stroke. In addition to them, quantitative outcome assessment was feasible for arterial diseases and 12 other types of cancer. The assessment was based on the calculation of gender specific disease burden measured in attributable death (AD) and disability adjusted life years (DALY) applying the methodology of the WHO Global burden of disease study, 2004 for a baseline (2006) and for a predicted situation after the proposed changes take place (WHO 2008b). Three percent discount rate was used without age-weighting. Gender and age-specific frequency measures of exposures and diseases were taken from the most reliable Hungarian sources available. Association measures (relative risks) for active and former smokers were acquired from the literature. Taking into account that risks to develop various diseases gradually decrease after quitting smoking, short-term effects were assessed by using intermediate risk levels for those quitting as a consequence of policy introduction, while long-term effects were modeled without this consideration. The results revealed substantial annual reduction both in AD (633 lives) and DALY (8,309 life years) related to decreased smoking prevalence in the long term. Ádám et al. (2013) provide detailed description of the methodology.

Health Effects of Passive Smoking

Health effect observed in smokers may develop in passive smokers, too; although components are typically in lower concentrations. Stronger impact or effects not seen in smokers are, however, unlikely (IARC 2004).

ETS is a proven human carcinogen that can cause lung cancer (IARC 2004). It induces middle ear and lower respiratory tract infections, and impaired pulmonary function in exposed children. There are data about its relation with chronic obstructive pulmonary diseases. The thrombotic and atherosclerotic effects of passive smoking are well known, exposure significantly increases the morbidity and mortality of coronary heart diseases and stroke. Passive smoking increases the frequency of sudden infant death and ETS exposure of the mother causes low birth weight (U.S. DHHS 2006).

Outcome assessment proved to be feasible for the same four priority diseases as found with active smoking. The assessment was carried out in the same way as with active smoking except that the impact was only considered for nonsmokers and different association measures were used for ETS exposures suffered during spare time activities, at workplaces and at home. For those nonsmokers exposed to ETS at various places, only benefit from the least reduced exposure level was taken into consideration. The effect of reduced ETS exposure proved to be higher than that of the decreased prevalence of active smoking (1,052 AD and 13,627 DALY).

Health Effects of Other Factors

The identified positive effects on built environment and land use, family income, and recreation can improve mental health, while the impact on social contacts such as the increasing stigmatization and social exclusion of smokers has an opposite outcome. Nevertheless, assessment of such indirect effects is rather difficult due to the diverse interactions among the various health determinants and risk factors.

Summary

The proposal results in a significant, quantifiable reduction in the disease burden related to active and passive smoking (Table 3.2).

Conclusion

Beyond conducting a regular qualitative assessment, the authors attempted to quantify all causal pathways where it was feasible. According to the results, the proposal has a definite positive impact on the health of the population. Mechanistic toxicological studies on the health effects of tobacco smoke components, as well as epidemiological observations in countries after introducing similar restrictions all support the favorable effects. The study revealed that reduction in active and passive smoking results in an annual health gain of 1,685 lives and 21,936 DALYs. According to observations, the main concern regarding the fallback of trade and the consequent increase of layoff in the hospitality sector is rather unlikely; the reduced state income from taxes on tobacco production and trade is much compensated by the benefits.

Observations made in other countries were used in the quantitative exposure assessment; however, the limitations to extrapolate data derived in a society to another must be acknowledged. Applying the precautionary approach in our professional consensus, typically the lowest levels of changes reported by various sources were used in the model. To find valid data for quantitative assessment proved to be difficult. Nevertheless, quantitative outcome assessment was feasible for 17 and 4 diseases influenced by the changes in active and passive smoking, respectively. Despite the uncertainties regarding some input values of the model and that

Table 3.2 Health outcomes predicted to be influenced by the tightening of the Hungarian anti-smoking regulations, presented by determinants of health

Health determinant	Effect on health outcomes
Lifestyle Substance use (smoking)	Positive effect on the incidence of smoking-related diseases (633 AD and 8,309 DALYs saved annually)
Physical environment Air	Significant positive effect among nonsmokers on acute respiratory symptoms, pulmonary functions, chronic respiratory diseases, lung cancer, coronary heart diseases, and stroke (1,052 AD and 13,627 DALYs saved annually)
Built environment and land use	Slight positive effect on mental diseases
Working environment and housing conditions	Significant positive effect among nonsmoker employees and family members (see Air)
Socioeconomic environment Income and social status	Moderate positive effect on mental health, improved quality of life
Employment and working conditions (job safety)	No effect (perhaps slight negative effect in the catering and tobacco industry)
Social contacts	Slight negative effect on the smokers' mental health and quality of life
Culture	Moderate positive effect on smoking-related diseases and on quality of life
Recreation	Moderate positive effect on mental health and on quality of life

horizontal interactions between qualitatively and quantitatively assessable causal pathways of the impact scheme were only qualitatively evaluated, the presented assessment process provides an applicable example for the assessment of health risks related to policies.

The Danish Energy Policy 2008–2020

Introduction

Due to the complexity of environments and people, policies can have immediate short-term and long-term intended and/or unintended effects. The intended effects of an energy policy, for example, can be to reduce greenhouse gas (GHG) emission by a certain percentage within a defined period, promote the exploitation of cleaner energy sources and supply reliable and affordable electricity power to consumers. The intended effect of cheap electricity supply to consumers can be achieved within the short-term but in the long-term, novel exploitation technologies for (mostly) clean energy can lead to unintended consequences within the social, economic and/ or health sectors. The relevance of an energy policy at both the national and international scale need not be over emphasized; especially as reliable energy supply is central to economic development, and key to many social activities. Irrespective of how it is carefully structured and implemented, an energy policy, just like any other policy, can indirectly modify the determinants of health (environmental, social, behavioral), leading to the emergence or re-emergence of risk factors that can have potential health consequences on the population. This document details a top-down (policy, determinants of health, risk factors and health outcomes) risk assessment of the Danish Energy Policy 2008–2020.

Policy Description

The new Danish energy policy is timely and highly relevant at both the domestic and international levels. The policy is responsive to the changing external environment and strife to meet the energy needs of the population of Denmark. Primarily, it guarantees energy security and with it economic development as well as social well-being. The policy aims at cutting reliance on fossil fuels such as coal, gas, and oil which are known emitters of oxides of sulfur (SO_2), carbon (CO_2), and nitrogen (NO_x) into the environment. The policy's commitment to exploit more environmentally friendly energy sources portrays the diversity of energy resources in Denmark internationally and highlights the knowledge, skills, and capital capabilities of the country to exploit them.

It contains a range of initiatives: saving energy and improving energy efficiency, increasing taxes on the more traditional forms of energy, and promoting research and development of renewable energy sources and creating more effective energy technologies and transport. All these are aimed at ensuring that Denmark meets its obligations and pledges in relation to the integrated climate and energy proposal put forward by the European Commission in January 2008. Other ambitious targets within the initiatives will see higher energy efficiency for end users and a substantial reduction in energy consumption in new buildings.

Initiatives on renewable energy will encourage the use of energy from biomass (waste) and discourage the use of fossil fuels in central combined heat and power stations. Other initiatives will be geared towards programs to increase the deployment of wind turbines, both onshore and offshore. Substantial amounts of money will also be allocated for campaigns to promote the replacement of oil-fired furnaces with heat pumps and for subsidizing efforts towards renewable energy technologies such as solar and wave power. Energy tax initiatives include an increase in the existing CO_2 tax from 2008 and a new NO_x tax from the beginning of 2010. Initiatives at promoting energy technology will see a doubling of funding in energy research, development, and demonstration.

It is important to mention that the policy does not provide clues as to whether a health impact assessment (HIA) was carried out at any stage of its development nor provide information about the risk perception of those who were involved in drawing up the policy. Additionally, the policy does substantiate on how it might influence the determinants of health. However, fact sheets on the agreement between the Danish government and parliamentary political parties can be downloaded from the website of the Danish Energy Authority (www.ens.dk).

Table 3.3 Energy sources and determinants of health of potential influence

Energy source	Determinant of health of potential influence	References
Fossil fuel (oil, coal, gas)	Atmospheric pollution Water and land pollution Accumulation of solid waste	Speight (1996) Dincer and Rosen (1998) IEA (1998)
Biomass/ waste	Growth of specific high-energy crops High consumption of land and waste resources Loss of natural habitat and biota	Brower (1992) Grass and Jenkins (1994) Jenkins et al. (1998)
Wind	Scenic deterioration Land use Changes in landscape	Brower (1992) Coles and Taylor (1993)
Solar	See Wind Atmospheric pollution	Tsoutsos et al. (2005)
Wave	Physical effects of currents and waves Atmospheric and oceanic emissions	Boehlert et al (2008)

Determinants of Health and Risk Factors

Determinants of health such as air pollution, soil, and water contamination can interact to influence the health outcome of an individual and/or community depending on exposure scenarios and individual susceptibility (age, gender, etc.). The social and economic welfare benefits of energy security need not be over emphasized. However, extraction technologies can directly or indirectly account for conflicting health scenarios associated with the determinants of health. Energy sources such as fossil fuel, biomass/waste, wind, solar, and wave can directly or indirectly impact environmental determinants of health as shown in Table 3.3; through modifications of ambient and indoor air quality, soil nutrient cycle, texture, and quality and disruption of the hydrological cycle. Effects such as a drop in agricultural productivity will be obvious and others such as modification of the local vegetation can potentially lead to alterations in the dynamics of disease vectors. Initiatives of the policy geared towards promoting central heating systems and electric stoves in homes will potentially improve indoor air quality, which is vital as a proximal environmental health determinant (Table 3.3).

How energy sources impact determinants of health depend on issues related to modes of exploitation, transportation, and distribution. Consequently, energy production will always be associated with environmental impacts; making it tedious for policy developers to balance energy and environmental issues at same time. Social determinants are likely to be relevant too due to taxation, which could make energy efficient technology affordable to lower social groups.

In comparing risk factors inherent in different energy sources, controversy often surrounds activities to be included: accidents, routine operation, the fuel cycle, construction of the plant, and manufacturing the materials from which it is to be built (Bezdek 1993). Offshoots resulting from energy production, transportation and/or distribution including consumption are thus of growing concern as the dependence on fossil fuels and biomass accounts for high levels of gaseous

Table 3.4 Energy sources, health determinants, and associated risk factors

Energy source	Determinant of health of potential influence	Risk factors	References
Fossil fuel (oil, coal, gas)	Atmospheric pollution Water and land pollution Accumulation of solid waste Land degradation	PM levels SO_x, CO_x, and NO_x levels Ground level ozone GHG Lead and Mercury	Speight (1996) Dincer (1999) Greenhalgh (2002)
Biomass/waste	Growth of specific high-energy crops High consumption of land and waste resources Atmospheric pollution Loss of natural habitat and biota	PM, CO_x, SO_x and NO_x levels Acid rain Food shortages	Brower (1992) Grass and Jenkins (1994) Jaakkola and Jaakkola (2006)
Wind	Scenic deterioration Land use Changes in landscape	Low-frequency noise and vibrations Shadow flicker Scenic quality Interference with electromagnetic radiation	Brower (1992) Coles and Taylor (1993) Seifert et al. (2003)
Solar	See Wind Atmospheric pollution	Scenic quality PAC emissions Emission of trace metals	Gekas et al. (2002) Tsoutsos et al. (2005) Cocarta et al. (2008)

emission and PM levels in the atmosphere (Dincer and Rosen 1998). Combustion products cause visibility reductions in some areas of the world, produce acid rain, and cause or exacerbate multiple diseases over short and long time periods in others. Categorizing risk factors from energy generation, supply, and utilization should be carefully considered, as this may have an impact on the decision-making and/or implementation process. In particular, grouping or splitting them into several subcategories such as long-term low-dose radiation exposure from over-head power distribution lines, ground level ozone concentration, and atmospheric SO_2 build-up may seemingly reduce or increase their significance especially when other nonenvironmental risk factors such as extremes of age (very young and elderly), smoking, alcoholism, immune-suppression, and comorbid conditions are considered (File 2000). The Comparative Risk Assessment module of the global burden of disease is suitable for describing population exposure to risk factors and, their consequences for population health is an important step in linking the growing interest in the causal determinants of health across various public health disciplines from natural, physical, and medical sciences to the social sciences and humanities (Ezzati et al. 2002). Table 3.4. shows risk factors as a consequence of energy source (production, transportation, and utilization) and impact on the determinants of health.

Health Outcomes

Figure 3.1. shows the interactions within the top-down risk assessment model. It is important to remember that interactions within the model are not as direct and specific

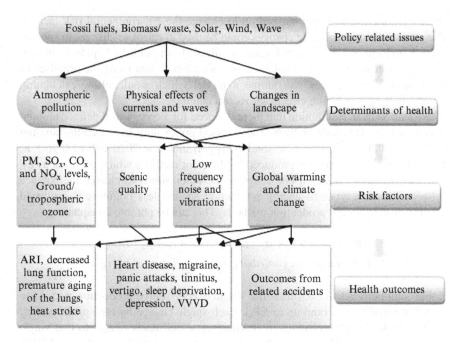

Fig. 3.1 Interaction of factors within a top-down risk assessment model

as depicted. Environmental determinants are more obvious since the policy under case study addresses priority energy sources which are all related to the environment. Each of the energy sources will affect determinants of health within the environment at different extents. Fossil fuel and biomass combustion will directly affect atmospheric pollution while exploitation of solar, wind, and wave energy will modify the landscape and increase various forms of environmental pollution.

Atmospheric pollution will trigger risk factors such as PM levels and the physical effects of waves can be associated with low-frequency noise and vibrations within the environment. Exposure duration and susceptibility of individuals are important considerations before health outcomes can be associated with risk factors. In cases such as air pollution, risk factors for a single health outcome do not occur individually. Excluding pre-existing conditions, asthma, for example can be associated with more than one risk factor (noxious gases and PM). Therefore, as one moves from top to bottom, the interactions of the factors become more and more complex as they tend to be interdependent on each other. Careful analysis through well designed dose-related studies is necessary to isolate evidences of the interactions for robust policy development.

A major issue of any risk assessment is quantification. In presented case it seems to be quite straightforward to conduct full chain quantification for individual policy priorities. For example the energy consumption target can easily be (re)calculated in decreased amount of air pollution in total per individual pollutants and type of energy production and summarized up to change the environmental risk factors. The same individual pollutant changes could be used to calculate changes in specific disease incidences via use of risk ratios available from published epidemiological research. Instead of such a calculation for a single pollutant using the premises of the Danish energy policy we outline a model which would allow calculating expected changes in health effects across full chain.

We start with an assumption that there is a need for a certain well defined amount of energy E for Denmark in 2008. The assessed policy aims to reduce this amount by 4 % until 2020. This leads to total energy available in 2020 will be 0.96 * E. This total energy available is produced by different methods which we mark as E_1, E_2 ... E_n. Besides decreased consumption the other aim is to change the balance between different types of energy production so that less pollutant is produced through diverse energy production methods. This can be put into an equation:

$$0.96 * E = \mu_1 * E_1 + \mu_2 * E_2 + \mu_3 * E_3 + ... + \mu_n * E_n$$
$$\mu_n = percentage\ contribution\ of\ a\ single\ type\ of\ energy.$$

For simplicity let us substitute the single energy source production $\mu_1 * E_1$ in 2020 by a marker EP_1 (and up to EP_n). Each single change by type of the energy production will lead to changes in environmental pollutants related to that single type of production. Mathematically we can expect the energy production EP_1 to produce a certain amount of specific pollutants, for example air pollution products P_1, P_2, P_3... P_n. The change in that single type of energy production will affect changes in production of each single pollutant. It is important to note that at this point one should not sum up the change in total pollution across pollutants but across energy production type. For risk assessment it is more important to know how production of single pollutants will change in total across different types of production rather than the total of pollutants linked to a single type of production. So, to get this number we need to sum up amount of pollutants produced via different types of production

$$\sum P_1 = P_{1EP1} + P_{1EP2} + P_{1EP3} + ... + P_{1EPn}$$

After one gets $\sum P_1$ a coefficient to calculate ambient air parameters needs to be applied followed by application of a risk ratio from epidemiological research to a specific subpopulations (or even total population) which allows us to calculate the changes in potential health effects. Once such an algorithm is developed and data is available the health effects of any energy policy could be quantified. Of course this simplified description does not contain formulas and considerations related to statistical uncertainties of individual steps. It is obvious that their inclusion is very important and necessary and they should come from basic epidemiological or technology research providing baseline information for individual steps of the calculation.

Summing up changes in pollution across pollutants and types of energy production might lead to quantification of changes in one single, in our case environmental, determinant of health. This kind of quantification is important to estimate interaction in between different determinants of health. There is no doubt about interaction of environmental and social determinants for example leading to changes in income, education, and health at the end. Similar mathematical modeling can lead to quantification of those interactions.

Conclusion

The exploitation of sustainable, competitive, and secure sources of energy, including transportation and utilization is a key policy objective of the European Union and its member states. A low-carbon energy policy such as the Danish Energy Policy 2008–2020 will not only decrease the emission of greenhouse gases, but also play an active role in the reduction of air pollutant emissions, improvement of air quality, and promotion of public health. Renewable energy sources have characteristically high capital costs relative to more conventional systems. Therefore, breaking into markets that have been dominated by traditionally large-scale fossil-fuel-based systems will be difficult. The determination of the government of Denmark to invest heavily in this sector as outlined in the energy policy is a step among many in the right direction.

The presented case study describes a full chain risk assessment of potential health impacts of the Danish energy policy and offers a kind of mathematical algorithm for calculation of overall changes in health effects related to energy policy. Statistical uncertainties around basic dose–response type relations needs to be taken into account in every single step of the model. Yet, despite the many uncertainties the case study and the mathematical models show the possibility to quantify health effects of an energy policy in top-down direction and therefore to conduct scientifically sound risk assessments of energy policies.

Quantification of Selected Health Impacts of the North Rhine-Westphalia Housing Subsidy Program 2010

Introduction

Housing conditions can have an enormous influence on people's health, in both positive and negative ways. Issues that need to be considered in this context are home safety and accidents, indoor air quality, thermal comfort and energy, residential environments and physical activity, and effects on mental health, especially with respect to aging populations (cf. WHO housing and health program, WHO Regional Office for Europe 2010).

There are many programs and strategies worldwide for improving housing with very different aims and objectives, depending on the regional housing situation. Housing subsidy programs have a long tradition in Germany. They aim to provide adequate housing for people with limited means.

Policy Description

For development and testing RAPID top-down methodology, the NRW housing subsidy program for 2010 (WoFP 2010, Ministerium für Bauen und Verkehr NRW: Düsseldorf. Runderlass IV.4-250-01/10) and, especially, the part of the programme that promotes age-appropriate housing fits well for a pilot study.

The *selection of this policy* was led by a set of criteria we established: localization (a national or regional policy should be selected), size (policy needed to be of a manageable size but not too small), and feasibility (selected policy should be attractive and up-to-date; furthermore verifiable objectives and sufficient data should be available). Most important criterion regarding content of selected policy was that the chosen policy should not be developed in the health sector, but had potential impact on human health.

Based on this, several potential policies were sought in a first step. The decision which one should be assessed was supported by six experts in an internal expert workshop held at our public health institute. They preselected three policies. These three preselected policies were tested for their suitability for risk assessment. Contents of this "screening and scoping" process were data sources, verifiable objectives, target groups, health determinants, and health effects influenced by the chosen program, existence of dose–response-functions for the health determinants and health effects, time frame of the program, and the connection with focal working areas in our public health institute.

National Background: Social Housing Subsidies in Germany and NRW

In addition to general regulatory conditions for the housing markets (state measures to maintain, adjust, and improve economic stability), depending on the objective, a variety of subsidy mechanisms are used in Germany to secure the appropriate supply of housing, e.g. social housing subsidies. The target group for social housing subsidies are households that cannot independently provide themselves with housing in the free housing market, e.g. due to low income, social characteristics, or special needs. Sources and original texts of listed laws and regulations can be found at website of the NRW Housing Ministry (http://www.mbwsv.nrw.de/wohnen/wohnraumfoer-derung/index.php).

The German federalist reforms of 2006 meant that sole legislative competence for social housing subsidies was transferred to the federal states, i.e. the states were given the right to legislate and provide funding in the area of social housing subsidy. In *North Rhine-Westphalia*, the state legislative exercised this competence on 1 January 2010 and replaced the federal Housing Subsidy Act with the Law on the Subsidising and Utilisation of Housing in North Rhine-Westphalia (WFNG NRW). This WFNG provides the basis for the Housing Subsidy Program for 2010 (WoFP) which offers one billion euro for loans for 2010. Each year a new housing subsidy program is published in North Rhine-Westphalia, so that the next program is expected at the beginning of 2011. In addition, when considering the WoFP 2010, it is also necessary to take account of the housing subsidy provisions for 2010, the subsidy provisions for housing for people with disabilities and the guidelines for subsidizing investment measures in the housing stock in North Rhine-Westphalia. The basis for the current decisions in relation to housing subsidies in North Rhine-Westphalia is provided by assessments commissioned by the state government of North Rhine-Westphalia. Key results of existing assessments are that, because of demographic change, age-appropriate housing for the elderly will become increasingly important not only in urban but especially in rural districts (F+B 2008).

The NRW Housing Subsidy Program for 2010

The Housing Subsidy Program for 2010 (WoFP) contains five key objectives, which are outlined in the first chapter:

1. The concept of generation-appropriate (fixed demographic) housing development as a response to changes in demand due to an aging population
2. Location-appropriate, integrative subsidy strategies as a response to the heterogeneous nature of regional and local housing markets and their predicted development
3. Subsidies available for necessary adaptations to existing housing stock on the basis of changes in household structures and utilization requirements
4. Continuation of the climate offensive for more climate protection in housing construction and for reducing housing ancillary costs
5. Utilization of housing subsidies to develop innovative solutions in the rented housing construction sector and in the owner-occupier sector for the purpose of experimental housing construction

For an adequate assessment of the policy it was necessary to narrow the objective down and *to focus on health relevant sections of the policy*. For this purpose, a keyword search was used to identify the references to health in WoFP 2010 and the associated statutory sources. The keywords used in relation to the consequences for health of lifestyle and housing conditions and the determinants in this area were identified in an expert meeting on the topic of "lifestyle and health" and were supplemented with a thematic search of the literature. From these, "barriers" are mentioned with particular frequency. The term occurs in the main analysis document, WoFP 2010, particularly in section "Generation-appropriate (fixed demographic) housing construction". In addition, this section also emphasizes the importance of the infrastructure. Generation-appropriate building means "planning and equipping buildings in such a way that people who are young and old, healthy and ill, with and without disability, can feel at home" (MMI 2011).

One of the key aspects of planning buildings is the lack of barriers. Since 1998 it is required that all subsidized new homes must be planned and built with no barriers under the terms of DIN 18025 Part 2, which contains minimum planning requirements that enable homes to be created for a large group of users at limited expense. These barrier-free homes are not intended explicitly as homes for the disabled, but rather as "universal homes" that can be used by young and old alike, whether or not they have physical impairments, and that will be viable properties in the real estate and rental markets long into the future. In the case of "special housing" suitable for disabled use, the requirements of DIN 18024 and of the first part of DIN 18025 must be met, whereby the relevant homes are tailored specifically to the needs of the residents.

The minimum planning requirements for barrier-free "universal homes" according to DIN 18025 Part 2 contain detailed specifications in relation to fittings, movement areas, doors, barrier-free accessibility, lower door handles and thresholds, lifts, ramps, and steps. Compliance with all these requirements in already existing housing is very difficult. Subsidies are also paid for existing housing stock if as many barriers as possible are removed. These homes are referred to as "lower-barrier" rather than "barrier-free".

Determinants of Health and Risk Factors

Housing is one of the key social determinants of health, as most people spend a lot of time at home. Due to this fact, housing is related to many other subordinated determinants and risk factors, for example thermal comfort, indoor air quality (dampness, molds, indoor emissions, infestations), noise, environmental barriers, home safety, the social and physical quality of the housing, and the immediate environment (WHO Regional Office for Europe 2007).

Because of this assessment's focus on "generation-appropriate (fixed demographic) housing construction" only determinants and risk factors related to this topic, such as *environmental barriers* and *home safety* and *accidents, esp. falls* will be further explored. These determinants belong to the most relevant housing and health relevant factors (LARES study, WHO Regional Office for Europe 2007).

The home is a major site of accidental injuries such as falls and fires. Besides children, the elderly are particularly at risk (Thomson and Petticrew 2005). A representative survey among adults in Germany shows that 31.6 % of all injuries occurred at home. In higher age this percentage increases: 69.4 % of the persons 80 years and older experienced an injury at home during the last 12 months before the interview (Saß 2010). One of the main reasons for an injury is falling at home. Falls account for one third of total costs of medical treatment for all injuries and are the most common cause of death due to accident in older people (von Heideken Wagert et al. 2009).

Risk factors for domestic falls in the elderly are multifaceted, as "a fall is the result of an interaction between personal and environmental factors" (Thacker and Branche 2000). Older people experience a decrease of skills, e.g., in seeing (limited visual field, lowering of visual acuity and color perception), hearing (hearing impairment), and a decrease of physical mobility (Saup 1993). Hence, risk factors for falling are often endogenous or personal risk factors, such as gait, balance, and functional impairments or diseases (Icks et al. 2005). Former falls are endogenous risk as well; furthermore iatrogenic risk factors (drugs) can lead to falls (Icks et al. 2005). Beside these personal or intrinsic factors, environmental factors (extrinsic factors) play a large role in triggering falls, especially domestic hazards, such as clutter, loose rugs, poor lighting, no stair railings, no grab bars, slippery surfaces, and steps (Icks et al. 2005; Thacker and Branche 2000).

In addition to all these risk factors, the behavior of the person who is at risk to fall is an important factor. These situational risk factors cover for example working with hazardous utilities and the unsuitable storage of everyday objects (Icks et al. 2005).

Exposure Assessment

To assess health-related consequences due to construction-related barriers in homes of the elderly which may occur each year in North Rhine-Westphalia, we first need to estimate the exposure distribution of the elderly population living in homes with barriers.

The number of older people who suffer a fall each year is difficult to assess, as not every fall leads to a documented treatment. Most reviews and studies estimate that about one third or 30 % of older people in ordinary housing fall each year (e.g. Stevens et al. 2008; Towner and Errington 2004; von Heideken Wagert et al. 2009).

For Germany, exact numbers for incidences of falls are also still unavailable (Icks et al. 2005). Therefore, the international estimates (30 % of people older than 65 years living at home fall one or more times per year) are used as default values for Germany (DEGAM 2004; Icks et al. 2005).

In the year 2009, 3,637,438 people were aged 65 years and older in North Rhine-Westphalia (population structure provided by the NRW statistical office IT.NRW). It is estimated by Pappert (2010) that approximately 95 % of all persons aged 65 and older are living in homes with barriers. Applying this proportion to the elderly population in NRW, this means that in the year 2009 approximately *3455 thousand persons aged 65 years and older* are living in such homes.

Health Outcomes

Analogue to health determinants and risk factors many health outcomes are connected to poor housing conditions: general physical symptoms, infectious and chronic diseases, such as respiratory symptoms, asthma, and lung cancer. Furthermore, mental health may be affected, depression and anxiety may occur. Injuries and deaths are also possible effects (Krieger and Higgins 2002; Thomson and Petticrew 2005).

Due to our main focus on environmental barriers, home safety, and accidents, esp. falls it was possible to prioritize health outcomes towards *"falls and consequences of falls in the target group of the elderly"*. Fall-related injuries are the leading cause of injury deaths and disabilities among persons aged 65 years and more (Thacker and Branche 2000). Falls can result in major injuries such as fractures, head injuries, and serious soft tissue injuries. Major injuries increase the risk of institutionalization and mortality. Furthermore, fear of falling, functional limitations, and the increased risk of being placed in a nursing home may reduce well-being in older people (von Heideken Wagert et al. 2009). The following list summarizes different estimates and ratios derived from international literature to describe the different health outcomes of falls:

- *Injuries requiring medical treatment*: about 10 % of all falls lead to injuries requiring medical treatment (DEGAM 2004; Icks et al. 2005). Others estimate that about 20 % of falls require medical care (Towner and Errington 2004). In a study assessing the incidence of falls and fall-related injuries of very old people (85 years and older) 40 % of all falls led to injuries (von Heideken Wagert et al. 2009);
- *Fractures*: fewer than 10 % of all falls result in fractures (Gillespie et al. 2009; Towner and Errington 2004); DEGAM (2004) and Icks et al. (2005) estimate that about 5 % of all falls lead to fractures. Regarding very old people (85 years and older) 8 % of all falls lead to a fracture (von Heideken Wagert et al. 2009);
- *Hip fractures*: about 1–2 % of all falls lead to hip fractures (DEGAM 2004; Icks et al. 2005). Fall-associated fractures in older people are a significant source of morbidity and mortality (Gillespie et al. 2009). As a consequence of a hip fracture 50 % of persons (>65 J) did not regain their former level of function (Thacker and Branche 2000); 20 % of all older adults who fracture a hip die within a year (Costello and Edelstein 2008). In Germany the perioperative lethality of hip fractures is 10 % (DEGAM 2004);
- *Loss of functionality*: 85 % of all fallers suffer loss of functionality, and, as a consequence, need a walker for example (DEGAM 2004). 25 % of all older fallers are in nursing homes within a year (Costello and Edelstein 2008);
- *Fear of falling*: 70 % of fallers fear further falls, and, as a consequence, lose their self-confidence and are restricted in activities of their daily life. These restrictions lead to further decrease of locomotive abilities (DEGAM 2004).

Altogether, the most common serious injuries are hip fractures (Thacker and Branche 2000).

Outcome Assessment (Quantification)

To assess health-related consequences due to construction-related barriers in homes of the elderly which may occur each year in North Rhine-Westphalia, we decided to estimate the number of falls, the number of hip fractures as one of the most important consequences and the number of resulting deaths. Based on exposure assessment, we know that approximately 3,455 thousand persons aged 65 years and older are at risk, that means exposed to barriers in the home in NRW in the year 2009 (see "determinants of health/risk factors" section).

For estimating the number of falls, we use the reported percentage of people aged 65 years and older that fall at least once a year: 30 %. In addition, we assume that 50 % of these falls occur in the homes or adjacencies (DEGAM 2004; Icks et al. 2005; Thacker and Branche 2000). We make a basic assumption that these falls are due to barriers in and around the houses. Applying these percentages, more than *518 thousand persons older than 65 years were estimated to fall* in 2009.

Two percent of all fallers aged 65 years and older suffer a hip fracture (Frick et al. 2010). Applying this percentage to the North Rhine-Westphalian fallers in this age group, this would result in *10366 estimated hip fractures* in the year 2009. A hip fracture at older age may cause in 20 % of all cases death within a year (Costello and Edelstein 2008). This would result in *2,073 estimated deaths due to barriers in homes of the elderly* in the year 2009.

As discussed, many factors influence the risk of falling at home. Not all falls in homes with barriers will be induced by construction barriers, and therefore this assumption will be an overestimate. Our literature review did not reveal any study on the impact of barrier-free construction on falls, injuries, or deaths. In absence of such evidence we assume, that 30–70 % of falls in homes are induced by construction barriers. This means, that *potentially 3110–7257 hip fractures and 622 to 1,451 deaths resulting from hip fractures could have been avoided in the year 2009*, if all homes of people aged 65 years and older in North Rhine-Westphalia were barrier-free.

Conclusion

We estimate that approximately 3,000–8,000 hip fractures and 600–1,600 resulting deaths may occur each year in North Rhine-Westphalia due to construction-related barriers in homes of the elderly. These health impacts can potentially be reduced by construction of barrier-free housing or modification of existing housing stock towards "lower-barrier" housing. The NRW housing subsidy program is focusing on the construction of barrier-free housing. Depending on the implementation success of the NRW subsidy housing program, the actual health impacts might be lower. On the other hand, other health impacts of the housing subsidy programme are not modeled here. They are likely to have substantial health impacts too.

28,120 hip fracture cases (persons 65 years and older) were treated in NRW hospitals in 2007 (LIGA.NRW 2009). Our estimate of 3,067–7,156 hip fractures for 2007 due to construction-related barriers in homes of the elderly seems to be a realistic estimate.

Our quantitative estimates show the potential for improving the housing conditions and the resulting health improvement of a considerable amount of people. However, the housing subsidy programme is covering only a small part of the housing stock in NRW. Each year around 3 % of the subsidiary housing stock is modified into barrier-free housing.

The effect of barrier-free housing construction on falls in the elderly is not subject of housing intervention studies until now. Therefore we applied a wide range for the exposure-response function based on expert judgment. The resulting estimates reflect the uncertainty related to this aspect in the modeling of the health impacts.

At this point of time, there are, of course, numerous open questions, e.g., regarding adequate modeling, understanding of the causal chain, selection of stakeholder, validation, communication of results, chances of influencing the decision-making process, uptake of the quantification part in HIA, possibilities to link to prevention programs like the NRW program on "fall prevention".

Falls and injuries in the elderly is a complex phenomenon. In addition to "environmental housing modifications", further interventions are needed to prevent falls and injuries in this vulnerable group

Estimates of the Health Risk Reduction Associated with Attainment of the New Particulate Matter Standards in Poland

Introduction

Airborne suspended particulate matter can be either primary or secondary in nature. Primary particles are emitted directly into the atmosphere by natural and /or anthropogenic processes whereas secondary particles are predominantly of man-made origin and are formed in the atmosphere from the oxidation and subsequent reactions of sulfur dioxide, nitrogen dioxides, ammonia, and volatile organic compounds.

Since 1990 size fractionation of total suspended particles (TSP) was attempted by measurement of airborne particles with aerodynamic diameter $d \leq 10$ µm (PM10). The major part of PM10 may have a natural origin (sea spray and mineral dust), and it is therefore also important to measure PM2.5 or even PM1 (Fenger 2009).

There is also growing concern related to the health effects of airborne, especially fine particles. Toxicological and epidemiological studies demonstrate positive association between ambient concentrations of airborne particulate matter and increased adverse respiratory and cardiovascular events (Dockery et al. 1989; Seaton et al. 1995; Chapman et al. 1997; Donaldson and McNee 2001; Boldo et al. 2006; Zhang et al. 2011), including morbidity and mortality (Samet et al. 2000; Samoli et al. 2005; Moreno et al. 2007).

Despite insufficient knowledge on the exact exposure-effect relationships between PM10 and human health, PM10 (thoracic fraction) standards have been developed. In 1999 the European Commission has included the PM10 monitoring and limits values in the Air Quality Directive. In 1987 the WHO guidelines, the recommended level was decided below which health effects were thought unlikely to occur (around 100 µg m^{-3} annual mean for both airborne particles and sulfur dioxide) and a safety factor of 2 was applied. It should be remarked, however, that the World Health Organization concluded that health risks are present at any level of particles. Therefore, beginning with the second revision of WHO guidelines for particulate matter in 2000 and continuing with the most recent guideline (WHO Regional Office for Europe 2006) the concept of no observed effect level was abandoned in favor of a model in which no threshold of adverse effect within the usual ambient range was assumed (Anderson 2009). Under this concept, the guideline, while set at a level that gave reasonable protection for public health, was higher than that at which effect could be observed. This shift in thinking was strongly influenced by the accumulating results of time-series studies of mortality, which tended not to observe a threshold of effect within the ambient range (Anderson 2009). The APHEA study of 29 European cities (Samoli et al. 2005) can be one of the examples. Authors of this study documented that no threshold appeared in the relation between the exposure to PM10 and daily mortality.

As a result of the recently approved European directive on air quality (99/30/ CE), new limiting values for several atmospheric pollutants have been met in 2005, and by 2010. The mass concentration level of PM10 has been established as the main parameter used for measuring and controlling the particulate pollution of ambient air. In addition, the measurement of PM2.5 (aerodynamic diameter d $\leq$ 2.5 μm) is at present required in the European Union at representative sites. These sites should coincide, wherever possible, with the PM10 sampling points.

To estimate the health risk reduction associated with attainment of the new particulate matter standards in Poland the outline of the top-down approach model has been developed. It should be noted that "the new particulate matter standards in Poland" means not only the new standard values but also establishing new parameters used for measuring and controlling the particulate pollution of ambient air, as well as, introducing the new measuring system. Also as a result of the new policy complex consequences should appear, especially a change in risk factors but also in the health outcomes.

Policy Description

International and National Background and Policy Context

Air pollution can basically be regulated in various ways (Fenger 2009): by setting emission standards, by air quality standards, by raising emission taxes and by doing cost-benefit analyses. The classical, and in principle soundest, way is to limit the emission from a source, a sector, or an entire country; the pragmatic way is to state how much pollution may be in particular ambient air and regulate the dispersion accordingly. The first approach has been attempted for centuries although with limited success. The second is fairly new being dependent upon more or less sophisticated measurements and computational techniques. In modern practice these two approaches are implemented simultaneously accompanied by rules and regulations for both emission and ambient air concentration. These two ways of regulation were used in Poland. Recently, the cost benefit analyses have become a new tool in the air pollution policy.

Our analysis concentrated on the general population of Poland with target group of people living in Upper Silesia—the heavily industrialized and urbanized region.

Analysis of Affected Factors from the Historical Perspective

In the period of 1980–1990, the particulate pollution of ambient air has been assessed by the measurements of the concentration of total suspended particles (TSP) and the deposition level by using the Weck jar (the standard for the deposition $= 50$ ton/(km^2 year). In Upper Silesia the daily TSP levels were often between 500 and 1,000 μg m^{-3} while the deposition of particles was about 600 tons/(km^2 year) but in some areas, for example in Zabrze, even 800 tons/(km^2 year). The environmental data were confidential. No official information appeared about the possible health effects of the polluted environment.

Significant political and economic transformations in Poland changed the sources of the anthropogenic pollution from 1990. The reduction of emission of air pollutants from the metallurgical, chemical, and coal mining industries took place, especially, in Upper Silesia. Very soon it became clear that it was predominantly the reduction of emission of particles larger than 10 μm. Rapid decrease of the concentration of TSP and the deposition levels was observed: in Upper Silesia daily levels of TSP were less than 100 μg m^{-3} while the deposition level decreased below 50 tons/(m^2 year).

Polish regulations in force up to 1984 applied to TSP used extremely high limits when compared to annual and daily limiting values established by the Directive for PM10. In 2002 the Polish Ministry of Environment established new Polish regulation with following standards for PM10: 24-h standard $= 50$ μg m^{-3} with accepting tolerance 10 μg m^{-3} in 2003 and 5 μg m^{-3} in 2004, and the annual standard being equal to 40 μg m^{-3} with accepting tolerance 3.2 μg m^{-3} in 2003 and 1.6 μg m^{-3} in 2004.

Determinants of Health

In the period of 1990–2002 the beneficial influence of the changes on the public health did not appear. Especially, in Upper Silesia adverse respiratory and cardiovascular events still increased, including morbidity and mortality (see e.g. Pastuszka et al. 1993) although the concentration of all monitored pollutants, including airborne particles decreased during the 10 years 5–20 times. There were certainly a number of reasons for this situation, including the fact that rapid and drastic decrease of the concentration of TSP was related mainly to the reduction of the concentration of particles larger than 10 μm while the concentration of fine particles was only little reduced. Besides, in this period the exposure to pollutants in the indoor environment still remained very high, especially exposure to environmental tobacco smoke (ETS) was very high.

Actual monitoring data indicate an improvement of the air quality but there are a number of exceptions. Although significant political and economic transformations in Poland during the last 20 years changed the profile of the sources of anthropogenic pollution, and the traffic emission of particles is becoming a new important source of airborne particles, the industrial and municipal emission probably contributes the most to the aerosol particles in Polish territory (Pastuszka et al. 2010). However, this problem needs further studies.

Risk Factors

Categorizing risk factors, which should probably mostly decrease because of the implementation of the new particulate matter standards in Poland, the updated monitoring data must be carefully considered, as they may have an impact on the decision-making and/or the next steps of the change in the national particulate standards (also for the PM2.5). In particular, their grouping or splitting into several subcategories such as long-term exposure to PM10, additional exposure to environmental tobacco smoke (ETS) and atmospheric sulfur dioxide may reduce or increase their significance especially when other nonenvironmental risk factors such as smoking, alcoholism, or immune-suppression are considered (File 2000). Even considering only the environmental agents it can be found that exposure to different environmental factors associated with either outdoor or indoor air pollution at the same time can lead to the modification of health effects. For example, asbestos and the chemicals in cigarette smoke act together to produce more lung cancer than either exposure does separately. This "synergistic" response increases risks by multiples of the separate risks from each exposure, rather than by additions, giving very high risks of lung cancer to those who both smoke and breathe in asbestos dust (Gee 1997). It is likely that the higher lung cancer rate in urban areas is due in part to traffic fumes, as well as to domestic coal burning, industrial pollution, and smoking, causing possibly several thousand extra cancer deaths a year (Gee 1997).

Such synergistic response was also found for other adverse health effects generated by a set of factors. Pastuszka et al. (2003) examined the relationship between the levels of airborne particulate matter (solid particles, bacteria and fungi), and asthma in the children population in Sosnowiec, Upper Silesia. The results show that the averaged concentration levels of total suspended particles (TSP), respirable particles less than 5 μm in diameter (PM5), as well as of the studied bioaerosols (fungi, bacteria, Gram-negative bacteria) were higher in the group of homes with asthmatic children than in the group of reference homes although in each home with asthmatic children only concentration of some of these pollutants (sometimes only one) exceeded the appropriate level determined in the reference homes.

The integrated exposure to both biological and nonbiological air pollutants probably significantly elevates health risks. A meta-analysis of 11 epidemiological studies (Romieu 1992) yielded an estimate of a 20 % increase in respiratory infection occurrence for an increase in NO_2 exposure of 30 μg m^{-3}.

Health Outcomes

The risk factor and estimated health outcome should be described and evaluated in a systematic and comparable way. Airborne particles, including not pathogenic bioaerosol particles, have various acute and longer-term adverse health effects. Short-term exposure can impair lung function, cause mucosal inflammation, increase tissue sensitivity to repeated exposure, and cause respiratory symptoms. Long-term or repeated exposure to air pollutants can cause chronic bronchitis, emphysema, and lung fibrosis. Generally, exposure to aerosol particles is related with a number of adverse health effects, causing increased morbidity and mortality (Samet et al. 2000; Samoli et al. 2005; Moreno et al. 2007).

Recently, Kowalska and Zejda (2012) confirmed that the daily risk of death and hospitalization due to cardio-respiratory diseases in Upper Silesia increases with the concentration of airborne particles. This risk is at the level similar to the values estimated for other regions in the world. Especially, they found that a 24-h increase of PM10 concentration by 10 μg m^{-3} causes 0.3 % increase of the risk of death.

Our task is to use the health impact assessment (HIA) methodology to estimate the number of health events attributable to air pollution in the target population (5 Polish cities) assuming that there is a causal relationship between particulate pollution and the observed health effects. Such health impact assessment of long-term exposure to PM2.5 in 25 European cities has recently been published by Boldo et al. (2006). However, it is important to note that there are always uncertainties in the estimated benefits of removing a particular exposure. In addition, the benefit may be achieved much later than predicted (Boldo et al. 2006). On the other hand, it is difficult to fully identify and assess the airborne particles—health links because many environmental factors act simultaneously and many diseases have multiple causes, including nonenvironmental factors. Therefore, new tools to create appropriate environmental health policies are still needed, for example the method using environmental health indicators (EHIs). These indicators are presented in the form facilitating their interpretation for effective decision-making. Such indicator-based approach has been used by Wcisło et al. (2002) to assess the environmental hazards and related health effects in population of industrial cities with more than 100,000 inhabitants in Upper Silesia, Poland.

Conclusion

Clean air is considered to be the basic requirement for human health and well-being. Therefore, the Polish government has been concerned with air pollution and its impact on human health for about 30 years. The environmental policy in Poland has been significantly changed during this period. On the other hand, significant political and economic transformations in Poland during the last 20 years changed the profile of the sources of anthropogenic pollution and it is important that the new standards seem to be appropriate for the new hierarchy of the emission sources.

It should be emphasized that in contrary to the previous standards, the new Polish standards for airborne particulate matter are health based or based on environmental effects. However, in the future also other factors such as prevailing exposure level, technical feasibility, source control measures, abatement strategies, as well as social, economic, and cultural conditions must be taken into consideration.

Methodological Considerations

To estimate the influence of the new regulations on public health not only the actual exposure of the general population to PM10 should be known, but also this exposure in the past, as well as, in the future. The detail analysis should respect the following problems:

First problem is the access to the historical data. Up to the political and economic changes in Poland in the 80s, all environmental data were confidential. Access to these historical documents (reports and papers) is now unlimited but the analysis of the published and unpublished data should be carried out carefully.

Finding the local conversion factor to convert TSP to PM10 is another problem. Pastuszka et al. (1999) found that in Poland it is possible to use the existing/reported PM concentration data to predict the historical values of PM10 but only for selected areas and for selected periods during the past 30 years. Besides, it should be noted that the PM10/TSP ratio has been changing significantly with time.

Valid assessment of the exposure of the whole Polish population to PM10 is the third problem. The existing monitoring network should be extended by adding the new monitoring stations near the busy roads and the crossroads. In fact, the managers of the national monitoring system have recently been establishing some new stations oriented towards measurement of the levels of PM10-traffic origin but additionally at least 20 such stations should appear in Poland. The exposure to PM10 indoors should also be included into the monitoring reports.

The Slovak National Action Plan on Alcohol Problems for the Period 2006–2010

Introduction

In any given society, levels of alcohol-related deaths and diseases tend to rise and fall with rises and falls in overall levels of consumption. The world health report 2002 (WHO 2002) estimated that 4 % of the global burden of disease is attributable to alcohol and, as such, alcohol was the fifth leading risk factor among the 26 selected risk factors for mortality and morbidity globally. As a response to this, the 57th World Health Assembly in 2004 adopted resolution WHA57.16, which urged Member States to give attention to the prevention of alcohol-related harm and promotion of strategies to reduce the adverse physical, mental, and social consequences of harmful use of alcohol.

The State health policy of the Slovak Republic (Ministry of Health 2007) perceives health as the basic human right. Its objective is to direct the interests and endeavor of all the society units towards health as the key factor in society's development and to create an environment, in which the citizens' preconditions for support, protection, development, and restoration of health would be secured regardless of age or social group. When determining the public health priorities, a holistic approach to health should be taken and it needs to accentuate cooperation between the health care providers, institutions developing their activities in the field of public health (including the institutions dealing with research within the public health and education) and the people taking decisions. There are four priorities identified in the new wording of the State Health Policy of the Slovak Republic:

1. Chronic diseases
2. Infectious diseases
3. Environment and health
4. Tobacco and alcohol

As it is visible from the structure of the State Health Policy of the Slovak Republic one of the crucial action plans is National Action Plan for the problems with alcohol (Institute of Drug Addiction 2008).

Policy Description

The history of alcohol control policy dates back more than 3,000 years (Bruun et al. 1975). After World War I, many countries initiated and soon repealed laws prohibiting the sale of alcoholic beverages. Modern efforts to prevent alcohol problems through public policy received wide recognition with publication of a 1975 monograph, Alcohol Control Polices in Public Health Perspective, sponsored by the World Health Organization (Bruun et al. 1975).

The framework of the alcohol control policy in Slovakia is defined by the WHO European strategy for alcohol control policy and the EU strategy for decreasing the scope of damage relating to alcohol consumption. At present, Slovakia has an up-to-date action plan for the problems caused by alcohol adopted by the Government in 2006. According to the action plan, the Ministry of Health of the Slovak Republic bears the responsibility for implementation of the alcohol control policy, and it should submit a report about fulfillment of the action plan tasks to the Government to discuss it every 3 years.

The 10 areas for action and the identified outcomes in the European Alcohol Action Plan (EAAP) continue to be of central importance for the implementation of the Slovak National Action Plan on Alcohol Problems and have been an integral part of the framework. These areas are:

- Information and education
- Public, private, and working environments
- Drink-driving
- Availability of alcohol products
- Promotion of alcohol products
- Treatment
- Responsibilities of the alcoholic beverage industry and hospitality sector
- Society's capacity to respond to alcohol-related harm
- NGOs
- Formulation, implementation, and monitoring of policy

With the aim to assist public health leaders and policymakers, Brand et al. (2007) developed a composite indicator—the Alcohol Policy Index—to gauge the strength of a country's alcohol control policies. The Index generates a score based on policies from five regulatory domains—physical availability of alcohol, drinking context, alcohol prices, alcohol advertising, and operation of motor vehicles. The Index was applied to the 30 countries that compose the Organization for Economic Cooperation and Development and regression analysis was used to examine the relationship between policy score and per capita alcohol consumption. Countries attained a median score of 42.4 of a possible 100 points, ranging from 14.5 (Luxembourg) to 67.3 (Norway). The analysis revealed a strong negative correlation between score and consumption ($r=-0.57$; $p=0.001$): a 10-point increase in the score was associated with a 1-L decrease in absolute alcohol consumption per person per year (95 % confidence interval, 0.4–1.5 l).

Slovakia belongs to the "Top Ten" countries together with Norway, Poland, Iceland, Sweden, Australia, Hungary, Finland, Japan, and Canada. Still, the major limitation of the Alcohol Policy Index is that it does not value the policy effects, nor link them to any of the above potential measures of policy impact (Ritter 2007). In addition, as Brand et al. (2007) note, it does not accommodate the implementation or enforcement of alcohol policies.

The Slovak National Action Plan on Alcohol Problems includes interventions on all elements of the alcohol policy index (see Table 3.5.below).

Determinants of Health

There are quite a lot determinants of health linked to the National Action Plan on Alcohol Problems identified. Behavioral determinants are linked to the well-known and quite generally accepted fact that drinking customs and habits are deeply rooted in many European cultures including the Slovak one. Czech Republic and Slovakia are part of the group of traditional beer drinking cultures, with many people drinking daily with meals. However, in the last two decades, beer consumption in Slovakia has decreased significantly from over 8 L per capita aged 15+ years in 1983 to 5.4 L in 2003, with its pattern becoming closer to that of northern Europe with spirits consumption and binge drinking (Zatoński 2008). Age as an independent determinant of health is very important especially regarding to alcohol-related harm to vulnerable groups such as children. The more frequently a child or adolescent drinks to excess, and the younger he or she is, the greater is the risk of developing an alcohol-related disorder—alcohol misuse or dependence syndrome (Stolle et al. 2009).

On border of behavioral (culture, habits), environmental (availability of alcohol in shops, availability and access to shops) and social (poverty lack of purchase power, education) determinants of health is the long tradition of homemade alcoholic beverages. This is not a Slovak phenomenon only; it includes illegally produced vodka in Poland and the Baltic Countries, and homemade fruit brandies which in

Table 3.5 Interventions in the Slovak national action plan on alcohol problems

Domain	Intervention
Physical availability of alcohol	Creating an environment that promotes underage drinking
	Reducing sales and provision of alcohol to children and youth
	Controlling the supply and availability of alcohol, especially for children
	The introduction of licensing (license trade) on the sale of alcohol and spirits
	Reducing the number of outlets for alcoholic beverages and restrictions for its sale
Drinking context	Create coordinating body at national level (potentially at lower levels) with the aim to implement National Action Plan on Alcohol Problems
	Education and access to relevant information via public and private educational agencies targeted at children, youth, parents, prisoners, employees, pregnant women, etc.
	Facilitating effective communication between GPs and patients related to alcohol problems, intensification of early diagnosis
	Ensuring equal opportunities for patients with mental disorders associated with excessive alcohol consumption to be treated in specialized mental health care services
	Shaping positive attitudes towards health, raising awareness of pupils, students, and teachers regarding healthy lifestyle and risks of excessive drinking
Alcohol prices	Effective taxation policy
Alcohol advertising	Creating a safe social environment with no alcohol advertisement in events organized in terms of institutions and organizations, targeted at children and young people
	Avoiding of alcohol advertising targeted at youth
Operation of motor vehicle	Reducing the number of alcohol-related traffic accidents by ensuring the control of alcohol consumption

some countries (e.g. Bulgaria, Romania, Hungary, Slovenia, and to an extent in Slovakia), can be legally produced at home in large amounts (Zatoński 2008). Importance of this habit is underlined by recent evidence of higher hepatotoxicity of homemade beverages, for example, in Hungary (Szűcs et al. 2005). According to the Behavioral Risk Factor Surveillance System (BRFSS) survey, more than half of the adult U.S. population drank alcohol in the past 30 days. Approximately 5 % of the total population drank heavily, while 15 % of the population binge drank (CDC, 2010). According to the Alcohol-Related Disease Impact (ARDI) tool, from 2001 to 2005, there were approximately 79,000 deaths annually attributable to excessive alcohol use. In fact, excessive alcohol use is the third leading lifestyle-related cause of death for people in the United States each year (CDC, 2010).

While alcohol consumption is an intermediate factor in the causal chain linking social determinants to a variety of end-point health conditions, including cancer, tuberculosis, HIV/AIDS, and cardiovascular disease, it also has its own end-point disease states, including alcohol dependence and other alcohol use disorders. In most cases, alcohol consumption has deleterious effects on other disease outcomes, but in some, most notably heart disease, moderate consumption may be protective of health (Schmidt et al. 2010).

Social Class (Socioeconomic Position, Socioeconomic Status)

Social class is a strong determinant for heavy alcohol consumption and alcohol-related mortality. Register-based follow up study was used to estimate the contribution of excessive alcohol use to socioeconomic variation in mortality among men and women in Finland (Mäkelä et al. 1997). Alcohol-related mortality constituted 11 % of all mortality among men aged ≥20 and 2 % among women and was higher among manual workers than among other classes. It accounted for 14 % of the excess all-cause mortality among manual workers over upper nonmanual employees among men and 4 % among women and for 24 % and 9 % of the differences in life expectancy, respectively. Half of the excess mortality from accidents and violence among male manual workers and 38 % among female manual workers were accounted for alcohol-related deaths. The contribution of alcohol-related deaths to relative mortality differentials weakened with age.

Alcohol-related mortality rates are higher for men in the manual occupations than in the nonmanual occupations, but the relative magnitude depends on age (Harrison and Gardiner 1999). British men aged 25–39 in the unskilled manual class are 10–20 times more likely to die from alcohol-related causes than those in the professional class. For women in paid employment there is no consistent class gradient; younger women in the manual classes are more likely to die from alcohol-related causes.

In Sweden, for both genders manual workers, lower nonmanuals, entrepreneurs and unclassifiable groups had significantly higher alcohol-related mortality than did upper nonmanuals (Hemström 2002).

These results suggest that social interventions aimed at reducing poverty and inequality have the potential to reduce levels of alcohol-related harm among the poorest groups in the community.

Health Care

A particularly important consequence of alcohol stigmatization may be reduced access to health and welfare services. In many parts of the world, those perceived as "drunks" have difficulties obtaining health care services (Strong 1980), and a summary of six studies from Australia, the United Kingdom, and the United States reported that respondents felt that heavy alcohol users should receive less priority in health care (Olsen et al. 2003).

Risk Factors

Binge drinking (drinking five or more drinks on an occasion) is an important risk factor and public health problem as well but quiet a little is known about which beverage types are consumed by binge drinkers. As beer, wine, and liquor are taxed, marketed, and distributed differently, knowledge about which beverage types are consumed by binge drinkers is very important. According to Naimi's et al. study (2007) beer accounted for two-thirds of all alcohol consumed by binge drinkers and accounted for most alcohol consumed by those at greatest risk of causing or incurring alcohol-related harm. Lower excise taxes and relatively permissive sales and marketing practices for beer as compared with other beverage types may account for some of these findings.

Consumption of homemade spirits is an additional risk factor for the development of alcohol-induced cirrhosis and may have contributed to high level of liver cirrhosis mortality in Central and Eastern Europe Comparing the concentration of short-chain aliphatic alcohols in spirits from illegal and legal sources in Hungary led to the findings that the concentrations of methanol, isobutanol, 1-propanol, 1-butanol, 2-butanol, and isoamyl alcohol (potentially hepatotoxic substances) were significantly higher in homemade spirits than those of from commercial sources (Szűcs et al. 2005).

Consumption of different beverage types. The library research and analysis of the various published articles relating to experimental and survey studies lead to the results indicating that (1) after spirits consumption blood alcohol concentrations rise more quickly than after beer; (2) for most behavioral tasks beer creates less impairment than brandy at the same dose levels; (3) brandy also leads to more emotional and aggressive responses; (4) those who drink beer or beer and spirits have more alcohol-related problems than others; and (5) beer drinkers are more likely than others to drink and drive, to be arrested for drinking-driving and to be in alcohol-related accidents (Smart 1996). Consumption of alcohol in the Slovak adult population in 2002 was estimated at 10.8 l/year/person. Beer contributed 48 % of total alcohol consumption, wine 16 % and spirits 36 %.

Drinking during pregnancy is fairly common, three times the levels reported in surveys that ask only about drinking during the month before the survey. Women who binge drink before pregnancy are at particular risk for drinking after becoming pregnant (Ethen et al. 2008). Binge drinking during pregnancy can lead to Fetal alcohol syndrome. Women who drink during pregnancy risk giving birth to a baby with behavior problems, growth deficiency, developmental disability, head and facial deformities, joint and limb abnormalities, and heart defects. The risk of bearing a child with these birth defects increases with the amount of alcohol consumed. The first trimester may be a time of greatest risk for the fetus, although there is no time during pregnancy when it is known to be safe to drink alcohol.

Health Outcomes

A complete list of causes of death attributable to alcohol exposure, according to the International Classification of Disease, Tenth Revision (ICD-10 codes) from the year 2001, is presented in Table 3.6.

In addition there are diseases with some level of casual relationship to alcohol consumption. Beside the causes already included in the table above alcohol has been demonstrated to be associated with a proportion of deaths from other causes, including hemorrhagic stroke and cancers of the mouth, esophagus, and liver. Some of the diseases associated with alcohol consumption could, however, be considered for inclusion in a wider definition of alcohol-related deaths. Medical literature suggests that five groups of malignant neoplasm (Table 3.7) have an association with alcohol (Room et al. 2005).

Table 3.6 Underlying causes of death related to alcohol consumption

Description	ICD-10 codes
Alcohol-related pseudo-Cushing's syndrome	E24.4
Mental and behavioral disorders due to alcohol use	F10
Degeneration of nervous system due to alcohol	G31.2
Alcoholic polyneuropathy	G62.1
Alcoholic myopathy	G72.1
Alcoholic cardiomyopathy	I42.6
Alcoholic gastritis	K29.2
Alcoholic liver disease	K70
Chronic hepatitis, not elsewhere classified	K73
Fibrosis and cirrhosis of liver	K47
Alcohol-related chronic pancreatitis	K86.0
Finding of alcohol in blood	R78.0
Toxic effect of alcohol	T51
Accidental poisoning by and exposure to alcohol	X45
Intentional self-poisoning by and exposure to alcohol	X65
Poisoning by and exposure to alcohol, undetermined intent	Y15

International Classification of Diseases, Tenth Revision

Table 3.7 Malignant neoplasm associated with alcohol consumption

Description	ICD-10 codes
Malignant neoplasm of lip, oral cavity, and pharynx	C00-C14
Malignant neoplasm of esophagus	C15
Malignant neoplasm of liver and intrahepatic bile ducts	C22
Malignant neoplasm of breast	C50
Malignant neoplasm of colon, malignant neoplasm of rectum	C18, C20

Conclusion

To draw the full chain pathway from an alcohol policy to health outcome is apparently not a simple task. The Slovak national action plan on alcohol problems does aim to tackle relevant determinants of health according to the main elements of OECD alcohol policy index, yet fails to establish systematic and to aim linked data collection system. Consequently data are available only on the level of risk factors (alcohol consumption data as surrogate for drinking habits of population) and of some health outcomes.

Since the time of introduction of the Slovak alcohol policy it shows at present clearly a small effect; of course it needs to be mentioned that time is a very important variable and it is rather unlikely to achieve quick effects in alcohol consumption.

The alcohol policy seems to have a clear effect on health care system preparedness to deal with the problem; both selected disease indicators show consistent increase after introduction of the policy. Concrete quantification of other health effect was not possible due to lack of data by appropriate population groups. There is some data on consumption (risk factors) as presented above but it is for the whole population, not stratified by social groups, certain environment and income or education categories. Similarly, health data is available also only for the whole population, making application of risk ratios presented in the literature of little use.

Road Traffic Legislation in Slovakia

Introduction

Road safety and related adverse health effects such as injuries are an urgent public health issue worldwide. Slovakia is no exception. After the transition of political system in 1989 and subsequent changes in economy and social structures a fast development in motorized road traffic has been observed. The number of motor vehicles is growing constantly and the density of traffic is increasing in urbanized areas especially. However, the road system in Slovakia was not designed to hold such a burden. As a consequence—new safety issues have emerged recently such as increased risk of traffic accidents of bikers and pedestrians as well as drivers or passengers. The governmental structures designed a new legislation where one of the goals was to increase safety and decrease the number of accidents and deaths. A key issue which also emerges here is an evaluation of the impact of these new measures on health. We will employ the top-down risk assessment procedure to evaluate the impact of these legislative changes on concrete health effects.

Policy Description

The new legislation on road traffic was accepted by the parliament of the Slovak Republic and is in effect from 1 February 2009. A similar legislation existed in Slovakia before but new developments in road traffic such as rapid increase of traffic density and intensity and high number of traffic-related injuries and fatalities lead to a need to reconsider existing rules and introduce new ones. The legislation covers the whole range of rules concerning traffic. It is divided into eight chapters:

- Chapter 1: Basic statements
- Chapter 2: Rules of road traffic
- Chapter 3: Road traffic accidents and their registration
- Chapter 4: Enforcement of rules
- Chapter 5: Driving of vehicles
- Chapter 6: Registration of vehicles and registration numbers
- Chapter 7: Responsibilities for not complying to the rules
- Chapter 8: Final statements

The legislation introduces (compared to the legislation in effect previously) a number of key rules with potential impact on public health. We identified the most important ones. The identified policy elements of interest in the case of the road traffic legislation are as follows:

- Introducing speed limit in town from 60 to 50 km/h
- Bus speed reduction on highway to 100 km/h
- Reduction of truck speed to 90 km/h
- Obligation to turn on lights while driving
- Obligation of use of winter tires
- Helmets are to be worn by adults while riding bicycles outside of towns and by children while riding outside and inside towns
- Reflection accessories for bikers in low visibility

Determinants of Health

The impact of policies or strategies on health could be assessed through the concept of determinants of health. The process of linking the selected elements of the policy to health determinants could be seen as a two-step process.

Within the first step a link of the selected policy to the broader groups of health determinants as they are defined for example by the WHO was established. The main groups of health determinants considered by us were socioeconomic, environmental, behavioral, biological determinants, and health care.

In step 2 the broader groups of health determinants are "broken down" to determinants more specific to our case. A clear link should be apparent between the elements of the policy and the respective health determinants.

This phase of the establishment of the "full chain" of the impact process is crucial since here the direct impact of the policy is presented which serves as a basis for identifying the risk factors and thus the effects on health. Therefore attention needs to be paid to this process and some specific rules should be followed.

Socioeconomic Determinants of Health

The obligation of use of winter tires for a specific period of time during the year can be linked to this group of health determinants in general (step1). Describing the relation and specifying the determinants in more detail linked this part of the policy to income and subsequent quality of vehicle and tires available respectively. Another specific health determinant which can be linked to this element of the policy is driving skills and experience (relating to different styles of driving with winter and summer tires).

Environmental Determinants of Health

Quality of road, level of road, number of cars on road and type of cars on road can be affected by the reduction of maximum speed of vehicles in town to 50 km/h, trucks to 90 km/h in general and buses on highways to 100 km/h. These limits will affect the quality of the roads through change in structural deployment of the road and will change the numbers of different types of cares (automobiles, trucks, buses, etc.) on different types of roads.

Behavioral Determinants of Health

The fact that helmets are to be worn by adults while riding bicycles outside of towns and by children while riding outside and inside towns and that reflection accessories for bikes in low visibility conditions are obligatory, will influence the behavior of drivers and/or bikers.

Although other links might be possible to establish in this case, our findings are that the above described links are the strongest and the most comprehensive. Therefore the other groups of determinants are not listed here.

Risk Factors

Defining the link of health determinants to policy components is crucial to establish the mechanism of impact of the policy on health considered here in the broader meaning. Coming down to specific health effects, a defined relationship with specific risk factors need to be in place. To keep the "full—chain" model in place there is a need to link the policy-health determinant part of it to the risk factor-health effect part. This can be done by deriving specific risk factors from the determinants of health where we previously have established a link to the policy. Ensuring this, a clear line of impact can be drawn from the level of policy to the level of health outcomes.

In the first step a list of concrete risk factors was created which were considered as eventually linkable to parts of the assessed regulation and to health effects, respectively. Below are the clusters of populations at risk and the respective identified risk factors.

- Factors influencing the health of pedestrians: fast driving motor vehicles, fast riding bicycles, fast driving motorcycles, narrow roads crowded with vehicles, not complying to rules for pedestrian walking on roads, driver fatigue
- Factors influencing the health of drivers or passengers of motor vehicles: driving over the speed limit, distraction by external factors, use of drugs. not wearing a seatbelt, technical status of the vehicle, driver fatigue
- Factors influencing the health of persons riding bicycles: not complying to the rules for riding a bicycle on roads, not wearing a helmet, technical status of the bicycle, fast driving motor vehicles, fast riding bicycles, fast driving motorcycles, driver fatigue
- Factors influencing the health of persons driving motorcycles: driving over the speed limit, distraction by external factors, use of drugs, not wearing a helmet, technical status of the vehicle, driver fatigue

- Factors influencing the health of persons otherwise being part of road traffic: fast driving motor vehicles, fast riding bicycles, fast driving motorcycles, narrow roads crowded with vehicles

The above listed factors within the clusters are considered to be risk factors which could seriously impact the health of people. All of these are directly or indirectly linked to the assessed legislation and thus could be modified by the effectiveness of the implementation of the regulation (e.g. effectiveness of law enforcement and compliance).

Furthermore, the above-mentioned factors are confirmed as risk factors for health in scientific literature. The WHO considers the majority of these factors to be a serious risk for health and supports this by scientific evidence (in some cases more in some cases less relevant) (Peden et al. 2004). The Center for Disease Control and prevention (CDC) of the government of the USA also reports evidence supporting the risk posed by these factors (Schrieber and Vegega 2001; U.S. DHHS 1995).

After listing groups of risk factors an assessment was done to analyze which risk factors would fulfill the conditions of linking to the identified health determinants on one hand and to specific health outcomes on the other hand. Our consideration gave us the following risk factors which could be used as part of the "full chain" assessment procedure:

- Insufficient driving skills and insufficient technical state of vehicle are risk factors which can be linked to socioeconomic determinants on one side and to health outcomes on the other side
- Poor quality of roads within towns and overcrowded roads can be linked to environmental health determinants (road quality, number of cars, and type of cars on the road)
- Risky driving (speeding, not using lights, etc.); not respecting rules of traffic (such as not wearing helmets and speeding) can be related to behavioral health determinants.

Health Outcomes

The main health outcome of exposure to risks factors related to road traffic is injuries or fatalities. According to the WHO, every day around the world, more than 3000 people die from road traffic injury. Low-income and middle-income countries account for about 85 % of the deaths and for 90 % of the annual disability adjusted life years (DALYs) lost because of road traffic injury (Peden et al. 2004). These figures illustrate the seriousness of the issue for public health. Projections show that, between 2000 and 2020, road traffic deaths will decline by about 30 % in high-income countries but increase substantially in low-income and middle-income countries (Peden et al. 2004).

For the purposes of this case study one risk factor—health outcome relationship was chosen to demonstrate the methodology of quantifying or approximating the effect or the relationship. Bicycle driver injuries were chosen as the health outcome and not wearing a helmet was chosen as a risk factor.

Effect Quantification

A quantified relationship between the defined risk factors and health outcomes should be a main outcome of the policy risk assessment. Such information will provide good arguments and evidence to describe the potential effects of the policy once implemented (positive or negative).

In optimal case a well-designed epidemiological study is conducted to analyze the relationship between the risk-factors and health outcomes. As a result clear and valid evidence would be presented for the risk assessment. However, considering the need for quick answers and conclusion on one side and lack of resources on the other side a simpler approach must be in place.

A scientific literature review on the topic of the risk factor-health outcome relationship analyzed could in most cases provide decent approximation of the effect of the implementation of the policy. Measures such as odds ratio, risk ratio, attributable risk fraction derived from studies conducted on the topic could serve to calculate the approximate effect of policy implementation on incidence or prevalence or other frequency measures of the health outcomes of interest.

In cases where such an approach is not feasible, an expert consensus or expert opinions could be used as a surrogate measure. It is obvious that this approach is the least valid but in many cases could be the best quantification tool possible.

For the purposes of our case study we demonstrate the approach of approximating the effect of the policy implementation based on evidence from scientific literature.

Our review of scientific literature was aimed at the effectiveness of helmets in bicycle riders as a protective measure against injuries. According to Thompson et al. (Thompson et al. 2000), the risk of head injury in helmeted vs. un-helmeted cyclists adjusted for age and motor vehicle involvement indicate a protective effect of 69–74 % for helmets for three different categories of head injury: any head injury (OR=0.31; CI 0.26–0.37), brain injury (OR, 0.35; CI 0.25–0.48), or severe brain injury (OR, 0.26; CI 0.14–0.48). In their study, helmets were equally effective in crashes involving motor vehicles (OR, 0.31; CI 0.20–0.48) and those not involving motor vehicles (OR, 0.32; CI 0.20–0.39).

The systematic review of Thompson et al. (Thompson et al. 1996) found no randomized controlled trials on the topic. Their review identified five well conducted case control studies suitable to be used in our case. Helmets according to them provide a 63–88 % reduction in the risk of head, brain, and severe brain injury for all ages of bicyclists. Helmets provide equal levels of protection for crashes involving motor vehicles (69 %) and crashes from all other causes (68 %). Injuries to the upper and mid facial areas are reduced by 65 %.

Coffman (2003) states that bicycle injuries are the most common cause of serious head injury in children, and most of these injuries are preventable.

The protective effect of bicycle helmets is well documented, but many child bicyclists do not wear them. This article summarizes the current state of research on bicycle injuries and helmet use and examines the effectiveness of legislation and injury-prevention strategies. Current studies according to Coffman indicate that children who wear helmets experience fewer head injuries and decreased severity of injury. Community-wide helmet-promotion campaigns combined with legislation are most successful in increasing helmet use and decreasing injury. Nurses can participate both at the institutional level and in community advocacy groups to promote bicycle safety for children.

Based on the above listed evidence for the relationship of not wearing a helmet and pertaining a head or brain injury it can be concluded that the reduction in risk by introducing obligatory helmet wearing can be approximated within the margins of 63–88 %.

Conclusion

Within the presented case study the full-chain approach was applied to evaluate the impact of the introduction of the new road traffic legislation on the health of the population. In all steps of the process (policy analysis, link to health determinants, risk factors, and identification and quantification of health outcome) the full chain approach has proven a suitable method to establish a link between selected parts of the policy, concrete determinants, and risk factors and quantifiable health outcomes. In the presented case study a specific relationship between obligatory helmet wearing (introduced by the new legislation) and risk of bicycle-related head and brain injuries was evaluated. Evidence from available scientific literature was used for the quantification. Using this method a prospective risk reduction of bicycle-related head and brain injuries within the margins of 63–88 % was estimated as an effect attributable to the introduction of the policy.

As a result of this case study a number of methodological considerations could be formulated for future use of the full-chain approach. On the level of policy selection it is crucial that the selected parts of the policy are clearly linkable with a specific group of health determinants so that the "causal chain" can be established and described in full extent. The established links should be clear, i.e. a pathway should be described in all cases as clear as possible including a description of the mechanism of the impact of the policy on particular determinants or groups of determinants.

On the level of risk factors it is essential that selected risk factors have an established link to at least one of the health determinants identified in the previous step, that they are clearly defined and if possible easily measurable. Same applies on the level of health effects where the possibility of effect quantification or at least approximation for the relationship of the risk factor and the health effect is important.

In general, steering committees or ad-hoc groups consisting of experts for the respective fields of interest should be used as advisory bodies wherever time and resources make this possible on virtually all levels of the assessment process.

The Lithuanian National Road Safety Program 2005–2010

Introduction

Traffic crashes cause about 127,000 deaths and 2.4 million injuries a year in the European Region. They kill more children and young people aged 5–29 than any other cause. Accidents remain the most important category of external cost of transport in Europe: 158 billion a year or 2.5–3.0 % of GDP in 17 Member States. The economic consequences of road insecurity have been estimated between 1 and 3 % of the respective GNP of the world countries (WHO 2010).

Road traffic injuries are one of the top three causes of death for people aged between 5 and 44 years, and a leading cause of death for people aged between 15 and 29 years (WHO 2008b).

Despite the significant growth in European road traffic volumes, it has been possible to reduce the total road death toll by 44 % between 1991 and 2006. While this positive trend can be seen across all countries in the European Union, there are significant variations between the different regions. Geographically, the highest rates of road deaths are to be found in eastern and south-eastern Member States of the European Union. Given the still lower level of vehicle ownership in most of these countries, the reasons behind these high values, compared to western Europe, can probably be found in the quality of infrastructure supply and less-developed awareness of road safety issues. Road traffic injury rates in Lithuania remain one of the highest in the European Union (WHO 2004b).

Road traffic injuries can be prevented. Experience suggests that an adequately funded lead agency and a national plan or strategies with measurable targets are crucial components of a sustainable response to road safety (WHO 2010).

Top-down approach was used for the case study and applied for the National Road SafetyProgramme 2005–2010. Top-down model implies that policy and certain targets set out in the policy as well as means to achieve these targets may have impact on certain determinants of health and cause direct and/or indirect changes in one, few, or all major determinants of health such as behavioral, environmental, socioeconomic, depending on the policy content. Modifications of the health determinants can than consequently cause changes in associated risk factors and they then cause changes in related health outcomes.

Policy Description

The National Road Safety Programme (further refered as Programme) for 2005–2010 has been adotped on 8 July 2005 by the Decision of the Government of the Republic of Lithuania No 759 (Government of the Republic of Lithuania 2005). It has been amended once in 2007 by the Decision of the Government of the Republic of Lithuania No 493 (Government of the Republic of Lithuania 2007).

The main intention of the Programme development was to create targeted and long-term conditions for improving traffic safety, to plan and implement relevant activities which would help to reduce accidents on the roads in order to reach road traffic safety without reducing mobility freedom but making it safer. By means of the Programme it was intended to implement the goal of the European Union—to reduce by half the number of people killed in road traffic events by 2010 (European Commission 2003).

The main target of the Programme is to reduce by half the number of people killed in road traffic events by 2010 in comparison with the year 2004. Other targets of the Programme are the following:

- By 2008 reduce number of killed on the roads by 25 %
- By 2008 reduce number of injuried during road traffic events by 10 %
- By 2010 reduce number of injuried during road traffic events by 20 %

Main objectives related to implementation of the above-mentioned targets are:

1. *related to human behavior*: by 2010 increase use of seat belts, special safety restraints, and safety chairs for children;reduce number of people driving under influence of alcohol, drugs, psychotropic, and other substances having mental impacts;make speed control more strict;improve education and examination of drivers;improve safety of pedestrians and cyclists;strengthen control of driver's work/rest regime;improve culture and education of traffic participants;improve the work of traffic control, medical care, and rescue services.
2. *related to road infrastructure*: eliminate causes of accidents in city and state road segments with high frequency of accidents;create a road safety audit;
3. *related to improvement of safety of vehicles*: improve visibility of heavy vehicles during the dark time of the day;improve safety of vehicles.
4. *related to legal basis improvement*: improve legal basis for safe traffic;develop a scientific study for establishment of insitution co-ordinating road safety.

Institutions involved in implementation of the Programme are the Ministry of Transport and Communications, the Ministry of Health, the Ministry of Education and Research, the Ministry of the Interior, the Ministry of Finance, Lithuanian Road Administration under the Ministry of Transport and Communications, Police Department under the Ministry of the Interior, Fire and Rescue Department under the Ministry of the Interior, head of counties' administrations, municipal authorities, other state authorities, nongovernmental organizations, and research institutions. The Ministry of Transport and Communications is holding the main responsibility andco-ordination function.

The permanently operating Road Safety Commission is monitoring implementation of the state policy in the field of traffic safety. Stakeholders invovled in implementation of the Programme are reporting to the Road Safety Commission. The Commission, approved by the Government, consists of state and municipal authorities, as well as representatives of nongovernmental organizations. Reflecting the high priority the Government gives to road safety, the Prime Minister chaired the Commission in 2008.

The Programme is directly accountable in terms of health consequences of crashes and collisions on the roads – fatalities and injuries. The main wider health determinants and risk factors are mentioned in the programme and linked to health outcomes.

Every year about 6,000 crashes happen on the roads where people are killed or injuried in Lithuania. Even more events happen in which road transport means, transport infrastructure objects are damaged.

Traffic intensity has increased on average by 3.8 % in the period 2002–2004. Number of people killed per 1,000 of vehicles was 0.46 in 2004.

In the period 2002–2004 2,155 persons were killed in road crashes (229—because of drunk drivers fault); out of them 717 pedestrians, 639 drivers; 504 passengers, 266 cyclists; and 22,585 (3,097 because of drunk drivers fault) were injuried.

In comparison with the other European Union countries in Lithuania fatality rates are very high for pedestrians and cyclists (50 % of all fatalities on the roads). 67.7 % of all traffic accidents happened because of the drivers' fault, and 20 % due to pedestrians´ fault.

For Lithuania the most frequent types of traffic accidents are collision with the pedestrian (35.5 % in 2002–2004;35.09 % in 2009); collision of vehicles (26.5 % in 2002–2004;33.39 % in 2009); collission with bycyclists (11.7 % in 2002–2004; 7.53 % in 2009), driving on an obsticle (11.3 % in 2002–2004; 7.66 % in 2009) and turning over (10.9 % in 2002–2004, and 9.25 % in 2009).

Determinants of Health

The Programme outlines four major determinants which all are related to health outcomes of road safety policy: related to human behavior, related to road infrastructure, related to improvement of safety of vehicles and related to legal basis improvement.

For the sake of this case study we used a modified Lalonde model of health determinants (Lalonde 1974) and identified the following wider determinants of health: biological, behavioral, environmental, socioeconomic, health care, rescue services accessibility, road safety culture.

Biological determinants include age and sex, as evidence shows that road users of certain age, especially young and elderly ones, are more vulnerable to exposure of different risk factors. Vulnerability to road crash deaths increases with age, being highest among people 20–24 years old. Three fourths of the people 0–24 years old killed in road crashes are male, and the increased risk for males relative to females increases with age. The increase with age reflects changes in exposure to risk resulting from differences in travel patterns (Sethi et al. 2007). Due to their greater frailty, the elderly are more likely to be seriously injured in any given accident than younger people (SafetyNet 2008). The ratios of elderly to middle-aged and of elderly to all fatalities clearly show that the risk of being killed in an accident is higher for the elderly than for the middle-aged and that the elderly have a higher fatality risk than the average in almost all EU-14 countries. Among the elderly, women are more likely to be killed in road accidents (36 %) than within the whole population (23 %) (SafetyNet 2008).

Behavioral determinants of health constitute one of the major groups of health determinants related to road safety policy. It is closely linked to biological, cultural, socioeconomic determinants. One of important aspects of behavioral determinants is the road safety culture described as the overall attitude of citizens to road safety, overall attitude towards the idea that safer is better than risky/fancy/"cool" which sometimes are used as synonyms. It is also related to values within the society determining choices between vehicle, public transport, walking, and cycling. Respect and understanding of other road users as full members of traffic process might change exposures to risk factors related to road traffic crashes.

Environmental determinants are related to physical environment features such as road infrastructure, modal mix, safety measures implemented on the roads, types of roads (urban, suburban; highways and other types of the roads). We considered vehicle design in this category too.

Socioeconomic factors are related to income, education, and well-being. We have also attributed legislation and enforcement, political will, media campaigns to socioeconomic determinants though in the literature they are also named as risk factors (or positive factors in case they exist and are implemented properly) (WHO 2004b). Allocation of funds necessary for implementation of evidence-based practices is one of major prerequisite for successful interventions.

Timely and qualified health care and rescue services accessibility has a major impact on the consequences of road crashes. It has recently been demonstrated that an inclusive trauma care system is associated with a significant risk reduction of mortality of 16 % (Lunevicius and Rahman 2012).

Risk Factors

Several risk factors increase the likelihood of road traffic injury. This include: inexperienced or novice drivers; excessive speed; not using helmets; driving under the influence of alcohol; failure to use seat-belts and child passenger restraints in cars; unsafe road design; insufficient vehicle crash protection; lack of conspicuousness (WHO Regional Office for Europe 2004).

Speed limits are set nationally, local authorities can set lower limits. Maximum limit on urban roads is 50 km/h. The level of enforcement of this regulation is graded as 6 on a 0–10 scale. The score represents consensus based on professional opinion of respondents of a WHO study (WHO 2009a). Drink-driving law exists. Blood alcohol concentration (BAC) limit for general population is 0,04 g/dl, and for young or novice drivers 0,02 g/dl. Random breath testing and/or police checkpoints are carried out periodically. Road traffic deaths involving alcohol was 12 % in 2006; the level of enforcement is graded 6 (WHO 2009a). Motorcycle helmet law exists; applies to all riders; helmet standards not mandate; helmet wearing rate is unknown; enforcement level is 6 (WHO 2009a). According to the same report seat-belt law exists; applies to all occupants; seat-belt wearing rate is unkown; enforcement level is 6, and child restraints law exists; level of enforcement is 5.

Study by Lunevicius and Rahman (2010) aimed to explore the epidemiology of road traffic injuries in Lithuania between 1998 and 2007showed that males, youth, pedestrians, and the elder suffer a significant burden of road traffic injuries. Since mortality rates are three to four times higher in male than in females, this may reflect a higher exposure to road traffic injury risk factors among males. Study showed one in every five road traffic injury deaths is related to alcohol consumption.

Lunevicius explored six data sources and pointed out that validity of each data source was not accessed independently but all of these data banks were used for national consumption. In some instances, such as determining the prevalence of alcohol in traffic crashes, data was not available for specific years. These datasets capture only alcohol as a risk factor for road traffic injuries; data for other risk factors, such as the use of seet belts, crash helmets, cell phones, and illicit drugs was not available. There is a lack of detailed data regarding specifix risks to different age groups, particulary youth and elderly, across various traffic settings.

Perceptions of different risks by different road users may have impact on effectiveness of interventions. They can be improved by taking recipients perceptions into account. Ramos et al (2008) studied young people perceptions of traffic injury rinks, prevention and enforcement measures applying quantitative method. Young people identified such determinants as driving under influence of drugs and alcohol; fatigue; night driving; unsafe infrastructures; age of drivers; lack of public transport alternatives. Young people admit the the following reduce risk driving: fines, speed kameras, alcohol breath testing. They prefer community work to fines. They have a poor image of public admisnitrations in charge of prevention of traffic injuries.

Health Outcomes

The main health outcome for the road safety policy is road traffic injury. It can be fatal or nonfatal.

Data on fatal road traffic injuries in Lithuania are based on the data recorded by the police. In this recording system persons killed in a road crash are persons who are injured in a road traffic crash and die within 30 days after the accident and are reported as road traffic deaths. Persons who are injured in a road traffic crash and need immediate hospital or inpatient treatment for at least 24 h are classified as seriously injured. Persons who are injured in a road traffic crash but don not need inpatient treatment are classified as slightly injured. However, official statistics differentiate only between fatalities and injuries, not specifying serious or slight injuries. Injuries are not properly recorded and might be substantially under reported.

Data from the Lithuanian Statistical Department even for fatalities differ from that of police, as it considers persons as killed in road traffic event as persons who are injured in a road traffic crash and die within 1 year after the accident.

Data used in this report is mainly based on police records 2010 (Table 3.8).

According to the data of Transport and Road Investigation Institute in 2009 losses due to road crashes were 1,558 million litas (approx. 450 million Euro), about 3 % of GDP (in other European countries these losses are about 1–2 % of GDP).

Starkuviene and authors evaluated the changes in years of potential life lost due to alcohol-related injuries in Lithuania for the "Year of sobriety" (2008) in comparison to the years 2006 and 2007 (Starkuviene et al. 2010). Age standardized rates of alcohol-related years of potential life lost (YPLL) per 100,000 population

Table 3.8 Change in number of deaths and injuries in Lithuania within the period of National Road Safety Programme implementation

Year/type of health outcome	2004	2010	Change, cases	Change, %
Fatalities	751	300	−451	−60 (goal of the programme−50)
Injuries	7877	4328	−3549	−45 (goal of the programme−20)

Source: Lithuanian Road Police Service (2010)

due to injuries (ICD-10 codes V01 − Y98) were calculated. Decline of YPLL/100,000 was observed for major types of injuries both for males and females, except suicides which increased from 2006 to 2008 by 17.7 % and reached 1133.8/100,000 population being the leading cause of YPLL among all alcohol-related injuries among males. The positive changes in YPLL due to alcohol-related injuries indicate successful implementation of evidence-based alcohol control measures (Starkuviene et al. 2010).

Lithuania has reached major achievements in reducing fatalities and injuries while targeting at substantial change in road safety in the country. In comparison with 2001 number of fatalities in road traffic events has been reduce by more than half. To a major extent the National road safety program 2005–2010 has contributed to these achievements, as substantial changes were reached during the last 3 years (2008–2010). Indicators related to all road traffic participants have improved. However, Lithuania is still among the ten European Union countries with the worst road fatality rates.

The new National road safety program for 2011–2017 sets more ambitious vision of long-term road safety in Lithuania with no fatalities and no serious injuries on the roads of Lithuania (Lithuanian zero vision). Based on the achievements of the analyzed Program, the main target for the new Program is to achieve a fatality rate that put Lithuania among the first ten countries with the best figures in the European Union. Based on the 2009 data of the European Transport Safety Council the best countries were Sweden, United Kingdom, the Netherlands, Malta, Germany, Finland, Ireland, Denmark, Spain, and France with number of deaths /1 million inhabitants ranging from 39 to 66 (average 51.2). There is room for improvement; the number of deaths per one million inhabitants in Lithuania was 110 in 2009.

Conclusion

The Programme is directly accountable in terms of health consequences of crashes and collisions on the roads causing fatalities and injuries. The main wider health determinants and risk factors are mentioned in the programme and linked to health outcomes. Programme measures are based on evidence of best practice and effective interventions.

Programme has fully achieved its targets and contributed to the reduction of fatalities by 60 % and of road traffic injuries by 45 % in 2010 compared to 2004.

Additional data on relations between policy options and wider health determinants would help to identify driving forces and pressures influencing health outcome.

Data regarding age-specific patterns and injury-related risk factors are needed to further inform effective prevention strategies in Lithuania. Further, prospective studies are also necessary to evaluate the extent to which these risk factors affect injury incidence.

The Slovenian National Strategy on Wine Production

Introduction

The wine production and consumption has great tradition and importance in Slovenia. Slovenia is a net importer of grapes and wines. More stable development in vineyard areas, but decline in yields, are found for Slovenia. Exports and imports of wines are approximately at similar levels, but relations between export and import wine prices are rather unstable (Bojnec 2006).

The wine production represents important share of agricultural economy in Slovenia. Around 100.000 people live at least partially from wine production. Wine production represents 9.9 % of total domestic product in agriculture, which represented the second largest single share of crop production in 2008 (Žavcer 2010).

Policy Description

Policies affecting wine production are of importance for sector, national economy, and well-being. Strategy on wine production in Slovenia has been drafted in August 2009 by Ministry of Agriculture, Forestry and Food of the Republic of Slovenia, Directorate for Agriculture. The main aims of the Strategy are the following: preservation of present surface area of vineyards by improvement of knowledge of wine producers, use of environment friendly technologies including biological wine growing, preservation of domestic market share for wine production by means of production of wines of better quality, marketing campaigns, education of wine producers and wine consumers, and increase the share of export.

In April 2008 the European Commission adopted regulation 479/2008 which reorganizes the EU wine market and replaces the previous regulation EC 1493/1999 which was reaction to not stable balance between supply and demand in late 90s when wine consumption in EU has been decreasing and the wine exports has been increasing at a much slower rate than the imports. The purpose of the new regulation is to ensure that EU wine production matches demand, to eliminate public intervention in EU wine markets and to make the European wine more competitive. According to the new EU legislation, Strategy on wine production falls well into new EU legislation. National legislation is in compliance with EU legislation.

The driving force for the new Strategy is European legislation and need in the country to turn trends of wine production and wine market. There are three main population groups that this policy could affect. Wine growers are the main group that are going to be affected. The new Strategy on Wine Production brings mostly new quality standards, what means that that growers will need to comply with them, the anticipated result is likely growth of sale. It is expected that the policy will have impact on workers in wine production. Occupational health is expected to improve; introduction of new technologies to reduce exposure to pesticides will result in decreased number of occupational diseases. The Strategy could have an impact on consumers of wine, too. An increased consumption of high-quality wine in moderate amount and a decreased consumption of low-quality wine is expected (Grønbaek et al. 2001).

Implementation of the Strategy is at most parts very likely. It is difficult to predict whether such kind of Strategy can increase export of wine, this will depend mostly on situation on global market.

Determinants of Health and Risk Factors

The Strategy was discussed with representatives of all involved sectors and groups at stakeholders meeting. There is a difficulty to make a clear comprehensive selection of health determinants on which the policy could have an impact.

There is no good precise tool and therefore selection is based on input of stakeholders and good knowledge and experiences of the assessing team. Impact on the following health determinants and related risk factors was identified.

Environmental Determinants

The Strategy states demand for using "environment friendly technologies—including biological wine growing". The main aim of new Strategy is to avoid excessive use of pesticides and fertilizers and go for the use of environmental friendly products. Pesticides are a cause of pollution, affecting land and water in particular. The acute effects of pesticide exposure are well known, particularly through certification procedures and reports of epidemics of poisoning, occupational accidents, and suicide attempts. Besides cancers and reproductive effects, nervous system damage has been reported in terms of peripheral neuropathy and central nervous degenerative disease, with special emphasis on Parkinson's disease (Checkoway and Nelson 1999, 327–336). It is expected that new Strategy on Wine Production will cause preservation of land, reduce the amount of used pesticides and fertilizers and have an overall positive impact on environment. The risk for environment and exposure of workers to pesticides will decrease.

Socioeconomic Determinants

The aim of the Strategy is "preservation of present wine production," what means present or possibly increased tax revenue.

The new Strategy on Wine Production will not have important impact on tax revenue and common welfare. The main aim is to preserve present production and present tax revenue which represents very small part in budget revenue.

Employment has positive effect on health in any society. It is well known that societies with high unemployment rate have very high rate of ill- health. Unemployment leads to social deprivation, poor income (need for social support), and poor mental health of unemployed and to disparity in society. Result is usually unhealthy lifestyle (smoking, drinking), which is the main risk factor for many chronic diseases. Wine production is a source of living for 5 % of total population in the country. A drop of wine production would result in decrease of unemployment rate.

Risk related to unemployment is alcohol abuse. Unemployment rates in alcohol treatment programs are strikingly high, yet the drinking behavior of unemployed populations has been neglected by alcohol researchers. Stress-based and socio environmental theories of alcoholism coupled with empirical research on the health and social costs of unemployment have suggested that the unemployed may be "at risk" for abusing alcohol. Specifically, the unemployed are said to abuse alcohol as a means of coping with financial stress triggered by job loss. The study, "The public health effect of economic crisis and alternative policy responses in Europe: an empirical analysis," found that a rise of 3 % in unemployment is associated with a 28 % increase in deaths from alcohol abuse and a 4.5 % increase in suicides in the population younger than age 65 (Stuckler et al. 2009). Unemployment is a main risk for social exclusion and deprivation and consequently for risks such as alcohol abuse. Different components of social exclusion influence each other, thus creating a spiral of insecurity, which ends in multiple deprivations. Deprivation usually begins with the loss of employment, which in turn leads to a significant degradation in living standards, that is, increased risk of poverty.

The risk factors related to social exclusion and deprivation are alcohol abuse, drug addiction, heavy smoking, unhealthy diet, poor living conditions (damp).

Behavioral and Personal Determinants

Price of wine has impact on wine consumption. There is pretty good negative correlation between alcohol—wine consumption and price. For example, a price elasticity of alcohol demand of −0.5 means that a 1 % increase in price would reduce alcohol consumption by 0.5 % (or a 10 % increase in price would reduce consumption by 5 %) (Chaloupka et al. 2002). The Strategy is emphasizing production of high-quality wines what means average rise in price. Consumption volumes may reduce as a result of increased cost of quality wines. Changes in wine drinking habits may also initiate positive alterations in the composition and consumption habits of diet (Ruidavets et al. 2004).

For the prioritization of health determinants easily usable table was developed with a scoring system. The following criteria were used in the prioritization process: number of people affected, quality of life affected, national expenses affected, and literature evidence. The most important health determinant is the employment rate. The criteria were assessed on very broad way and must be considered with big uncertainty.

Exposed Groups

The Strategy affects mostly people working in wine industry and to some extent the whole population. Fulfillment can prevent loss of jobs in the wine sector and dependant sectors and prevents further national financial burden for social benefits. There will not be important impact on wine consumers and general population as the consumption of wine is just partly determined by price and quality.

Horizontal Interactions

The most important determinant of health is socioeconomic. The group of socioeconomic determinants has few subdeterminants, such as trading, sales, income, common welfare the most important for public health is employment rate. There is a hierarchy in the group of socioeconomic determinants, one having impact on the other. For example good sale and good production are having positive impact on employment rate and the latter on education. On the other hand good education, knowledge of production, and sales, have impact on production and sale and consequently on employment rate. It seems like subdeterminants influence each other, not that much as top-down model but more as a circle model. Behavioral and personal determinants (wine consumption) are not expected to undergo big change. It is likely that price of wine (socioeconomic determinant) will have impact on consumption of wine (behavioral and personal determinant). But on the other hand, consumption of wine has impact on production, sale, and employment rate (socioeconomic determinants) in the sector. Socioeconomic determinants of health are having impact on behavioral and personal determinants and other way around.

Summary

The impact on environmental determinant of health is not of big importance. The main aim of Strategy is to preserve production and sales what would have positive impact on employment rate which is far the most important health determinant for public health. There is strong connection between the determinants of health.

The following main risk factors were identified: alcohol abuse, social exclusion, and deprivation, exposure to pesticides at work place, increased amount of manual work. Most risk factors are influenced by poor implementation or failure of the Strategy.

Health Outcomes

Alcohol abuse causes a number of diseases and conditions that are solely attributable to alcohol. These include alcoholic psychoses, as well as some diseases affecting the nerves, degeneration of nervous system due to alcohol, alcoholic myopathy, alcoholic gastritis and pancreatitis, alcoholic liver cirrhosis, and number of other conditions.

There are also a number of diseases and conditions which are only partially attributed to alcohol. For instance alcohol can contribute to a number of different cancers. The risks of developing lip, tongue, throat, esophagus and liver cancer increases proportionally with the amount of alcohol consumed. Even moderate alcohol consumption can increase the likelihood of breast cancer, according to recent research, and a series of studies confirm that the risk increases with the amount consumed (WHO 2004a).

Alcohol consumption is also strongly associated with intentional injuries caused by aggressive behavior leading to violent crime.

Social exclusion and deprivation leads to alcohol abuse, drug addiction, heavy smoking, unhealthy diet, and poor living conditions. Risk factors deriving from social exclusion and deprivation can cause alcohol abuse that causes all diseases related to alcohol consumption mentioned above. Another consequence is heavy smoking. Cigarette smoke contains several carcinogenic pyrolytic products that bind to DNA, causing lung cancer, cancer of the mouth, larynx, possibly cancer of pancreas, bladder, and breast. Cigarette smoke causes chronic obstructive lung disease, emphysema, impairment of lung function, exacerbation of asthma, chronic heart disease, heart attack, stroke, and peripheral vascular disease and hypertension. A result of social deprivation is unhealthy diet that is important risk factor for heart disease, vascular diseases, metabolic disorders and diseases, some cancers (colon, rectum, and pancreas). Poor living conditions can also cause some diseases, such as respiratory diseases, allergies, and mental disorders due to overcrowding.

Occupational health problems in wine production sector are commonly reported. Viticulture workers are at risk of work-related musculoskeletal problems, especially of the wrists and hands, from vine pruning work, and can develop allergic diseases, including occupational asthma, from exposure to insect pests growing on vines (Youakim 2006).

The Strategy aims not to use chemicals in wine production but mostly organic substances. Therefore from the point of view of pesticide exposure at work place, it is very likely to expect less disease caused by pesticide exposure. On the other hand manual work will increase what means more injuries and absenteeism due to injuries.

Outcome Assessment

At this stage due to lack of background data, it is speculative to assume the number of new cases of diseased people who will face social exclusion and deprivation and consequently alcohol abuse, unhealthy diet and adopt other risk factors because of possible loss of job, due to failure of implementation of the new Strategy.

Summary

There are number of diseases with well-known and established etiology that can be ascribed to failed implementation of Strategy. Most of them are related to increased unemployment rate and pathology deriving from poor social conditions of people.

The most known risk factors are alcohol abuse, heavy smoking, unhealthy diet, and poor living conditions, all of them leading to a number of diseases.

There is a massive body of literature on different risk factors described above and possible health outcome.

Conclusion

The selected policy is a sectoral policy prepared by the Agricultural sector with the aim to preserve present production of wine. It is a result of on-going decrease of wine production and wine sales.

The assessment was made in direction what would be if proposed Strategy would not be implemented. The Strategy is a policy that has the intention to save and preserve the present situation from on-going decline.

The most important determinants of health are socioeconomic. It has subdeterminants, such as, trading, sales, income, common welfare, and most important one for public health issue — employment. It seems like subdeterminants influence each other, not that much in top-down direction but more as a circle. Therefore one policy with just one positive impact on one subdeterminant can have a chain reaction on a couple of determinants and the other way around.

The risk factors affected by increased unemployment rate are alcohol abuse and social deprivation and exclusion. Alcohol abuse is also an outcome of broader social deprivation and exclusion. The other risk factors in that group are unhealthy diet, heavy smoking, and poor living conditions.

What is still not available is reliable data on diseases and risk factors, on some exposures/intakes, and time of exposure needed for development of diseases. That makes quantification difficult. The other problem is lack of information about people who are affected by the policy in such way that health can deteriorate, leading to development of disease.

That was the main obstacle in the study. Even whether a part of quantification was possible (like number of people who could lose jobs) quantification of risk affecting people to develop disease was impossible to calculate.

There are still a lot of uncertainties. They could get overcome in the future with the availability of more sophisticated methods and when the picture of impact of any policy on disease development will get clearer.

Research Need and Feasibility of the Health Impact Quantification of Policies for Medical Uses of Radiation in Tuscany, Italy

Introduction

Over the last 30 years imaging techniques have become indispensable as an aid in diagnosis, prognosis, monitoring of disease, and the implementation of interventional procedures (both diagnostic and therapeutic). Among medical imaging techniques radiological and nuclear medicine examinations are based on the use of ionizing energy ("Ionizing Radiations" IR). Medical Imaging (MI) exposes the patient and the operator to physical hazard and confers a definite (albeit low) long-term risk of cancer. Computed Tomography (CT) procedure has grown exponentially by 7.8 % annually between 1996 and 2010 in the USA. In particular, in 2006 CT for cardiovascular clinical test accounted for 12.1 % of the collective radiation dose used in a wide variety of cardiovascular conditions (NCRP 2009). The American National Cancer Institute researchers estimated that radiation from more than 70 million CT scans performed in the United States in 2007 would ultimately cause 29,000 cases of cancer that could lead to 15,000 deaths (Berrington de González et al. 2009). Therefore imaging testing is a significant source of radiation exposure of a not negligible proportion of the general population.

The achieved results support EU and the Member States to increase and reinforce public health interventions in the radioprotection policy area preventing unnecessary exposure due to increasing trends in prescriptions of radiological exams. In general, literature findings point out the need for better guidelines for health professionals based on evidences balancing benefits of imaging use against financial costs and long-term health risks. Moreover, although the legislation has set limits to the dose per exams, no indications are provided to strictly control on factors responsible for avoidable irradiation, mainly associated to unawareness about the risk induced by IR in medical imaging testing. Precautionary policies should address efforts toward monitoring the accordance between medical practice and interventions based on integrated risk assessment.

Context and Aims

Within the RAPID project, the present case study has tested a full chain approach for the assessment of health impacts due to the use of IR under the current guidelines, with a focus to the use of medical imaging testing in cardiovascular diseases. The level of the determinants of health has been of particular interests as for clarifying up streaming dependence from policy and down streaming modification of the exposure to the risk factors.

The impact assessment was performed to enlighten determinants of health actually modified by the current policy and to evaluate the feasibility of quantification of cancer cases attributable to useless exams in the current "unawareness scenario". Overexposure mainly depends on useless medical imaging testing, which relates to one-third of all CT scans, according to Brenner (Brenner and Hall 2007).

The tertiary care cardiological department of the Institute of Clinical Physiology of the National Research Council in Pisa, (IFC CNR) made available its expertise and clinical practice either to define priorities for different health determinants and also to estimate the attributable cancer incidence and mortality for cardiological patients admitted in the IFC clinical ward. A preliminary investigation on exposure patterns, according to interventions targeted to reduce useless exams, had been carried out at a regional level.

Assessing the health impact of the medical imaging testing under the Tuscany regional radioprotection regulation, would supply a comprehensive knowledge for decision maker. The description of the full chain of the causal pathway, proceeding from the legislation (top) to the selected health outcome (down), would enhance those policies targeted to reduce the irradiated dose, therefore contributing to decrease the number of future potential cancers due to ionizing radiation testing.

Policy Description

National Legislative Decree 187/00, issued to implement the European directive 97/43/Euratom, regulates protecting the patient from ionizing radiation. The International Commission on Radiological Protection sets recommended dose limits in planned occupational and public exposure situations. As for patient's context, guidelines indicate limits of radiological examinations for different parts of the body.

In accordance with the implementation of Euratom Directive, Tuscany Regional Law N. 32, 2003, disciplines the assessment of exposures for medical purposes with regard to the regional population and concerned groups. According to the implementation of Decree 187/2000, the Tuscany Regional Health Plan 2008–2010 recommends the definition of protocols and best practices addressed to reach a significant reduction of ionizing radiations in medical practice. In particular, the Plan acts in accordance with local initiatives conveying towards industrials, physicians, and patients awareness with the aim of modifying cultural and socioeconomic health determinants.

Underpinning Motivations for the Case Study and Background Knowledge

Selection of the policy was based on the consideration that the inappropriate use of ionizing imaging testing, fueled by radiological unawareness, is a significant source of useless radiation exposure of patients often creating a risk without a commensurate benefit. The links between the regional legislation on population radioprotection and the research focus in the Institute are more specifically described below.

- At first, according to programs endorsed by the Food and Drug Administration in 2010, the Tuscany Regional Council has taken a commitment to monitor the radiation exposure of the population and medical workers due to medical examinations, and to promote a widespread communication campaign for Tuscany citizens including a training pathway on risks from exposure to IR.

  Therefore, the regional government funded the project "Stop Useless Ionizing Testing in Heart Disease—primary prevention of cancer through reduction of inappropriate ionizing testing" (SUIT-HEART Project) to the Institute of Clinical Physiology and Istituto Toscano Tumori.

- Secondly, the Institute research activity is mainly targeted to support local and national policy maker to promote and adopt healthier plans by increasing the current base of knowledge. Among the issues of IR, a clinical research branch is aimed to improve knowledge in radiation-related risks of cardiologists, patients, technologists, medical physicists, and radiologists. Furthermore, a specific attention is pointed towards general practitioners and public administrators. Generally, most of cardiologists and other specialists share a lack of knowledge concerning the risk of commonly performed imaging tests using ionizing radiation, and they do not fully disclose risks and alternative indications to patients (Correia et al. 2005). The need of training on updated imaging techniques is also common among physicians. Therefore, specific goals of IFC are to train and inform specialists and practitioners, inform users, to help patients in understanding the implications of the informed consent, and to program interventions for reducing the radiation release in medical practice.

Worldwide, policies will enhance the knowledge of risks by monitoring the radiation exposure, and the adequate use of devices. Recently, Halliburton and Schoenhagen (2010) have described specific areas of policy interventions to reduce the inappropriate use of imaging techniques. They include promoting the patient awareness about the radiation risks, expanding the appropriateness criteria into clinical decision making, incorporating safeguards into scanner designs, developing radiation dose reference values for specific procedures, incorporating radiation dose values into the electronic medical records, creating a national dose registry, establishing minimum standards for training and education of imaging personnel, and expanding mandatory accreditation for advanced imaging facilities.

Particularly, for the Tuscan regional context, political actions should be enhanced to balance the criteria of justification of radiological medical procedure with the health care system strategy, actually based on reimbursement per number of exams performed. Based on this strategy the use of medical imaging tests in the diagnostic and therapeutic pathway is indirectly favored.

Further strategies, within other political sectors, have been highlighted to be cross-linked to radioprotection issues, indirectly affecting the distal determinants of health. Mainly they regard the passenger safety in air travels, the management of radioactive hazardous waste, the disposal of contaminated equipment, the occupational safety, new health technologies cost-benefit analysis, the manufacturers' profit, and the medico-legal issues.

Determinants of Health and Risk Factors

Determinants of health are personal, social, biological, economic, and environmental factors that are responsible for the distribution of risk factors in the populations and interact with each other. These factors are affected by decisions and choices that connect the health sector to other sectors. In this sense, they weave a dependency with judgments not based on health benefit but rather on convenience for the health care system, for the economic or commercial context or for the interests of lobbies (academics, enterprises, etc.). Generally, the distal factors, depending on the socio-economic, the general cultural and political context are considered as the wider determinants of health. Determinants of health that have been included here, are the sharp rise in the number of medical imaging testing, the level of technological updating, the public strategy for the reimbursement of healthcare services, patient expectation to be assisted, underestimation of risks by practitioners and physicians, training strategies for practitioners, referral guidelines effectiveness.

All these factors affect the dose to patients more or less indirectly. Differently the medical practice is a factor depending on physician abilities and awareness of risks. Therefore, it might largely determine the exposure more directly, playing a role similar to the risk factor itself.

Both natural and artificial radiations are risk factors and they directly increase the cumulative individual effective dose and, therefore, the possible risk of cancer. The current use of radiological imaging techniques is the major artificial source of radiation accounting for 150 % of natural radiation source, two-thirds coming from cardiovascular testing. Other patient-related co-factors are responsible for the increase of cumulative individual exposure. They are mainly: age, gender, suspected diagnosis as well as individual characteristics, and working within the staff of the interventional cardiology or previous exposure history (occupational or residential) and life activity patterns (number of aircrafts flights have shown to raise exposure to cosmic rays).

General Findings and Feasibility of Exposure Quantification

Within the case study, the health determinants were identified and prioritized in a desktop-based assessment. At first, an extensive review of recent evidence (high-impact factor journals, guidelines, and recommendations by scientific associations were analyzed) allowed the identification of factors to be included in the chain and of the principal connections, within levels and through the causal chain. Secondarily, a checklist was developed for the consultation of a multidisciplinary team made by eight experts in disciplines related to medical imaging (cardiology, radiology, hemodynamic, pulmonary, nuclear physic, genetic, general medicine, health care system management). Main determinants of the risk factor causing differential pathways of exposure in the medical setting were identified and classified by relevance from low to great. They are listed below in order of relevance:

1. "Experience and training" of technicians and physicians of the imaging groups. This factor strongly increases the appropriate use of medical procedures and optimization of radioprotection guidelines.
2. "Facility assets" including equipment and technological devices, which collectively affect the patient dose.
3. "Definition of operative protocols" (i.e. the adaptation of X-ray parameters to body characteristics) may significantly reduce the exposure when tailored to the patient characteristics.

4. "Justification for radiation-based examination", such as CT, has been considered crucial for unnecessary exposure avoidance. In particular, IFC researchers have shown that, in some contexts, clinical protocols with the lowest possible radiation dose can provide same information with a significant reduction of risk (Picano 2003).

In agreement with the general literature findings, experts have also highlighted specific actions conveying positive effects upon the current medical practice and the prescription standard. Specifically, they include an increased user's knowledge on imaging techniques and dose-risk relation (including the knowledge of the long-term risks and the downstream costs due to cancer, carried out with the risk-benefit analysis), the communication of radiological risk to the patient undergoing an exam.

However, currently, mainly qualitative and subjective metrics are available to highlight the impacts of the different interventions mentioned above. Attempts to quantify the effect of specific actions tailored to a reduction of dose have been shown in the literature, for example comparing scan protocols, primary health care systems, trained health operators, protocols for clinical diagnosis.

In consideration of the scarce quantitative information and the complex network regarding all the above detailed factors, the analysis of impacts has been narrowed to the consideration of the level of useless exams performed by the physicians within the clinical cardiology ward of the Institute.

The assessment focused the European and national indications for minimizing the number of CT by adhering more strictly to referral guidelines. Therefore, we evaluated the feasibility of comparing the current exposure scenario to a more conservative one, due to the implementation of an appropriate use of medical imaging testing. In cardiovascular disease, the impact of current guidelines has been quantified by IFC researchers in terms of useless exams performed by physicians ranging from about 20 to 40 %, depending on the type of radiological examination (Picano et al. 2007).

The health gain could be quantified in terms of number of cancer cases saved at the regional population level accounting for a medical practice based on risk awareness.

Apart from the interventional cardiologists, who are today the most exposed among health professionals (Venneri et al. 2009), IFC researchers have considered subpopulation of exposed man and women, aged 56–77 years, primarily admitted to the cardiological ward of the clinic for coronary artery disease, previous revascularization procedure, previous infarction, heart failure, or severe arrhythmias (Bedetti et al. 2008).

Assessing exposure would require defining opportunely the time window, standardize at regional level either the patients admissible to the cardiological ward and the procedures that they could be addressed to after the diagnosis has been done. Lastly, the dose irradiated by different medical imaging teams should be ascertained and a median value provided, controlling between machines variability. Additional limitation is carried by the measure of awareness which is subject to semi-quantitative measuring, and the average radiological awareness among physicians is currently ranked by a scoring system (Picano et al. 2007).

The evolving trend of multi-slice computed tomography use should also be reconsidered including costs and financial recession.

To enforce the regional radioprotection programmes, the impact of the above enlisted factors acting on the awareness scenario should be more calculation-based. Currently, no stable survey of the practice has been put in place to estimate the magnitude of inappropriate usage.

Health Outcomes

Ionizing radiation is known to cause harm. Some cardiological interventional procedures with long screening times and multiple image acquisition (e.g. percutaneous coronary intervention, and radio-frequency ablation) may give rise to deterministic effects in both staff and patients as skin lesions, erythema, ulcers, epilation, cataracts and permanent sterility. Damage at DNA level is a probabilistic effect (there is no known threshold dose) and is considered the main initiating event by which radiation damage to cells results in development of cancer. Laboratory studies have provided data on radiation induced genetic effects. The likelihood of inducing the effect increases in relation to dose and may differ among individuals.

While the effects of low-level exposure remain uncertain (Brenner et al. 2003), the associations between radiation exposure and the development of cancer are mostly based on populations exposed to relatively high levels of ionizing radiation.

The estimate of the attributable cancer incidences is based on the rates of cancer that occurred in people exposed to radiation from the atomic bombs dropped on the Japanese cities of Hiroshima and Nagasaki at the end of World War Two. However, many experts consider that model inadequate.

Attributable total cancer risk has been chosen as health outcome. It is statistically calculated combining evidence of dose estimates and cancer risk estimates. IFC researchers have recently assessed the cumulative effective dose as indicator of stochastic risk of cancer in adult patients admitted to the cardiology ward (Bedetti et al. 2008). The cumulative radiological history was collected from a structured questionnaire. The amount of cumulative risk for the patient and for subpopulations was calculated, based on the personal history of exposure to ionizing radiation (including three main subcomponents of exposure natural, diagnostic, professional). Current guidelines, dose references, and accepted evidence in BEIRVII were used to calculate risk. Results showed that three types of procedures were responsible for 86 % of the total collective effective dose and the median estimated extra risk of cancer was approximately 1 in 200 exposed subjects (Bedetti et al. 2008).

Therefore, risk quantification could be computed for the regional level by standardizing technological parameters determining the median irradiated dose among cardiovascular centers.

Conclusion

The case study has developed the assessment of a policy, actually addressed to protect health, introducing the full chain approach to fully disclosing factors that are indirectly connected to health and dependent from other sectors. Presentation of the full chain to the medical division personnel has highlighted a common stricter view of what is health. In addition, a methodological guide to support decision makers in the assessment the complex health impacts of policies has been tested, including the consideration of horizontal actions planned in different sectors. In particular, the analysis has disclosed different but contemporary strategies (i.e. manufacturers' business interests, financial trends orienting the healthcare system, incomplete developed scientific evidence for long-term risks) that modify the use of MI and the awareness of risk, indirectly determining the exposure to the risk factor.

Finally, ethical issues are to be stressed to enhance the awareness of risks, either targeting the educational upgrading of physicians and the communication of possible risks to patients. The local government commitment appears fundamental for driving local interventions and for targeting the issue of effective communication and information.

The quantification of the impact from single intervention could be crucial to develop strategies for risk reduction but it remains a challenge for future research. Further quantification could facilitate the decision based on differential exposure scenarios.

In conclusion, cancer morbidity and mortality attributed to the medical imaging have been shown to be driven by a not satisfactory evaluation and monitoring of the current policy programs and guidelines.

When a top-down assessment of a policy is approached, the opportunity for expanding the analysis beyond conventional or proximal health determinants by involving actors within policies connected with public health actions should be explored.

Direct effect is observed for single location initiatives (i.e. those promoted within the IFC research programs on awareness). The public health authority together with medical corporate, manufacturers, business innovators, and product developers in the imaging sector, could lead the efficacy of interventions to a higher regional and national scale, collectively driving the understanding about the risks from medical devices using IR.

The Influenza Preparedness Plan of Romania

Introduction

The case-study is a top-down analysis of Romania's National Plan for Intervention in Influenza Pandemics based on a theoretical model/framework as per guidelines and standard set of health measures prescribed by the European Centre for Disease Prevention and Control (ECDC) and WHO. The case study analyses the existing policy and suggests two alternatives also.

Romania's existing policy on influenza pandemic preparedness is discussed keeping in perspective data based on the outbreak in 2009. The data were collected based on the following parameters: improvement in the population health, utilization of healthcare system, and years of potential life lost before age 65.

Policy Description

The case study discusses the current policy as well as two alternative policies covering in detail content, strategy, output analysis, policy implementation aspects, stakeholder analysis, health determinants analysis (socioeconomic, lifestyle and behavior, access to services, environment), and finally, the health status impact assessment. The current policy for preventing and limiting illness A/H1N1 was prepared by the Romanian Ministry of Health (order nr.1094/10.09.2009) under the guidance of the European Union. The first alternative policy focuses on proactive school closure (Electronic school absenteeism surveillance, Manual setting supervision in schools, Education delivery strategy). The second alternative policy focuses on prevention and preparedness for influenza pandemic, by increasing the vaccination rate among people of all age groups.

The case study is based on literature review of various relevant research articles, observational papers, and modeling studies, which aimed to gather the most significant information and data appropriate for the study.

ECDC Reports and WHO guidelines concerning pandemic influenza were the basic information sources and moreover, the standard recommendation for comparing national plans and strategies regarding school closures in different countries which decreased the spread of the virus.

The ECDC (2009) defines social distancing as a collection of measures intended to decrease the frequency of contact among people, therefore possibly reducing influenza transmission. Another definition which in meaning is similar to the first one says that social distancing is a term applied to certain actions that are taken by health officials to stop or slow down the spread of a highly contagious disease.

According to these, the school settings and day care interventions are measures included in this category and these may have some positive impact by reducing transmission of human respiratory infection spreading from person to person.

The key words used for the study were social distancing measure, school closure, and influenza pandemic, reactive/proactive school closure intervention, from the National Library of Medicine and other online libraries from different university web sites.

Data were collected for four measures of the impact of pandemic influenza on the population (both as case count and rate per 100,000 population): infected cases, hospitalizations, deaths, and years of potential life lost by the age of 65 (YPLL65).

The influenza that the AH1N1 virus brought caused many controversies in Romania both on international and national level. Following the discovery of this virus, the most important question which was raised was what solutions and strategies are needed in order to lower as much as possible the infection rates on national level.

Based on a research in France on the cause of the outbreak of the virus and the willingness of the population to get vaccinated against pandemic influenza, the following criteria were found to be most relevant:

- The level of worry and experience of seasonal influenza vaccination (came out to be the strongest factors predicting vaccination intention against A/H1N1 influenza)
- The low-level perception of risk (at the beginning of the pandemic influenza it is perceived to have similar risks as seasonal influenza does, becoming a factor of refusal to get vaccinated)
- The increase of vaccination depends a lot on the perception factor, which needs a change by using the Health Belief Model (Setbon and Raude 2010).

The Romanian Ministry of Health developed two series of campaigns for promoting the vaccination process against pandemic influenza; the first vaccines were administrated to students, pregnant women, and medical system employees on the 1st of December 2009, being one of the strategies regarding priority groups.

The pandemic influenza info's as part of the second campaign spread as fast as the disease itself, in the mass-media in order to convince Romanian population to get vaccinated: TV news, newspapers, and the Ministry of Health internet site. The accent was on increasing the idea of risk related to this new influenza, since the general opinion of the population was to relate it to a seasonal influenza risks and not believing on its high level of risks proven worldwide.

With more than 60 % of cases aged 18 or younger in some influenza pandemics, children appear to be important vectors of transmission, and are more infectious and susceptible to most influenza strains than are adults (Cauchemez et al. 2009).

High-risk groups must be considered when vaccination starts because these individuals have high complications risk and must be vaccinated earlier:

- All children aged 6–23 months
- Adults aged 65 years and older
- Person aged 2–64 years with underlying chronic medical conditions
- Pregnant women
- People who live together in large numbers in an environment where influenza can spread rapidly, such as prisons, nursing homes, schools, and dormitories
- Healthcare workers
- Patients who are immunosuppressed

As per the case study respiratory infections are always observed to spread easily in day care and school settings.

School closure can operate as a proactive measure, aimed at reducing transmission in the school and spread into the wider community. School closure can also be a reactive measure, when schools close or classes are suspended because high levels of absenteeism among students and staff make it impractical to continue classes.

The main health benefit of proactive school closure comes from slowing down the spread of an outbreak within a given area and thus flattening the peak of infections.

Vaccination is the most effective method for preventing influenza infection. Trials have been conducted to demonstrate that vaccines offer protection for population and calculated effectiveness has ranged between 30 and 70 % in preventing hospitalization (WHO 2006).

The main economic cost arises from absenteeism of working parents or guardians who have to stay home to take care of their children. Studies estimate that school closures can lead to the absence of 16 % of the workforce, in addition to normal levels of absenteeism and absenteeism due to illness. Decisions also need to consider social welfare issues. Children's health and well-being can be compromised if highly beneficial school-based social program, such as the provision of meals, are interrupted or if young children are left at home without supervision. The estimated costs of school closure are significant, at £0.2 bn—£1.2 bn per week. School closure is likely to significantly exacerbate the pressures on the health system through staff absenteeism (Sadique et al. 2008).

Determinants of Health and Risk Factors

The determinants of health and related risk factors identified to be influenced by the assessed policy are as follows:

- Social distancing and quarantining: internal travel restrictions, isolation and quarantine, workplace closures, avoiding personal contact, cancel public events
- Travel and trade restrictions: travel advice, entry screening, border closure, international travel restrictions
- Community infection control: animal and bird surveillance, prophylaxis, prisons, military barracks, and home for elderly surveillance
- General personal hygiene: self-hygiene hygiene, respiratory hygiene, mask wearing, regular hand washing

Based on the identified determinants of health and risk factors the case study gives a comparison of the existing policy vis-a-vis the two alternatives.

Status Quo: Under the European Union guidance, Romanian Ministry of Health developed an action plan for preventing and limiting illness by influenza A/H1N1 in public and private school systems (order nr.1094/10.09.2009).

- The action plan for preventing and limiting illness by influenza A/H1N1 in the public and private school units shall be updated according to the epidemiological situation at national and international level in accordance with the recommendation of European and International organizations
- The County Departments of Public Health will allocate to the School Authorities materials on influenza and preventive measures to inform students, parents, and teachers on the effects of this issue

- The school directors are responsible for the information circuit and for the implementation of the measures in compliance with the suspected cases of influenza illness
- The school directors have to create a database with all the important service telephone numbers and with the all parent's telephone numbers
- In the school institution a place have to be organized with toilet access for those who are suspected having influenza-like illness
- They must have mask, soap supplies
- When some of the children are sick, the teacher is required to wear a mask for protection
- Every morning the teacher must evaluate the children's health condition and then report the possible cases to the authorities
- There are some temporary suspension measures regarding when the school needs to be closed and these are
  - in the situation of one confirmed A/H1N1 influenza case in one class, the courses of this class will be suspended for 7 days (1 week period)
  - in the situation of 3 confirmed A/H1N1 cases in different classes, the courses of this school will be suspended for 7 days (1 week period)
  - The suspension decision regarding the school closure at local level should be taken into account by the County Department of the Public Health

Proactive School Closure

Developing an electronic school absenteeism surveillance system could lead to an early reactive supervision regarding the closure of schools. This tool will be used for monitoring influenza pandemic A/H1N1, detecting the early outbreaks which will help us also seeing the rate of school absenteeism.

Manual setting supervision in schools: The manual setting supervision in schools would be developed at national level. A staff composed of four people will work a period of 3 months each year (according to the sentinel supervision statement from the National Preparedness Plan in case of Influenza Pandemic A/H1N1) when it is supposed that the peak attack rates could occur (December, January, and February).

Education delivery strategy: The purpose in this second approach is that students should be provided with a reasonable degree of teaching and learning if schools close for an extended period in an influenza pandemic. This may include information on the curriculum, or hints about how to use a child's home surroundings—or programs on television or radio—to inform their work. Therefore, parents could rely on the online or TV lessons and it would not be necessary to stay home for educating them. In this matter, the parents would not be so stressed and the children would not feel the loneliness and boredom generated by the social disruption phenomena.

Campaign for Increasing Pandemic Influenza Vaccination Rate

Because immunization is the most effective means of preventing influenza transmission, pandemic strategies must include ways of increasing vaccination rate. Campaigns for increasing influenza vaccination rates must be suitable for every high-risk group because their incentives are diverse. Moreover, campaigns need to consider three strategies: education, information, and communication.

Communication campaign can include posters that promote personal protective measures, social distancing measures, and pandemic vaccination. Moreover, information about the pandemic influenza vaccine can be incorporated into a specific website that will include:

* Questions and answers about pandemic influenza
* Questions and answers about pandemic influenza vaccine
* Photos and videos related to pandemic influenza
* Stories about people who have suffered or died from pandemic influenza
* Official recommendations, schedules for vaccination
* Additional information about influenza, including links to other resources

Additional strategies that can be implemented for healthcare workers include the following: conducting an employee survey about influenza knowledge, providing employee education, making employee vaccines readily available and free of charge, designating immunization nurses to serve as clinical champions, monitoring and reporting the employee influenza vaccination rate, and recognizing the clinic with the highest employee vaccination rate.

Romania has the manufacturing capacity for influenza vaccine (Cantacuzino Institute). High-risk groups were defined for pandemic vaccination. There is no plan for increasing vaccination among health care workers and essential service workers. There are plans for storage, distribution, and safe administration. Storage and distribution is arranged by the epidemiology department of public health authorities. The administration is done mainly by family physicians. Vaccination is, by name of the family physician, reported numerically in the county's Department of Public Health. The plan has a legal framework for implementation. The country will be divided in three regions and the vaccination strategy will be according to the attack rates of the regions. There exists a methodology for reporting of adverse reactions to vaccination. Thus, we used the methodology described by Reed and collaborators (Reed et al. 2009) and latest demographic data (Source: National Institute of Statistics, year 2008) to estimate the real morbidity and mortality of pandemic influenza cases in Romania

Exposed Groups

Data from several sources, including the National Health Interview Survey, suggest that immunization rates are lower in racial/ethnic minority groups. Disparity exists for all age groups in the Hard-to-reach (HTR) groups such as the housebound elderly, disenfranchised groups, people living in disadvantaged urban communities and undocumented immigrants which have low immunization rates.

Exposure Assessment (Quantification)

Status Quo: The most affected were people in the age group 5–24 years old (median number of hospitalized cases = 168.4 per 100,000 population) and the least affected were people in the age group 65 and older. The estimated median number of deaths was 321 (lower limit = 205; upper limit = 503). The most affected age group was 50–64 years old (median = 2.4 deaths per 100,000 population) and the least affected was 0–4 years old age group. Median estimation of YPLL65 was 15,195 years of potential life lost before the age of 65 (lower limit = 9,672.5; upper limit = 23,852.5). The heaviest impact was put by the deaths on the age group 25–49 years old, the active population age group.

Horizontal Interactions

Strategies to increase pandemic immunization rates are strategies at the individual level, at the provider level and at the structural level. Studies show that churches were particularly successful collaborators in strategies to increase immunization rates at the individual level. Moreover, mobilizing trustworthy spokespeople (local sports figures or members of the clergy) to recommend vaccination is a successful strategy for increasing immunization. There is evidence suggesting that patient reminders, provider education and prompting, physician incentives, and standing orders are effective ways to increase adult immunization coverage, increasing immunization rates at the provider level. At the structural level, increasing health care insurance may increase immunization. Because combination of strategies increases the effectiveness of individual strategies, vaccination can be combined with school closure measure in order to reduce the impact of an influenza pandemic.

Summary of Affected Factors and Risks

Social and economic factors (Poverty / Financial hardship / Social disruption)

- Lack of supplies and medical care
- Wage losses, unemployment
- Self-isolation lifestyle, loneliness

Fixed

- Aging

- Children under 6 months old cannot be vaccinated
- Elderly have priority on vaccination as other special population (disabled, minorities, etc.)

Access to services

- Education / Health services / Transport
- Lack of education and lack of ——school lunch and breakfast program
- No access to health care services
- Internal and international travel restriction

Health Outcomes

Influenza is a public health threat, unpredictable and with an important impacts both on individual and society level. The severity of a pandemic virus can be evaluated from these two perspectives: individual/patient who has been infected and from the population level—that is, how many complications and deaths might be expected as a whole.

Increasing vaccination rates for pregnant women, a group especially vulnerable to the risks from seasonal influenza and also had excess mortality during the influenza pandemics: Strategies for increasing vaccination rate may include: assessing baseline immunization rates for obstetric providers, active education and offering vaccination training to obstetricians and nurses, implementing standing orders for influenza vaccination in pregnancy. Pregnant women should also be provided with clear, easy-to-understand information about vaccination.

Increasing vaccination rates for children: Different countries will be in different positions regarding the amount of pandemic A/H1N1 2009 vaccine in their possession and the timing of delivery of the vaccines. Romania has in country vaccine production capabilities but nevertheless, vaccine supplies are limited. The trade-off between reducing transmission and targeting high-risk groups depends on whether herd immunity can realistically be achieved. In order to achieve herd immunity, the pandemic influenza coverage should be in the range of 50–70 % among children, the most efficient age group at transmitting influenza viruses (WHO 2009b). A successful vaccination strategy that will achieve this target will have not only direct effect on a vulnerable population, but also an indirect effect through herd immunity effect. However, this target is difficult to reach.

Outcome Assessment

Policy Alternative 1: Closing schools will help reduce the spread of the pandemic. If these strategies will be put into action and children will receive online lessons, the impact on public health will be to some extent quite large in a positive way. The study estimated that the heaviest burden of pandemic influenza cases would be in 5–24 year old group and the lowest number was in the age group of 65 years and older. The study estimate the median number of hospitalizations = 12,829 (lower limit=8,176; upper limit=20,062). The most affected would be people in the age group 5–24 years old (median number of hospitalized cases=134.7 per 100,000 population) and the least affected would be people in the age group 65 and older (median number of hospitalized cases=16.8 per 100,000 population). The estimate median number of deaths is 283 (lower limit=181; upper limit=443). The most affected age group would be 50–64 years old (median=1.6 deaths per 100,000 population) and the least affected would be 0–4 years old age group (median=0.1 deaths per 100,000 population). Median estimation of YPLL65 would be 13,387.5 years of potential life lost before the age of 65 (lower limit=8,545; upper limit=20,918). The heaviest impact would be put by the deaths on the age group 25–49 years old, the active population age group.

Costs of the electronic absenteeism surveillance system: First of all there will be major planning costs regarding the infrastructure and logistic part for the school institution. The costs of implementing this card access system will be around 10 mil €, considering that in Romania there are 6,150 schools where the costs for the system itself will be approximately 1000 €/schools and the price of the each card will be around 1 € (taking into account that in Romania are 3.300 mil. pupils).

Costs of the manual setting supervision in schools: Considering that the entire investment will cover a period of 3 months, including four people who will work full time in this period on the website designing, the study assumes that the costs will be around 10.000 €/ year, including the staff monthly payment.

Costs related to education delivery strategy: Costs will involve planning and infrastructure, financial, logistics, and staff availability. As a result, designing the online lessons, financial expenditure involving the broadcasting of the lessons at the local Television and staff costs might be expensive. The costs cannot be estimated without knowing the broadcasting strategy. If the lessons will be broadcasted on the National Television, they will be free of cost, but only if this measure will be adopted in a legislative manner.

Policy Alternative 2: If the strategies designed for education, information, and communication are put into action and are successful, the impact on public health will be significant: the more people will get vaccinated, the lower transmission rate will be. An increased rate of vaccination will make people feel more relaxed because the stress and fear getting the influenza virus will be diminished knowing that many people are vaccinated.

The study estimated that the heaviest burden of pandemic influenza cases would be in 5–24 year old group and the lowest number was in the age group of 65 years and older. The study estimate the median number of hospitalizations=6,887 (lower limit=4,389; upper limit=10,770). The most affected would be people in the age group 5–24 years old (median number of hospitalized cases=50.5 per 100,000 population) and the least affected would be people in the age group 65 and older (median number of hospitalized cases=13.1 per 100,000 population). The estimated median number of deaths would be 250 (lower limit=159; upper limit=393). The most affected age group would be 50–64 years old (median=2.2 deaths per 100,000 population) and the least affected would be 0–4 years old age group (median=0.1). Median estimation of YPLL65 would be 11,535 years of potential life lost before the age of 65 (lower limit=7327.5; upper limit=18,060). The heaviest impact would be put by the deaths on the age group 25–49 years old, the active population age group.

Costs of the campaign for increasing pandemic influenza vaccination rate: Costs involve planning and investment in infrastructure for designing and timing of the campaigns, call and mail reminders distribution, education provision. These costs will be approximately 3 mil. €. The TV campaigns will be the most expensive part of the whole set of campaign measures because of the broadcasting price. Moreover, the staff costs will be significant, considering the amount of work that needs to be done: delivering posters/flyers, home visits, home calls.

Summary of Health Outcomes

The most effective transmission of the influenza virus occurs in schools settings, among children and the best strategy for reducing influenza transmission at the population level is vaccination. Both proposed strategies have a direct and indirect impact on influenza virus transmission rates. In the case of school closure, the direct effect is transmission within the school age children and the indirect effect is the same effect on older population groups. In the case of vaccination, an individual protection is achieved but also a herd immunity effect would lower the transmission of the influenza virus in the given population.

Conclusion

Influenza is a global health problem that requires solutions on global scale. Both pharmaceutical and nonpharmaceutical interventions are required in order to lower the impact of this disease on the population health. The study analyzed the health policy regarding the influenza epidemic—Romanian National Plan for Intervention in Influenza Pandemics with a top-down approach focusing on two interventions: increase social distancing by proactive school closure and increase vaccination coverage, especially among children. The study used official surveillance information and published epidemiological studies to estimate the impact of proposed measures on public health. A reduction in total cases and hospitalized influenza cases was estimated for both interventions. The economic and social cost of interventions is high. Estimates for total cases decrease from status quo (15,195 YPLL65) to alternative policy 1 (13,387 YPLL65) and further decrease in the case of alternative policy 2 (11,535 YPLL65) which means an improvement.

The most common measures of severity from the individual's perspective are the case-fatality rate (CFR) and the hospitalization rate. However, there are challenges associated with estimating these rates in practice.

Mortality reduction due to vaccination is difficult to assess.

If schools close too late in the course of a community-wide outbreak, the resulting reduction in transmission is likely to be very limited. Policies for school closure need to include measures that limit contact among students when not in school. If students congregate in a setting other than a school, they will continue to spread the virus, and the benefits of school closure will be greatly reduced, if not negated.

There are three key issues affecting equal access to vaccines: manufacturing capacity, cost and delivery. Equal access to pandemic vaccine is important in situations where there are many poor countries that do not have the necessary technology for producing the vaccine or resources for buying it.

Methodological Recommendations

Guidance for the Top-Down Assessment of Population Health Risks of Policies

Systematic review, integration and summarization of the practical considerations relating to the advantages, disadvantages and limitations of applying various approaches and methods during preparation of case studies formed the basis for the development of a methodological guidance. It summarizes those methodological elements that were found most expedient in the discussion process aiming to reach a consensus. The guidance is structured and the recommendations are presented by the main levels of the impact chain that takes the top-down direction proceeding from the policy level through related health determinants and risk factors to health outcomes. At each level, typical examples from the case studies are quoted as recommendations for applicable practice. Finally, cross-level issues are discussed that may relate to different levels of the impact chain or reflect universal, overarching phenomena.

Policy

The policy, related health risks of which are to be assessed, can be a strategy, program, or regulation, including any kinds of legal instruments. It is a crucial requirement for the policy to be of recognized importance from a population health point of view. This prerequisite stands regardless of the level and sector of initiation that can be either central, regional, or local government, industry or other organizations.

In an ideal situation the commission for the conduct of an assessment comes from policy makers. The request for assistance in decision making justifies the need for the assessment even if it does not necessarily assure the public health importance of the impact that can, however, be judged upon in the initial phase of the assessment process. If the task is commissioned there is no special need for a self-initiated selection to find a suitable policy to assess related health risks. An example for commissioned work is provided by the Hungarian case study, where the Hungarian Ministry of Health entrusted the HIA workgroup of the University of Debrecen with the preparation of the assessment. If not given at forehand, a transparent selection process that identifies a policy suitable for assessment is important. Similar considerations apply when a policy is very comprehensive and consequently its causal web is too complex so that the assessment should focus only on a part of the policy to assure feasibility. A good example for the methodology of policy selection is found in the German case study. First, authors set clear preferential criteria for the preselection of policy, such as level (national or regional preferred), sector (nonhealth), size (manageable) and relevance (attractive, up-to-date) of policy, feasibility of its assessment (verifiable objectives, availability of data), and most importantly its potential to have considerable impact on human health. They sought for expert opinion about importance to narrow down the selection and analyzed the remaining policy choices by feasibility issues such as availability of valid data and dose–response functions, verifiable objectives, definable target group, time frame, identifiable health determinants and risk factors, and availability of expertise.

In summary, during the selection of a policy to carry out assessment on, the following issues should be taken into consideration: the importance of the topic, the need of policy makers for assistance in the decision-making process and the feasibility of assessment.

After the policy was selected for assessment, the policy document is to be thoroughly studied. A good understanding of the policy context allows for the identification of the policy impact on health and health inequalities. The review of policy context is of utmost importance so that one can draw up the impact structure, prioritize causal pathways, and recognize challenges in the assessment process.

First of all the problem addressed by the policy should be identified. The driving forces of policy formulation, the demand for action should be revealed and explained in a concise way. Describing the position and role of a national policy in an international context assists the identification of the driving forces of policy development, meanwhile allows for finding similar policies implemented in other places. The experiences gained during the preparation and implementation of similar policies can provide useful information, even essential input data that may prove very helpful in the risk assessment process. Good examples for the description of the international policy context are found e.g. in the Hungarian and Slovenian case studies. In the Hungarian case, the international actions implemented to control environmental tobacco smoke exposure are thoroughly described with a focus on the legal instruments of the European Union that can urge the member states to formulate adequate national legislations. Examples of national policies on restricting smoking in public places are quoted and the information they provide and lessons learned during their implementation are utilized in the assessment process. The Slovenian case study analyses the European regulation of the wine market, its driving forces, and its influence on the preparation of the Slovenian Strategy on Wine Production.

It is worthwhile to explore the history of the policy, how it has evolved with time, as seen, among others, in the Polish and Slovakian studies. Authors provide a detailed description of the air pollution levels in Upper Silesia in the last 30 years and the changes in the Polish regulation of air hygiene standards in the same period. The Slovak case study on alcohol control also nicely explains the evolution of alcohol policies and places the Slovak National Action Plan on Alcohol Problems in the historical perspective.

The understanding of the legal environment and the relationships between the studied and other related policies enables the assessors to consider policy interactions. The presentation of a map of policy context can effectively assist the assessment process, like in the German case study which describes the links from the federal Housing Subsidy Act to the Housing Subsidy Program in North Rhine-Westphalia. In order to explain the development and main drivers of the policy in an objective manner, besides the links to other policies, the context regarding stakeholders and interests should also be explored. This aspect of the Danish Energy Policy is clearly described in the respective case study. As stated, "The relevance of an energy policy at both the national and international scale need not be over emphasized; especially as reliable energy supply is central to economic development and key to many social activities". According to the analysis the policy is relevant at both domestic and international levels, and it is timely and responsive to the changing external environment. Its significance is justified by its goal to ensure the supply of the needs of the Danish population by guaranteeing energy security and consequently economic development and meanwhile cutting reliance on fossil fuels.

After all the above issues are addressed, a detailed description of the policy content should be prepared that will demonstrate the main goal and objectives of the policy, tools of its implementation and methods for monitoring and evaluation of the impact. The identification of the target population and the time course of policy implementation require the examination of policy enforcement and effect. The poor implementation of a policy can dilute its impact even if the policy itself is carefully planned and well prepared. The feasibility of effectively implementing policy measures must also be taken into account when attempting to make predictions on possible health effects. The complexity level of required actions can influence effectiveness, especially if it is not adjusted to the institutional, human, and financial resources available for implementation. Apart from the effector side, success of a policy action also strongly depends on the acceptance and compliance of the public. It is easier to assess the feasibility of policy implementation if a policy has clear implementation plan. The estimation of costs of implementation gives information not only for the evaluation of feasibility but also allows for a cost-benefit analysis in a later phase of the assessment process. The Romanian case study included estimations for the costs of implementing the analyzed policy alternatives (see also next paragraph).

Sometimes there is more than one policy plan. Even if there is only one option, the alternative scenario is to reject it and keep the status quo. The assessment of alternatives can effectively assist the decision-making process by supplying direct information for the selection between available policy options. A good example for examining different scenarios is provided in the Romanian case study. Authors analyzed three different options of health policy on preventing and limiting the effects of an influenza epidemic (A/H1N1). The first alternative was to maintain the status quo that is no change in the existing policy, in the implementation cost as well as in the expected health impact. The second analyzed option was to use proactive school closure as a policy measure and the third was to initiate campaign for increasing vaccination rate.

Determinants of Health

Determinants of health are defined by the WHO as "the range of personal, social, economic and environmental factors which determine the health status of individuals or populations" (WHO 1998). In the structure of a full impact chain, health determinants take an intermediate position between the policy and the risk factors that directly affect health. Those factors that are considered as determinants of health are further upstream from the health outcomes in the causal chain and consequently more abstract in nature. Other terms applied for health determinants in the literature, such as wider determinants, upstream determinants, causes of causes, all reflect these characteristics. Unlike risk factors the exposure levels of which can often be quantified, health determinants have typically rather qualitative features in the risk assessment process. The category of health determinants may, however, overlap with that of risk factors and it can be difficult to differentiate between them in many cases. There is an ongoing debate in public health about the similarities and differences of health determinants and risk factors and whether it is reasonable at all to strictly differentiate them in the assessment process. The authors argue that such a distinction can be favorable when the task is to map the complex impact schemes of policies. The challenges of recognizing factors that belong to the level of health determinants in practice can be overcome by using a model with a pre-set list of determinants. There are various models developed in the past decades that present an integrated structure of health determinants. Taking into consideration the need for a comprehensive approach in assessing the complex causal web of policies, the used model should preferably represent the holistic model of health. The Lalonde model is the first and still widely used model that addresses the importance of the socioeconomic determinants of health (Lalonde 1974). This model was the most frequently used in the case studies, too. Other scientifically recognized models can, however, also be applied, like the similarly acknowledged model by Dahlgren and Whitehead (Dahlgren and Whitehead 1991).

The main task at the level of health determinants is the identification of those determinants that are likely to be affected by the policy. The availability of evidence for causality is the key issue in the selection of influenced health determinants. Since the way by which affected determinants are recognized can vary, transparent description of the selection method is obligate. The way of selection can be based on the information gained from the literature or provided by experts. Certainly all the case studies used the scientific literature related to the topic as a source of information. Extensive literature review was carried out, among others, in the Danish and the Hungarian assessments. These case studies reviewed the broad literature available on the wide-scale impacts of energy and anti-smoking policies, respectively, ranging from environmental to economic and social determinants. Danish authors indicated the references of literature sources from which information was used to find health determinants influenced by the assessed energy policy in the list of identified determinants. The other possible source of information used for selection purposes is expert opinion. A multidisciplinary team made by eight experts in disciplines related to medical imaging was asked by the Italian assessors to prioritize previously identified factors responsible for the final dose irradiated to patients. The Slovenian study sought not only for information from experts but also for opinions of representatives of involved sectors and groups of stakeholders to gain valuable insight in the broad impact scheme of the Slovenian National Strategy on Wine Production.

Apart from the method used, there can be two main strategic approaches distinguished in the identification process. The search may follow a broad perspective and try to find and consider all the relevant health determinants that can potentially be influenced by the policy, with the driving aim of not to lose any. The other approach focuses only on the most important health determinants the inclusion of which enjoys priority. Prioritization of health determinants can prove advantageous even in the broad approach, e.g. to narrow down analysis for quantitative assessment purposes. The prioritization process must consider important characteristics of the determinant and its position and interactions in the impact scheme. A critical aspect is the strength of evidence available on policy influence, which justifies the determinant's place in the causal web. The prioritization process should evaluate the feasibility to assess health outcomes linked to the determinant, through the assessment of exposure change of risk factors. Such a feasibility evaluation requires the assessors to think in advance and make internal loops of consideration between the levels of the causal chain. The possibility for quantitative assessment can be given high priority. If downstream assessment is deemed to be feasible, the anticipated magnitude of the health effects can also be a factor of priority setting. The significance of health effects mainly depends on the size of population affected, severity of health effects, and the magnitude of costs involved. Apart from the above issues, the focus of priority setting can also depend on the primary intention of the assessment, that is, what policy makers want to use the assessment for, as well as on the scale of human and financial resources available to carry out the assessment.

To conclude, a definite strategy for the identification and prioritization of health determinants is inevitable. The applied method, information sources, and evaluation criteria should be clearly described. The transparency of the prioritization process can be further increased by the use of a formal scoring system. Such a semi-quantitative method was developed and applied in the Slovenian case study (Table 3.9). The tool recognizes prioritization criteria by determinants of health and related risk factors, and requires the user to evaluate the effect size and strength of evidence by scoring them from 1 (no or minimal effect) to 5 (maximum effect expected).

Remarks:

- Add as many lines (determinants of health or risk factors) as necessary
- Scoring is from 1 (no or minimal effect) to 5 (maximum effect expected)

Table 3.9 Tool for horizontal prioritization

Determinants of health	Risk factors	Number of people affected	Quality of life affected	Related national expenses	Strength of literature evidence	Sum
Determinant of health I.						
	Risk factor I.1.					
	Risk factor I.2.					
Determinant of health II.						
	Risk factor II.1					
	Risk factor II.2.					

Risk Factors

Compared to health determinants, risk factors have a closer relation to health effects. They are the factors of the impact chain that directly affect health, that is the reason why they are also called proximal factors counter to the distal determinants of health. The more direct nature of risk factors is also reflected in their WHO definition: "social, economic or biological status, behaviors or environments which are associated with or cause increased susceptibility to a specific disease, ill health, or injury" (WHO 1998). The term risk factor carries a negative sense as it implies related harm, although protective factors that have a positive effect on health can also be referred to as risk factors in a broad understanding, having an opposite direction of effect. The term exposure denotes the frequency or level of contact of risk factors with individuals. From a practical point of view it is worthwhile to make a distinction between the risk factors that are influenced by the policy through health determinants and consequently play a direct role in the impact chain and the risk factors that modify individual susceptibility without being influenced by the policy. The consideration of susceptibility factors proves to be useful when sensitive subgroups of the affected population should be identified.

Linking health determinants to health outcomes in recognized causal pathways requires the identification and enlistment of all influenced risk factors. As risk factors directly expose people, the elements of the exposure event should be described, such as characteristics of the exposed population and the routes and pattern of exposure in different population groups. Recognizing differences of exposure in different population groups enables the assessors to carry out health outcome assessment specifically for subpopulations. Such a stratified assessment allows for considering equity issues. The Hungarian case study provides an example for calculating age- and sex-specific burden of disease related to active and passive smoking that is justified by the fact that the prevalence of exposure shows age and sex specificity, as well as that the strength of association between tobacco smoke exposure and various related health outcomes is different for females and males.

Prioritization may be necessary at the risk factor level, similarly to that with health determinants. The prioritization process should be based essentially on the same principles and criteria at both levels. An important criterion of consideration is the strength of evidence for causality that implies both the reliability of information source and biological plausibility. The other main issue is the significance of induced health effects. It depends on the extent of change the policy induces in the frequency or level of exposure, the size of population affected and the severity of related health outcomes. Unlike with health determinants, the extent of being exposed to a risk factor can often be assessed not only qualitatively but measured in a quantitative way. Since quantification is an important issue in several contexts, the consideration of selecting risk factors for detailed analysis can include the feasibility of quantitative exposure assessment.

The possibility that an exposure assessment can be carried out in a quantitative manner depends on the availability of various input data. To quantify exposure change as an effect of policy implementation needs first of all applicable exposure measure. The assessment requires numerical data on the baseline level or prevalence of exposure, and information about the magnitude of change of exposure policy implementation is expected to induce. The effect size of the policy on exposure is either provided by observational studies that examine the consequences of similar policies previously introduced in other populations or rely on expert judgment. The reliability of observational data can be regarded higher. Experiences from other places or times were used e.g. in the Romanian, German, and Hungarian case studies to estimate impact on exposure. The Romanian case study used data of the 2009 A/H1N1 influenza pandemic in Romania obtained from the National Center for Surveillance and Control of Infectious Diseases to establish the baseline values for the assessment. The German authors analyzed the theoretical effect of making all homes of people aged 65 years and older in North Rhine-Westphalia barrier-free. For that, they needed the baseline frequency of falls elderly people suffer in ordinary housing. Due to the lack of German data, they used international estimate of 30 % as default value. The Hungarian exposure assessment applied separate values for the reduction in the prevalence of active smoking, decrease in the prevalence of ETS exposure in the hospitality sector, workplace, and household as the consequence of banning smoking in closed public places and workplaces. The estimates were set by considering reported reductions from various countries, such as Italy, Ireland, and Finland. Besides the availability of necessary information, a major driving force of quantification is the demand determined by the interest of policy makers and other stakeholders. Quantitative estimates of exposure change have limited value if not used for the quantification of related health outcomes; therefore, when evaluating the feasibility of quantitative exposure assessment in the prioritization process of risk factors, one should also consider the availability of valid data and dose/exposure-response coefficients that will be used in the quantitative health outcome assessment. This anticipatory thinking with loops of consideration between the levels of the causal chain can prove to be useful when selecting impact pathways for detailed assessment.

Health Outcomes

Health outcomes form the bottom level of the impact scheme. They represent those health states, mainly diseases and injuries, that are the direct effects of the risk factors involved in the causal chain. There can be multiple stages in the pathomechanism of a disease. An elderly person can have osteoporosis as well as increased risk to fall. These factors can result in falls and consequent bone fractures that may eventually lead to death. It is context specific which stage is the most optimal to be considered as the health outcome in the assessment process. In the German case study, for example, three endpoints, falls, hip fractures, and death were chosen for assessment as health outcomes of the impact scheme. Due to this variability of endpoints, clear definition of the assessed health outcomes is inevitable. A good strategy is to identify ill-health states with ICD codes as seen in most of the case studies.

If assessment needs to be limited, health outcomes should be prioritized based on the same principles as applied in the prioritization of risk factors and health determinants. The significance of a health outcome in the assessment is determined by the strength of evidence for causality, as well as by its public health importance. The latter can be evaluated by considering the frequency of occurrence (incidence or prevalence) in the population and the severity of the ill-health state that is characterized by its chronic development, irreversibility, disabling potential, and lethality.

To be able to evaluate the size of health effects, the affected population has to be clearly identified. A detailed assessment should pay special attention to the varying exposure status and susceptibility of subgroups in the population. If the outcome assessment takes into consideration the differences in susceptibility, the evaluation of policy impact on health inequalities becomes possible.

Health outcomes are assessed most frequently in a qualitative way; however, quantitative estimates may be given priority where feasible. Qualitative evaluation can indicate the direction of effect and describe the effect size in categorical terms. Due to the subjective nature of qualitative statements, a significant issue in the assessment of health outcomes is the feasibility of quantification. Examples for quantitative outcome assessment are found in the Romanian, German, and Hungarian case studies. Romanian authors calculated age-specific incidence rates for hospitalization and death, as well as potential years of life lost as a measure of disease burden caused by pandemic influenza in the country in two alternatives of preventive policy measures. The German study estimated the number of hip fractures and deaths resulting from hip fractures that could have been avoided in the year 2009, if all homes of people aged 65 years and older in North Rhine-Westphalia were barrier-free. The Hungarian analysis calculated disease burden measures, including the combined measure of disability adjusted life years to estimate the impact of banning smoking in closed public places and workplaces in Hungary.

When set out for a quantitative outcome assessment, first decision must be made on the types of applied health measures that are typically epidemiological frequency measures. Those measures are adequate that can be feasibly used to supply input and output data for the calculation process. Whatever method is used, the availability of baseline frequency data of the health condition is indispensable for a successful assessment. Values of frequency measures of both health conditions and exposures should be available for the same, affected population. Such data are usually supplied by routine statistics, population-based registries, or surveys. Apart from availability, a crucial issue is the validity of data that should be carefully evaluated and clearly described. The modeling of changes in health outcome induced by changing exposure requires adequate dose/exposure-response functions. The scientific literature can provide the coefficients of these functions that can be traditional dose–response coefficients in case of environmental exposures or estimates of relative risk derived from epidemiological studies. The simplest output of a quantitative outcome assessment can be a frequency measure, such as the frequency of occurrence, incidence of morbidity, hospitalization, mortality, etc. Such endpoints were used in the German study. More sophisticated outcome measure can be a measure of disease burden, such as attributable death, potential years of life lost and disability adjusted life years (DALY). The Romanian assessment calculated potential years of life lost besides simple frequency measures. The Hungarian case study applied the most favorable choice of measure for expressing results of a risk assessment in a quantitative way, since the complex measure of DALY combines information about effect both on morbidity and mortality. Quantitative estimates of policy health impact provide not only easier understanding of assessment results for decision makers but also make cost-benefit analysis of policy introduction possible.

Cross-Level Issues

As discussed at the risk factor and health outcome level already, the intention and feasibility to provide quantitative estimates for health risks of policies are important aspects of the assessment process. An unequivocal definition helps to understand what *quantitative assessment* of health risks means. According to the agreed definition quantitative assessment can be perceived as the quantitative expression of expected changes in health outcome measures by using numerical information on how a policy affects health outcomes directly or through induced changes in exposure levels of risk factors. The provision of quantitative estimates as results of the assessment process has advantages to qualitative descriptions of health effects. Numerical information is usually welcomed in the policy making process, since it helps understanding the size of effect which is crucial for making comparisons, like in priority setting or cost-benefit analysis. Therefore quantitative predictions on health effects of policy alternatives can effectively assist bargaining and finding the optimal consensus. In practice, a clear understanding of the quantification process can be ensured if a logical algorithm for the assessment process is planned in advance from the policy level all along to health outcomes. The Danish case study provides an example for constructing an abstract plan for quantitative assessment. The authors modeled the aim of the Danish Energy Strategy to decrease energy demand by 4 % until 2020 and change the share of different production forms so that less pollutant is produced.

Although favorable in many ways, quantification also has some disadvantages that should be taken into account when intending to use quantitative methods in the assessment. A single numerical estimate of the health effect can be easily understood and dealt with, therefore very attractive for decision makers; however, a point estimate should never be the only disseminated result. A single number alone cannot reflect the complex structure of an impact scheme. Providing a sole point estimate fails to describe the magnitude of uncertainty of the estimation, too (detailed below). A perfunctory assessment may also overlook the problem of double counting that is the situation when the same health outcome is affected in various pathways that interact with each other, therefore effect sizes cannot be unconditionally added up. The characterization of *horizontal interrelations* between various causal pathways at different levels of the impact chain is an important element of a comprehensive assessment of policy-related health risks.

The scientific credibility and lucidity of a complex assessment process requires *transparency*. Authors have to plan, carry out, and report a study providing clear explanation of the work done at the various stages of the process. A detailed description on the method of information search and data collection, evaluation of strength of evidence and validity of data, prioritization of determinants of health, risk factors and health outcomes, selection of measures and functions applied in the assessment, and last but not least on the method of evaluating the reliability of results should be provided. The assessment and description of the *strength of evidence* for causality on different levels of the full impact chain requires special attention. The use of a guide, like those developed in the United Kingdom, can be helpful to review and grade evidence (National Institute for Health and Clinical Excellence 2005; Weightman et al. 2005). The acknowledgement and detailed description of the uncertainties and limitations of the assessment process are crucial factors of transparency, too.

Assessors always have to face some barriers, like the lack or questionable validity of baseline data that limit the potential achievements of the analysis. The acknowledgement of *limitations* in the use of methodology, and in the availability of resources is a serious issue of transparency. The admission that the assessment process cannot provide credible estimates for some health outcomes due to lack of data, functions, expert skills, etc., is a prerequisite of a scientifically correct process description. The existence of limitations in the assessment increases the level of uncertainty of its results. The statement that a health outcome cannot be assessed implies infinite uncertainty. Limitations that hindered the possibility to quantify health effects are addressed in some case studies.

Uncertainty is an inherent phenomenon of predictions. When an assessment produces effect estimates for a policy impact, especially if predictions for a future effect need to be provided, uncertainty is always involved. There are various elements of the assessment process that bear uncertainty. The evidence for causality can be questionable, just like the validity of applied data and functions. Baseline health and exposure data are usually provided by epidemiological studies that sample the source population. Therefore many input figures such as morbidity rates or prevalence of exposure are estimates themselves with inherent uncertainty due to random error of sampling. If the validity of the study is low, the level of uncertainty can be further enlarged by the presence of different biases of the study design and implementation. An additional source of uncertainty is when information attained in one context (situation/population) needs to be used and consequently extrapolated to another context, which is a quite regular practice in impact assessment. The Hungarian case study points out the importance to give preference to those sources that provide data from populations similar to that under study in order to assure the lowest possible level of uncertainty related to extrapolation. As one can conclude from the above arguments, uncertainty is always present in assessments; therefore it is not enough to state the existence of uncertainty since it has not got much added value, rather its level should be characterized at least in a descriptive manner. If quantitative assessment is carried out, the size of uncertainty can be specified by giving a range around the point estimate that can function as an interval estimate of the result. A good example for the indication of a range to characterize the size of uncertainty is found in the Romanian case study that provides lower and upper limits of estimation. Further information about how to describe uncertainties and the way to communicate them can be found in a WHO-IPCS guidance document on characterizing and communicating uncertainty in exposure assessment (WHO-IPCS 2008).

When making predictions on future health effects of policies, it is important to consider that the realization of impact needs time. Policy makers have to take into account when beneficial or adverse health effects will be experienced, therefore the description of probable *latency* of effects is important information for them to make good decisions. The length of the latency period has typically two components. There is time between the planning and implementation of a policy, and then time is needed for the development of health effects that may be determined by environmental and social factors, as well as by the biological factors in the pathomechanism of disease development (lag phase). An attempt to consider health outcomes dependent on time, is found in the Hungarian case study that modeled both short and long-term effects, taking into consideration the intermediate level of risk of former smokers.

Checklist for the Top-Down Assessment of Population Health Risks of Policies

The short extract of conclusions were used to prepare a unified set of recommendations in the form of a checklist that is intended be used for assessing health risks related to policies in the traditional top-down approach (Table 3.10).

Usability of the Combined Tool

One of the main goals of the RAPID project was to provide a methodological tool for those who want to carry out the comprehensive assessment of health risks related

Table 3.10 Checklist for the top-down assessment of health risks of policies

	Content of analysis	How to do
Policy	Place the policy into international, national, regional, or local context	The policy to be assessed is usually provided by policy makers
	Describe policy content (main goals, scope, implementation plan, methods of monitoring, and evaluation)	Read the policy and make a shortlist containing goals, actors, targets, tools, timeframe, implementation mechanisms and monitoring and evaluation mechanisms
	Identify the problem, demand for action, policy actors and ideas	
	Identify target population of the policy	Seek policy expert opinion if necessary
	Identify performance and outcome indicators in the policy	Consult authors/stakeholders of the policy
	Assess whether timeframe for goals and actions is set	Consider the entire policy making process in sociopolitical context
	Consider if cross-analysis across principles, goals, and actions could be conducted	Consider feasibility of assessment (verifiable objectives, definable target group of the policy, preliminary evidence for health impact)
	Assess the time course, feasibility, and cost of implementation	
	List information sources to do the assessment and description	
Determinants of health	Define the applied model of health determinants preferably presenting the holistic model of health (Lalonde, Dahlgren and Whitehead, etc.), use a pre-set list of health determinants	Extensive literature search, use available evidence summaries, reviews
	Identify which health determinants are influenced by the policy in a transparent way	Use expert opinion—public health and public health policy experts are recommended
	Decide upon using a full-scale or limited selection of health determinants for assessment; if limited selection is used, describe horizontal prioritization of health determinants, make internal loops of consideration between the levels of the causal chain in the prioritization process	Consult stakeholders
		Use a horizontal prioritization tool, for example:
		Score each of the following criteria: number of people affected, quality of life affected, related national expenses and strength of literature evidence from 1 (minimum) to 5 (maximum) for each relevant determinant of health
	Consider strength of evidence for causality/association/plausibility of the policy impact on determinants, importance of the related effect (size of population affected, severity of health effects, costs involved), feasibility of assessment favorably in a quantitative way, demand of policy makers, and extent of resources available	Place results into a table, summarize them by determinants and make a ranking
	Assess interactions between health determinants	
	List information sources used to make the assessment and description	

(continued)

Table 3.10 (continued)

	Content of analysis	How to do
Risk factors	Enlist all influenced risk factors by wider determinants of health	Literature search with focus on epidemiological literature
	Prioritize risk factors in a transparent way; make internal loops of consideration between the levels of the causal chain in the prioritization process	Database search (international and national statistics offices, environmental exposure databases, etc.)
	Consider strength of evidence (reliability of literature source, biological plausibility, etc.) and significance of induced health effects (size of exposure change influenced by the policy, size of population affected, severity of related health outcomes)	Qualitative assessment by indicating the direction of change or categorically describing its size Quantitative assessment by calculating frequency (prevalence) or level (dose, concentration) of exposure
	Consider feasibility of quantitative exposure assessment (availability of applicable exposure measures, numerical information on the baseline level/prevalence of exposure and on the expected change of exposure related to policy implementation)	If direct exposure measures are not available, use proxy measures Use a horizontal prioritization tool, for example: Score each of the following criteria: number of people affected, quality of life affected, related national
	Describe routes of exposure	expenses and strength of
	Describe exposed population and exposure pattern in different population groups (equity)	literature evidence from 1 (minimum) to 5 (maximum) for each relevant determinant
	Assess exposure	of health
	Assess interaction between risk factors	
	List information sources used to make the assessment and description	Place results into a table, summarize them by risk factor and make a ranking
Health outcomes	Define influenced health outcomes (apply ICD codes)	Literature search including medical, epidemiological and health economic literature
	Prioritize health outcomes in a transparent way	Database search (international and national statistics offices, other
	Consider strength of evidence for causality, severity (morbidity, disability, and mortality), reversibility, and frequency of occurrence in the population (in short the public health importance)	international, national, regional, local databases) Qualitative assessment by indicating the direction of change or by categorically describing the size of effect
	Identify populations affected with special attention to susceptible subgroups (equity)	Quantitative assessment by calculating simple frequency measures (morbidity,
	Consider availability and validity of baseline frequency data of the health condition and of dose/exposure-response functions applying dose-response coefficients or relative risk estimates	hospitalization, mortality, etc.) or measures of disease burden (attributable death, potential years of life lost and disability adjusted life years); give
	Assess change in health outcomes	preference to complex disease
	Determine cost related to health outcome if possible	burden measures (e.g. disability adjusted life years) if available and feasible

(continued)

Table 3.10 (continued)

	Content of analysis	How to do
Cross-level issues	Consider advantages and disadvantages of quantification (a single estimate may cover the complexity of the issue as well as the uncertainty of estimation, double counting)	
	There are likely to be many different full chain pathways within one case; if possible assess interrelations between various causal pathways	
	Indicate baseline scenario (what if current trends continue without policy change) at the various levels of the chain	
	Acknowledge limitations in the use of methodology	
	Describe uncertainty in a qualitative or quantitative way (provide ranges for estimates) at relevant points of the causal pathways as well as the overall uncertainty related to the full chain assessment	
	Consider latency period of the realization of health effects, differentiate short- and long-term effects	

to policy proposals. The structure of the top-down assessment of policy health effects fits the logical framework of the risk appraisal phase in health impact assessments. It starts with the policy in question, analyzes its impact structure through health determinants and risk factors to be able to assess the impact on health. Therefore the formulated guidance is able to provide assistance for the integration of risk assessment techniques into the HIA process, even in the challenging case when quantitative assessment shall be accommodated into the comprehensive impact assessment scheme of a policy proposal.

The developed combined tool includes guidance and a checklist. The guidance provides detailed description of the assessment process and explains critical theoretical and practical issues. By doing so, the guidance helps to understand and use the checklist in practice. The checklist offers a logical framework of assessment. It enlists the required steps and highlights the important issues that must be considered during the assessment process. The checklist addresses not only what to do but also how to do that by giving advice on practicalities of the assessment process.

The combined tool is expected to be used by public health professionals to assess health effects of policies, typically in the frame of health impact assessments. It is important to note that the guidance is not designed to fulfill the role of a cookbook. It can be effectively used only by professionals having practice with HIA and risk assessment; however, the tool can also provide assistance for those who have limited previous experience but would like to gain an insight in the process of assessing health effects of policies. The authors are convinced that the offered methodological assistance can contribute to the popularization of the concept that health issues should be routinely considered in policy development, as well as to the practical introduction of effective instruments of assessment that finally can provide help for the health-centered political decision-making process of any sector at local, regional, national, and international level alike.

References

Abrahams, D., Pennington, A., Scott-Samuel, A., Doyle, C., Metcalfe, O., den Broeder, L., Haigh, F., Mekel, O., Fehr, R. (2004). *European Policy Health Impact Assessment: A Guide.* Brussels, Belgium: Health and Consumer Protection Directorate General, European Commission. Available at: http://ec.europa.eu/health/ph_projects/2001/monitoring/fp_monitoring_2001_a6_frep_11_en.pdf. Accessed November 26, 2012.

Ádám, B. (2012). A model of health. *Public Service Review: Health and Social Care 32.* Available at: www.publicservice.co.uk/article.asp?publication=HealthandSocialCare&id=568&content_name=European Health and Social Care Focus&article=20175. Accessed November, 2012

Ádám, B., Molnár, Á., Gulis, G., & Ádány, R. (2013). Integrating quantitative risk appraisal in health impact assessment: Analysis of the novel smoke-free policy in Hungary. *European Journal of Public Health, 23*(2), 211–217.

Anderson, H. R. (2009). Air pollution and mortality: A history. *Atmospheric Environment, 43,* 142–152.

Basham, J. (2001). Application of COMEAP dose–response coefficients within a regulatory health impact assessment methodology. Committee on the Medical Effects of Air Pollutants. *Journal of Public Health Medicine, 23,* 212–218.

Bedetti, G., Botto, N., Andreassi, M. G., Traino, C., Vano, E., & Picano, E. (2008). Cumulative patient effective dose in cardiology. *British Journal of Radiology, 81*(969), 699–705.

Berrington de González, A., Mahesh, M., Kim, K. P., Bhargavan, M., Lewis, R., Mettler, F., et al. (2009). Projected cancer risks from computed tomographic scans performed in the United States in 2007. *Archives of Internal Medicine, 169*(22), 2071–2077.

Bezdek, R. H. (1993). The environmental, health, and safety implications of solar energy in central station power production. *Energy, 18*(6), 618–685.

Bhatia, R. (2010a). *A guide for health impact assessment.* Sacramento, California: California Department of Public Health. Available at: http://www.cdph.ca.gov/pubsforms/Guidelines/Documents/HIA%20Guide%20FINAL%2010-19-10.pdf. Accessed November 26, 2012.

Bhatia, R., Branscomb, J., Farhang, L., Lee, M., Orenstein, M., Richardson, M, (2010b). *Minimum Elements and Practice Standards for Health Impact Assessment, Version 2.* Oakland, California: North American HIA Practice Standards Working Group. Available at: http://www.humanimpact.org/doc-lib/finish/11/9. Accessed November 26, 2012.

Boehlert, G.W., McMurray, G.R., Tortorici, C.E. (Eds.), (2008). *Ecological effects of wave energy in the Pacific Northwest.* U.S. Department of Commerce, NOAA Tech. Memo. NMFS-F/SPO-92, p. 174.

Bojnec, S. (2006). Wine Markets in Central Europe. [online]. Available at: http://www.georgikon.hu/jcea/issues/jcea7-3/pdf/jcea73-14.pdf. Accessed October 8, 2010.

Boldo, E., Medina, S., LeTertre, A., Hurley, F., Mücke, H.-G., Ballester, F., et al. (2006). Aphesis: Health impact assessment of long-term exposure to PM2.5 in 23 European cities. *European Journal of Epidemiology, 21,* 449–458.

Brand, D. A., Saisana, M., Rynn, L. A., Pennoni, F., & Lowenfels, A. B. (2007). Comparative analysis of alcohol control policies in 30 countries. *PLoS Medicine, 4,* e151. doi:10.1371/journal.pmed.0040151.

Brenner, D. J., Doll, R., Goodhead, D. T., Hall, E. J., Land, C. E., Little, J. B., et al. (2003). Cancer risks attributable to low doses of ionizing radiation: Assessing what we really know. *Proceedings of the National Academy of Sciences of the United States of America, 100*(24), 13761–13766.

Brenner, D. J., & Hall, E. J. (2007). Computed tomography-an increasing source of radiation exposure. *The New England Journal of Medicine, 357*(22), 2277–2284.

Briggs, D. J. (2008). A framework for integrated environmental health impact assessment of systemic risks. *Environmental Health, 7,* 61.

Brower, M. (1992). *Cool energy: Renewable solutions to environmental problems.* Boston, MA: MIT Press.

Bruun, K., Edwards, G., Lumio, M., et al. (1975). *Alcohol control policies in public health perspective.* Helsinki: The Finnish Foundation for Alcohol Studies. 106 p.

Centre for Disease Control and Prevention. (2010). *Alcohol & public policy*. Atlanta, Georgia: CDC. Available at: http://www.cdc.gov/alcohol/index.htm.

Chaloupka. F.J., Grossman, M., Saffer, H. (2002). The effects of price on alcohol consumption and alcohol-related problems. *Alcohol Research & Health*, 26(1) 22–34. Available at: http://pubs.niaaa.nih.gov/publications/arh26-1/22-34.pdf Accessed November 8, 2010.

Chapman, R. S., Watkinson, W. P., Dreher, K. L., & Costa, D. L. (1997). Ambient particulate matter and respiratory and cardiovascular illness in adults: Particle borne transition metals and the heart-lung axis. *Environmental Toxicology and Pharmacology, 4*, 331–338.

Cauchemez, S., Ferguson, N. M., Wachtel, C., Tegnell, A., Saour, G., Duncan, B., & Nicoll, A. (2009). Closure of schools during an influenza pandemic. *Lancet Infectious Diseases, 9*(8), 473–481.

Checkoway, H., & Nelson, L. (1999). Epidemiologic approaches to the study of Parkinson's disease etiology. *Epidemiology, 10*, 327–336.

Cocarta, D.M., Badea, A., Apostol, T. (2008). Characterization of energy production and health impact in Romanian context. *Proceedings of the 3rd IASME/WSEAS international conference on Energy & environment*. World Scientific and Engineering Academy and Society (WSEAS), 198–203.

Coffman, S. (2003). Bicycle injuries and safety helmets in children. *Review of Research, Orthopaedic Nursing, 22*, 9–15.

Coles, R. W., & Taylor, J. (1993). Wind power and planning—the environmental impacts of wind farms in the UK. *Butterworth-Heinemann, Oxford, UK, 205–226*.

Correia, M. J., Hellies, A., Andreassi, M. G., Ghelarducci, B., & Picano, E. (2005). Lack of radiological awareness among physicians working in a tertiary-care cardiological centre. *International Journal of Cardiology, 103*(3), 307–311.

Costello, E., & Edelstein, J. E. (2008). Update on falls prevention for community-dwelling older adults: Review of single and multifactorial intervention programs. *Journal of Rehabilitation Research and Development, 45*(8), 1135–1152.

Council of the European Union. (2009). Council Recommendation of 30 November 2009 on smoke-free environments (2009/C 296/02). Available at: http://eur-lex.europa.eu/LexUriServ/LexUriServ.do?uri=OJ:C:2009:296:0004:0014:EN:PDF. Accessed January, 2013.

Dahlgren, G., & Whitehead, M. (1991). *Policies and strategies to promote social equity in health*. Stockholm, Sweden: Institute for Future Studies.

Dannenberg, A. L., Bhatia, R., Cole, B. L., Dora, C., Fielding, J. E., Kraft, K., et al. (2006). Growing the field of health impact assessment in the United States: An agenda for research and practice. *American Journal of Public Health, 96*, 262–270.

Dannenberg, A. L., Bhatia, R., Cole, B. L., Heaton, S. K., Feldman, J. D., & Rutt, C. D. (2008). Use of health impact assessment in the U.S. 27 case studies, 1999–2007. *American Journal of Preventive Medicine, 34*, 241–256.

Davenport, C., Mathers, J., & Parry, J. (2006). Use of health impact assessment in incorporating health considerations in decision making. *Journal of Epidemiology and Community Health, 60*, 196–201.

DEGAM. (2004). *DEGAM Leitlinie Ältere Sturzpatienten*. Düsseldorf, Germany: DEGAM und omicron publishing.

Dincer, I. (1999). Environmental impacts of energy. *Energy Policy, 27*(14), 845–854.

Dincer, I., & Rosen, M. A. (1998). A worldwide perspective on energy, environment and sustainable development. *International Journal of Energy Research, 22*(15), 1305–1321.

Dockery, D. W., Speizer, F. E., Stram, D. O., Ware, J. H., Spengler, J. D., & Ferris, B. G., Jr. (1989). Effects of inhalable particles on respiratory health of children. *American Review of Respiratory Diseases, 139*, 587–594.

Donaldson K., McNee W. (2001). Potential mechanisms of adverse pulmonary and cardiovascular effects of particulate air pollution (PM10). *International Journal of Hygiene and Environmental Health 203*, 411–415.

Eriksen, M., & Chaloupka, F. (2007). The economic impact of clean indoor air laws. *CA: A Cancer Journal for Clinicians, 57*, 367–378.

Ethen, M. K., Ramadhani, T. A., Scheuerle, A. E., Canfield, M. A., Wyszynski, D. F., Druschel, C. M., et al. (2008). National Birth Defects Prevention Study, Alcohol Consumption by Women Before and During Pregnancy. *Maternal and Child Health Journal, 13*, 274.

European Center for Disease Prevention and Control. (2009). *Guide to public health measures to reduce the impact of influenza pandemics in Europe*. 'The ECDC Menu', Stockholm, Sweden: ECDC.

European Commission. (2003). *European road safety action programme. Halving the number of road accident victims in the European Union by 2010: A shared responsibility* COM(2003)311 final, EC, Brussels, Belgium. Available at: http://ec.europa.eu/transport/roadsafety_library/rsap/rsap_en.pdf. Accessed January 2011.

Commission, E. (2007). *Green paper—towards a Europe free from tobacco smoke: Policy options at EU level*. EC: Brussels, Belgium.

Ezzati, M., Lopez, A. D., Rodgers, A., Hoorn, S. V., Murray, C. J. L., & Comparative Risk Assessment Collaborating Group. (2002). Selected major risk factors and global and regional burden of disease. *Lancet, 360*(9343), 1347–1360.

F+B, Forschung und Beratung GmbH. (2008). Optimierung der Gebietskulissen für die regionale Differenzierung der Wohnraumförderung in Nordrhein-Westfalen. F+B, Hamburg, p. 81.

Fenger, J. (2009). Air pollution in the last 50 years –from local to global. *Atmospheric Environment, 43*, 13–22.

File, T. M. (2000). The epidemiology of respiratory tract infections. *Seminars in Respiratory Infections, 15*(3), 184–194.

Fong, G. T., Hyland, A., Borland, R., Hammond, D., Hastings, G., McNeill, A., et al. (2006). Reductions in tobacco smoke pollution and increases in support for smoke-free public places following the implementation of comprehensive smoke-free workplace legislation in the Republic of Ireland: Findings from the ITC Ireland/UK Survey. *Tobacco Control, 15*(Suppl 3), 51–58.

Frick, K. D., Kung, J. Y., Parrish, J. M., & Narrett, M. J. (2010). Evaluating the cost-effectiveness of fall prevention programs that reduce fall-related hip fractures in older adults. *Journal of American Geriatrics Society, 58*(1), 136–141.

Gandini, S., Botteri, E., Iodice, S., Boniol, M., Lowenfels, A. B., Maisonneuve, P., et al. (2008). Tobacco smoking and cancer: A meta-analysis. *International Journal of Cancer, 122*, 155–164.

Gee, D. (1997). Approaches to Scientific uncertainty. In T. Fletcher & A. J. McMichael (Eds.), *Health at the crossroads: Transport policy and urban health* (pp. 27–50). Chichester, England: Wiley.

Gekas, V., Frantzeskaki, N., Tsoutsos, T. (2002). *Environmental impact assessment of solar energy systems. Results from a life cycle analysis*. Protection and Restoration of the Environment VI, Skiathos, 1–5 July.

Gillespie, L.D., Robertson, M.C., Lamb, S.E., Gates, S., Cumming, R.G., Rowe, B.H. (2009). Interventions for preventing falls in older people living in the community (Review). *Cochrane Database of Systematic Reviews* (2), John Wiley & Sons, CD007146. doi:10.1002/14651858.CD007146.pub2

Gorini, G., Chellini, E., & Galeone, D. (2007). What happened in Italy? A brief summary of studies conducted in Italy to evaluate the impact of the smoking ban. *Annals of Oncology, 18*, 1620–1622.

Government of the Republic of Lithuania. (2005). Decision on the National Road Safety Programme 2005–2010. *Official Gazette*, 84 (3117). Available at: http://www3.lrs.lt/pls/inter3/dokpaieska.showdoc_p?p_id=259383. Accessed January 2011.

Government of the Republic of Lithuania. (2007). Decision on the amendment of the National Road Safety Programme 2005–2010. *Official Gazette*, 59 (2297). Available at: http://www3.lrs.lt/pls/inter3/dokpaieska.showdoc_p?p_id=298103. Accessed January 2011.

Grass, S. W., & Jenkins, B. M. (1994). Biomass fueled fluidized bed combustion: Atmospheric emissions, emission control devices and environmental regulations. *Biomass and Bioenergy, 64*, 243–260.

Greenhalgh, R. (2002). *Fossil fuel and its impact on the environment*. Description of the harmful impact on the environment from the retrieval and conversion of fossil fuels to energy. http://www.pagewise.com. Accessed October 22, 2010.

Grønbaek, M., Becker, U., Johansen, D., Gottschau, A., Schnohr, P., Hein, H. O., et al. (2001). Type of alcohol consumed and mortality from all causes, coronary heart disease, and cancer. *Annals of Internal Medicine, 135*, 66–67.

Halliburton, S. S., & Schoenhagen, P. (2010). Cardiovascular imaging with computed tomography: Responsible steps to balancing diagnostic yield and radiation exposure. *Journal of the American College of Cardiology: Cardiovascular Imaging, 3*(5), 536–540.

Harris, P., Harris-Roxas, B., Harris, E., Kemp, L. (2007). *Health Impact Assessment: A Practical Guide.* Sydney, Australia: Centre for Health Equity Training, Research and Evaluation, University of New South Wales. Available at: http://hiaconnect.edu.au/old/files/Health_Impact_Assessment_A_Practical_Guide.pdf. Accessed November 26, 2012.

Harrison, L., & Gardiner, E. (1999). Do the rich really die young? Alcohol-related mortality and social class in Great Britain, 1988–1994. *Addiction, 94*(12), 1871–1880.

Health Canada. (2004). *Canadian handbook on health impact assessment.* Ottawa, Canada: Health Canada. Available at: http://www.who.int/hia/tools/toolkit/whohia063/en/index.html. Accessed November 26, 2012.

Hemström, O. (2002). Alcohol-related deaths contribute to socioeconomic differentials in mortality in Sweden. *European Journal of Public Health, 12*(4), 254–262.

Human Impact Partners. (2011). *A health impact assessment toolkit: A handbook to conducting HIA.* 3rd edn, Oakland, California: Human Impact Partners. Available at: http://www.humanimpact.org/doc-lib/finish/11/81. Accessed November 26, 2012.

Icks, A., Becker, C., & Kunstmann, W. (2005). Sturzprävention bei Senioren. Eine interdisziplinäre Aufgabe. *Deutsches Ärzteblatt, 102*(31–32), A2150–A2152.

Institute of Drug Addiction. (2008). *National Action Plan on Alcohol problems for the period 2006–2010.* Bratislava: Centre drug rehabilitation. ISBN 978-80-969196-2-8.

International Agency for Research on Cancer. (2004). *IARC monographs on the evaluation of carcinogenic risk of chemicals to humans* (Vol. 83). IARC, Lyon: Tobacco smoke and involuntary smoking.

International Energy Agency. (1998). *World energy outlook* (1998th ed.). Paris, France: IEA/OECD.

Jaakkola, M. S., & Jaakkola, J. K. (2006). Biomass fuels and health—the gap between global relevance and research activity. *American Journal of Respiratory and Critical Care Medicine, 174*, 851–852.

Jenkins, B. M., Baxter, L. L., Miles, T. R., Jr., & Miles, T. R. (1998). Combustion properties of biomass. *Fuel Processing Technology, 54*, 17–46.

Kowalska, M., Zejda, J.E. (2012). *Impact of air pollution (fine particles) on the health and quality of life in inhabitants of the Silesian Agglomeration.* Presented at the VII Conference Air Protection in Theory and Practice, Zakopane, Poland

Krieger, J., & Higgins, D. L. (2002). Housing and health: Time again for public health action. *American Journal of Public Health, 92*(5), 758–768.

Lalonde, M. (1974). *A new perspective on the health of Canadians: A working document.* Ottawa, Canada: Ministry of Supply and Services Canada. Available at: http://www.hc-sc.gc.ca/hcs-sss/alt_formats/hpb-dgps/pdf/pubs/1974-lalonde/lalonde-eng.pdf. Accessed January 2011.

Landesinstitut für Gesundheit und Arbeit NRW. (2009). *Landesinstitut für Gesundheit und Arbeit NRW, GBE-Stat 2009.* Annuß, R. (Ed.). LIGA.NRW, Düsseldorf, Germany.

Lhachimi, S. K., Nusselder, W. J., Boshuizen, H. C., & Mackenbach, J. P. (2010). Standard tool for quantification in health impact assessment: A review. *American Journal of Preventive Medicine, 38*, 78–84.

Lithuanian Road Police Service. (2010). Available at: http://www.lpept.lt/lt/statistika/2010/ Accessed February, 5 2011.

Lunevicius, R., & Rahman, M. H. (2012). Assessment of Lithuanian trauma care service using a conceptual framework for assessing the performance of health system. *European Journal of Public Health, 22*(1), 26–31.

Mäkelä, P., Valkonen, T., & Martelin, T. (1997). Contribution of deaths related to alcohol use to socioeconomic variation in mortality: Register based follow up study. *BMJ, 315*(7102), 211–216.

Mannheimer, L. N., Gulis, G., Lehto, J., & Ostlin, P. (2007). Introducing Health Impact Assessment: An analysis of political and administrative intersectoral working methods. *European Journal of Public Health, 17*, 526–531.

McCarthy, M., Biddulph, J. P., Utley, M., Ferguson, J., & Gallivan, S. (2002). A health impact assessment model for environmental changes attributable to development projects. *Journal of Epidemiology and Community Health, 56*, 611–616.

Metcalfe, O., Higgins, C., Lavin, T. (2009). *Health Impact Assessment Guidance.* Dublin, Ireland: Institute of Public Health in Ireland. Available at: http://www.publichealth.ie/sites/default/files/documents/files/IPH%20HIA_0.pdf. Accessed November 26, 2012.

Milner, S. J., Bailey, C., & Deans, J. (2003). 'Fit for purpose' health impact assessment: A realistic way forward. *Public Health, 117*, 295–300.

Mindell, J., Hansell, A., Morrison, D., Douglas, M., & Joffe, M. (2001). Quantifiable HIA Discussion Group. What do we need for robust, quantitative health impact assessment? *Journal of Public Health Medicine, 23*, 173–178.

Ministry of Health of the Slovak Republic. (2007). *State health policy concept of the Slovak Republic.* Bratislava, Slovakia: Ministry of Health of the Slovak Republic. Available at: http://www.health.gov.sk/redsys/rsi.nsf/0/F9D31C2B804C386AC12573A60037D67A?OpenDocument.

MMI. (2011). Volle Hallen—die BAU boomt. Presseinformationen der BAU 2011 (4/2011) p. 6.

Moreno, T., Querol, X., Alastuey, A., Ballester, A., & Gibbons, W. (2007). Airborne particulate matter and premature deaths in urban Europe: The new WHO guidelines and challenge ahead as illustrated by Spain. *European Journal of Epidemiology, 22*, 1–5.

Naimi, T. S., Brewer, R. D., Miller, J. W., Okoro, C., & Mehrotra, C. (2007). What do binge drinkers drink? Implications for alcohol control policy. *American Journal of Preventive Medicine, 33*(3), 188–193.

National Council on Radiation Protection and Measurements. (2009). *Ionizing radiation exposure of the population of the United States*, NCRP Report No. 160, NCRP, Bethesda, MD. Available from: http://www.ncrppublications.org/Reports/160. Accessed: December 12, 2012.

National Institute for Health and Clinical Excellence. (2005). *Guideline development methods. chapter 7 reviewing and grading the evidence.* London, UK: NIHCE

O'Connell, E., & Hurley, F. (2009). A review of the strengths and weaknesses of quantitative methods used in health impact assessment. *Public Health, 123*, 306–310.

Olsen, J. A., Richardson, J., Dolan, P., & Menzel, P. (2003). The moral relevance of personal characteristics in setting health care priorities. *Social Science & Medicine, 57*, 1163–1172.

Pastuszka, J., Zemła, B., Cimander, B., Sosnowska, M., Tyczyński, A., Górny, R., Lis, D., Lebecka, J., Chałupnik, S., Wysocka, M., Mielżyńska, D., Siwińska, E., Bubak, A. (1993). *Monitoring of carcinogenic risk for the general population of the Katowice District.* Part I, II and III In Sokal J (ed.), Report of the Institute of Occupational Medicine and Environmental Health, WHO Collaborating Centre, Sosnowiec, Poland (in Polish)

Pastuszka, J. S., Górny, R. L., Pajdo, S., Cimander, B., & Klinik, M. (1999). Studies of the relationship between concentration of the total suspended particles (TSP) and PM-10 in ambient air in 3 Polish towns. *Ochrona Powietrza i Problemy Odpadów, 5*, 179–182 (in Polish).

Pastuszka, J. S., Rogula-Kozłowska, W., & Zajusz-Zubek, E. (2010). Characterization of PM10 and PM2.5 and associated heavy metals at the crossroads and Urban background site In Zabrze, Upper Silesia, Poland, during the smog episodes. *Environmental Monitoring and Assessment, 168*, 613–627.

Pastuszka, J.S., Zejda, J.E., Wlazło, A., Lis, DO., Maliszewska, I. (2003). *Exposure to PM in Upper Silesia and results of the pilot study on the airborne particles, bacteria and fungi in homes with asthmatic children*, Proceeding of the 5th International Technion Symp. "Particulate Matter and Health", February 23–25 Vienna. Vienna, Austria: Austrian Academy of Sciences, pp. 95–99.

Peden, M., Scurfield, R., Sleet, D., Mohan, D., Hyder, A. A., Jarawan, E., et al. (Eds.). (2004). *World report on road traffic injury prevention: Summary*. Geneva, Switzerland: World Health Organization.

Picano, E. (2003). Stress echocardiography: A historical perspective. *American Journal of Medicine, 114*(2), 126–130.

Picano, E., Pasanisi, E., Brown, J., & Marwick, T. H. (2007). A gatekeeper for the gatekeeper: Inappropriate referrals to stress echocardiography. *American Heart Journal, 154*(2), 285–290.

Quigley, R., den Broeder, L., Furu, P., Bond, A., Cave, B., Bos, R. (2006). *Health impact assessment: International best practice principles*. International Association for Impact Assessment. Fargo, North Dakota. Available at: http://www.iaia.org/publicdocuments/special-publications/SP5.pdf. Accessed November 26, 2012.

Ramos, P., Diez, E., Perez, K., Rodriguez-Martos, A., Brugal, M. T., & Villabi, J. R. (2008). Young people perceptions of traffic injury risks, prevention and enforcement measures: A qualitative study. *Accident Analysis and Prevention, 40*(4), 1313–1319.

Reed, C., Angulo, F. J., Swerdlow, D. L., Lipsitch, M., Meltzer, M. I., Jernigan, D., et al. (2009). Estimates of the prevalence of pandemic (H1N1), 2009, United States, April–July 2009. *Emerging Infectious Diseases, 15*(12), 2004–2007.

Ritter, A. (2007). Comparing alcohol policies between countries: Science or silliness? *PLoS Medicine, 4*(4), e153. doi:10.1371/journal.pmed.0040153. Available at: http://www.plosmedicine.org/article/info:doi/10.1371/journal.pmed.0040153

Romieu, I. (1992). Epidemiological studies of the health effects of air pollution due to motor vehicles. In D. T. Mage & O. Zali (Eds.), *Motor vehicle, air pollution, public health impact and control measures*. Geneva, Switzerland: WHO.

Room, R., Babor, T., & Rehm, J. (2005). Alcohol and public health. *Lancet, 365*, 519–530.

Rose, G. A. (1992). *The strategy of preventive medicine*. Oxford, New York: Oxford University Press.

Ruidavets, J. B., Bataille, V., Dallongeville, J., Simon, C., Bingham, A., Amouyel, P., et al. (2004). Alcohol intake and diet in France, the prominent role of lifestyle. *European Heart Journal, 25*, 1153–1162.

Sadique, M. Z., Adams, E. J., & Edmunds, W. J. (2008). Estimating the costs of school closure for mitigating an influenza pandemic. *BMC Public Health, 8*, 135.

SafetyNet. (2008). *Traffic Safety Basic Facts*. Available at: http://ec.europa.eu/transport/wcm/road_safety/erso/safetynet/content/safetynet.htm. Accessed January 2011.

Samet, J. M., Domicini, F., Curriero, F. C., Coursac, I., & Zeger, S. L. (2000). Fine particulate air pollution and mortality in 20 U.S. cities, 1987–1994. *The New England Journal of Medicine, 343*, 1742–1749.

Samoli, E., Analitis, A., Touloumi, G., Schwartz, J., Anderson, H. R., Sunyer, J., et al. (2005). Estimating the exposure-response relationship between particulate matter and mortality within the APHEA multicity project. *Environmental Health Perspectives, 113*, 88–95.

Saß, AC. (2010). Unfälle in Deutschland. Ergebnisse des telefonischen Gesundheitssurveys "Gesundheit in Deutschland aktuell" (GEDA) 2009. GBE kompakt 2/2010. Robert Koch-Institut, Berlin. www.rki.de/gbe-kompakt.

Saup, W. (1993). *Alter und Umwelt: Eine Einführung in die ökologische Gerontologie* (p. 239). Stuttgart: W. Kohlhammer GmbH.

Schmidt, L. A., Mäkelä, P., Rehm, J., & Room, R. (2010). *Alcohol: Equity and social determinants. In Equity, social determinants and public health programs* (pp. 11–31). Geneva, Switzerland: WHO Press.

Schrieber, R. A., & Vegega, M. E. (Eds.). (2001). *National strategies for advancing child pedestrian safety*. Atlanta, Georgia: Centers for Disease Control and Prevention, National Center for Injury Prevention and Control.

Scott-Samuel, A., Birley, M., Ardern, K. (2001). *The merseyside guidelines for health impact assessment*, 2nd ed., International Health Impact Assessment Consortium, Liverpool, UK. Available at: http://www.liv.ac.uk/ihia/IMPACT%20Reports/2001_merseyside_guidelines_31.pdf. Accessed November 26, 2012.

Seaton, A., McNee, W., Donaldson, K., & Godden, D. (1995). Particulate air pollution and acute health effects. *Lancet, 345*, 176–178.

Seifert, H., Westerhellweg, A., Kröning, J. (2003). Risk analysis of ice throw from wind turbines. Paper presented BOREAS 6, 9–11 April 2003, Pyhä, Finland.

Setbon, M., & Raude, J. (2010). Factors in vaccination intention against the pandemic influenza A/H1N1. *European Journal of Public Health, 20*(5), 490–494.

Sethi, D., Racioppi, F., Mitis, F. (2007). *Youth and road safety in Europe. Policy briefing.* Copenhagen, Denmark: WHO Regional Office for Europe 34.

Smart, R. G. (1996). Behavioral and social consequences related to the consumption of different beverage types. *Journal of Studies on Alcohol, 57*(1), 77–84.

Speight, J. G. (1996). *Environmental technology handbook.* Washington, DC: Taylor and Francis.

Ståhl, T., Wismar, M., Ollila, E., Lahtinen, E., & Leppo, K. (Eds.). (2006). *Health in all policies. Prospects and potentials.* Helsinki, Finland: Ministry of Social Affairs and Health.

Starkuviene, S., Petrauskiene, J., & Kalediene, R. (2010). The effect of Lithuania's year of sobriety (2008) on losses due to alcohol related injuries. *The European Journal of Public Health, 20*(suppl 1), 176.

Steenland, K., & Armstrong, B. (2006). An overview of methods for calculating the burden of disease due to specific risk factors. *Epidemiology, 17,* 512–519.

Stevens, J. A., Mack, K. A., Paulozzi, L. J., & Ballesteros, M. F. (2008). Self-reported falls and fall-related injuries among persons aged > 65 years—United States, 2006. *CDC MMWR, 57*(09), 225–229.

Stolle, M., Sack, P. M., & Thomasius, R. (2009). Binge drinking in childhood and adolescence: Epidemiology, consequences, and interventions. *Deutsches Ärzteblatt International, 106*(19), 323–328.

Strong, P. M. (1980). Doctors and dirty work: The case of alcoholism. *Sociology of Health & Illness, 2*(1), 24–47.

Stuckler, D., Basu, S., Suhrcke, M., Coutts, A., McKee, M. (2009). The public health effect of economic crisis and alternative policy responses in Europe: An empirical analysis. *Lancet, 374*(9686), 315–323. Available at: http://www.cadca.org/files/resources/suicidestudy.pdf. Accessed 8.11.2010.

Szücs, S., Sárváry, A., McKee, M., & Ádány, R. (2005). Could the high level of cirrhosis in central and Eastern Europe be due partly to the quality of alcohol consumed? An exploratory investigation. *Addiction, 100*(4), 536–542.

Taylor, L., Blair-Stevens, C. (2002). *Introducing health impact assessment (HIA): Informing the decision-making process.* Health Development Agency, London, UK. Available at: http://www.nice.org.uk/niceMedia/documents/hia.pdf Accessed November 26, 2012.

Thacker, S.B., Branche, C. (2000). Reducing Falls and Resulting Hip Fractures Among Older Women. *MMWR Recommendations and Report, 49*(RR02), 1–12.

Thompson, D.C., Rivara, F.P., & Thompson, R. (2000). Helmets for preventing head and facial injuries in bicyclists. *Cochrane Database Syst Rev,* CD001855.

Thompson, D. C., Rivara, F. P., & Thompson, R. S. (1996). Effectiveness of bicycle safety helmets in preventing head injuries. A case–control study. *JAMA, 276,* 1968–1973.

Thomson, H., Petticrew, M. (2005). *Is housing improvement a potential health improvement strategy?* Health Evidence Network report. WHO Regional Office for Europe: Copenhagen, Denmark. Available at: http://www.euro.who.int/__data/assets/pdf_file/0007/74680/E85725.pdf

Thun, M. J., Apicella, L. F., & Henley, S. J. (2000). Smoking vs. other risk factors as the cause of smoking-attributable deaths: Confounding in the courtroom. *Journal of the American Medical Association, 284,* 706–712.

Towner, E., Errington, G. (2004). *How can injuries in children and older people be prevented?* Health Evidence Report. WHO Regional Office for Europe: Copenhagen, Denmark Access date: May 7, 2010.

Tsoutsos, T., Frantzeskak, N., & Gekas, V. (2005). Environmental impacts from the solar energy technologies. *Energy Policy, 33,* 289–296.

U.S. Department of Health and Human Services. (1995). *Injury-Control Recommendations: Bicycle Helmets.* Atlanta, Georgia: U.S. DHHS, Centers for Disease Control and Prevention, Public Health Service.

3 Top-Down Policy Risk Assessment

129

U.S. Department of Health and Human Services. (2004). *The health consequences of smoking: A report of the Surgeons General.* Atlanta, Georgia: U.S. DHHS, Centers for Disease Control and Prevention, National Center for Chronic Disease Prevention and Health Promotion, Office on Smoking and Health.

U.S. Department of Health and Human Services (2006). *The health consequences of involuntary exposure to tobacco smoke: A report of the Surgeons General.* Atlanta, Georgia: U.S. DHHS, Centers for Disease Control and Prevention, Coordinating Center for Health Promotion, National Center for Chronic Disease Prevention and Health Promotion, Office on Smoking and Health.

Veerman, J. L., Barendregt, J. J., & Mackenbach, J. P. (2005). Quantitative health impact assessment: Current practice and future directions. *Journal of Epidemiology and Community Health, 59,* 361–370.

Venneri, L., Rossi, F., Botto, N., Andreassi, M. G., Salcone, N., Emad, A., et al. (2009). Cancer risk from professional exposure in staff working in cardiac catheterization laboratory: Insights from the National Research Council's Biological Effects of Ionizing Radiation VII Report. *American Heart Journal, 157*(1), 118–124.

von Heideken Wagert, P., Gustafson, Y., Kallin, K., Jensen, J., & Lundin-Olsson, L. (2009). Falls in very old people: The population-based Umeå 85+ study in Sweden. *Archives of Gerontology and Geriatrics, 49*(3), 390–396.

Wcisło, E., Dutkiewicz, T., & Konczalik, J. (2002). Indicator-based assessment of environmental hazards and health effects in the industrial cities in Upper Silesia, Poland. *Environmental Health Perspectives, 110,* 1133–1140.

Weightman, A., Ellis, S., Cullum, A., Sander, L., & Turley, R. (2005). *Grading evidence and recommendations for public health interventions: Developing and piloting a framework.* London, UK: Health Development Agency.

World Health Organization. (1986). *Ottawa charter for health promotion.* Ottawa, Canada: World Health Organization.

World Health Organization. (1988). *Adelaide recommendations on healthy public policy.* Geneva, Switzerland: WHO.

World Health Organization. (1998). *Health promotion glossary.* Geneva, Switzerland: WHO.

World Health Organization. (2002). *The world health report 2002: Reducing risks, promoting healthy life.* Geneva, Switzerland: WHO. Available at: http://www.who.int/whr/2002/en/index.html

World Health Organization. (2003). *Framework convention on tobacco control.* Geneva, Switzerland: WHO.

World Health Organization. (2004a). *Global Status Report on Alcohol 2004.* Geneva, Switzerland: WHO. Available at: http://www.who.int/substance_abuse/publications/global_status_report_2004_overview.pdf. Accessed November 8, 2010

World Health Organization. (2004b). *World report on road traffic injury prevention: Summary.* Geneva, Switzerland: WHO.

World Health Organization. (2006). *Global pandemic influenza action plan to increase vaccine supply.* Geneva, Switzerland: WHO.

World Health Organization. (2008a). *Report on the global tobacco epidemic: The MPOWER package.* Geneva, Switzerland: WHO.

World Health Organization. (2008b). *The Global Burden of Disease: 2004 Update.* Geneva, Switzerland: WHO. Available at: http://www.who.int/healthinfo/global_burden_disease/2004_report_update/en/index.html. Accessed 20 January 2011.

World Health Organization. (2009a). *Global status report on road safety: Time for action, 135.* Geneva, Switzerland: WHO.

World Health Organization. (2009b). Mathematical modelling of the pandemic H1N1 2009. *Weekly Epidemiological Record, 84,* 341–352.

World Health Organization. (2010). *A decade of action for road traffic safety. A brief planning document.* Geneva, Switzerland: WHO. Available at: http://www.who.int/roadsafety/Decade_of_action.pdf Accessed January 25, 2011.

World Health Organization European Centre for Health Policy. (1999). *Health impact assessment: Main concepts and suggested approach.* *Gothenburg Consensus Paper.* Brussels, Belgium: WHO European Centre for Health Policy.

World Health Organization Regional Office for Europe. (2002). *European strategy for tobacco control.* Copenhagen, Denmark: WHO Regional Office for Europe.

World Health Organization Regional Office for Europe. (2004). *Preventing road traffic injury: A public health perspective for Europe.* Copenhagen, Denmark: WHO Regional Office for Europe.

World Health Organization Regional Office for Europe. (2006). *Air quality guidelines: Global update 2005, particulate matter, ozone, nitrogen dioxide and sulfur dioxide.* Copenhagen, Denmark: WHO Regional Office for Europe.

World Health Organization Regional Office for Europe. (2007). *Large analysis and review of European housing and health status (LARES): Preliminary overview.* Copenhagen, Denmark: WHO Regional Office for Europe.

World Health Organization Regional Office for Europe. (2010). *Housing and health.* Copenhagen, Denmark: WHO Regional Office for Europe. http://www.euro.who.int/en/what-we-do/health-topics/environmental-health/Housing-and-health. Accessed October 29, 2010.

World Health Organization, Government of South Australia. (2010). *Adelaide Statement on Health in All Policies: Moving towards a shared governance for health and well-being.* Geneva, Switzerland: WHO.

World Health Organization-International Programme on Chemical Safety. (2008). *Guidance document on characterizing and communicating uncertainty in exposure assessment. Harmonization Project Document No. 6 (Part 1),* Geneva, Switzerland: WHO.

Youakim, S. (2006). Occupational health risks of wine industry workers. *BCMJ, 48*(8), 386–391. Available at: http://www.bcmj.org/occupational-health-risks-wine-industry-workers. Accessed November 8, 2010

Zatoński. W. (ed.), (2008). *Closing the health gap in European Union.* Cancer Epidemiology and Prevention Division, The final publication of the project HEM—Closing the gap, p. 76, ISBN 9788388681493

Zavcer, I. (2010). *Rapid Reports. 2010,* Statistical Office of the Republic of Slovenia, Ljubljana, Slovenia. Available at: http://www.stat.si/doc/statinf/15-si-073-1001.pdf. Accessed November 8, 2010

Zhang, W., Lei, T., Lin, Z.-Q., Zhang, H.-S., Yang, D.-F., Xi, Z.-G., et al. (2011). Pulmonary toxicity study in rats with PM_{10} and $PM_{2.5}$: Differential responses related to scale and composition. *Atmospheric Environment, 45,* 1034–1041.

Chapter 4
Bottom-Up Policy Risk Assessment

**Peter Otorepec, Piedad Martin-Olmedo, Julia Bolivar, Odile Mekel,
Jutta Grohmann, Daniela Kállayova, Mária Kvaková, Jana Kollárová,
Ágnes Molnár, Balázs Ádám, Stella R.J. Kræmer, Mariusz Geremek,
Joanna Kobza, and Rainer Fehr**

Introduction

Chronic diseases, despite being largely preventable, account for 86 % of the premature deaths and 77 % of the overall disease burden in the World Health Organization (WHO)-European Region, with an impact on countries' economy ranking from 0.02 to 6.77 % of the gross domestic product (Suhrcke et al. 2006 cited by Busse et al. 2010). The unequal distribution of this burden of disease is also unfair and unjust (Metcalfe and Higgins 2009; Bambra et al. 2010). The beneficial influence that healthy public policies might exert directly or indirectly, on the population health is widely accepted. Factors such as the environmental, living and working conditions, access to education, or socioeconomic status, as well as the policies influencing those factors, are proved to be more relevant in determining population health than the weight of health systems, which contributes by about 25 % to the health outcomes. At the same time, it has being revealed that

P. Otorepec (✉)
National Institute of Public Health, Trubarjeva 2, SI 1000 Ljubljana, Slovenia
e-mail: peter.otorepec@ivz-rs.si

P. Martin-Olmedo • J. Bolivar
Escuela Andaluza de Salud Pública, Cuesta del Observatorio 4, 18080 Granada, Spain
e-mail: piedad.martin.easp@juntadeandalucia.es; Julia.bolivar@juntadeandalucia.es

O. Mekel
Unit Innovation in Health, NRW Centre for Health (LZG.NRW), Bielefeld 33611, Germany
e-mail: odile.mekel@lzg.gc.nrw.de

J. Grohmann
NRW Centre for Health (LZG.NRW), Bielefeld 33611, Germany
e-mail: jutta.grohmann@lzg.gc.nrw.de

D. Kállayova • M. Kvaková
Trnava University, Univerzitne namestie 1, 91701 Trnava, Slovakia
e-mail: daniela.kallayova@truni.sk; maria.kvakova@gmail.com

G. Guliš et al. (eds.), *Assessment of Population Health Risks of Policies*,
DOI 10.1007/978-1-4614-8597-1_4, © Springer Science+Business Media New York 2014

interventions leading to inequity or compromising future generations in meeting their needs (unsustainable) are likely to damage health (Kemm 2001; Metcalfe and Higgins 2009; Bambra et al. 2010; Solar and Irwin 2010; United Nations 2012). Therefore there is, a need for complex diagrams of causal pathways where a certain public policy might result in several health effects through different health determinants and related risk factors, or the other way round, the improvement of a socially determined health inequality requires different interventions throughout multifaceted pathways (Joffe and Mindell 2002, 2006). Metcalfe and Higgins (2009) exemplified this rationale looking at the problem of food poverty in Ireland which would require for being ameliorated of actions from several sectors such as transport, infrastructure, planning, education, agricultural and fiscal policies, all of them outside the health sector.

The top-down risk assessment that fits the classical HIA method and its application on policy was in depth presented in the previous chapter. Many public health experts find large policies difficult to assess as for their impact on health. People knowing well health outcome and it's societal burden may find it easier to find proper policies starting from the bottom line—from health outcome. The use of complex causal process diagrams for analyzing health impacts of policy interventions was already described by Joffe and Mindell (Joffe and Mindell 2006). The RAPID guidance based on bottom-up approach might be helpful to act more efficiently in reducing prevalence of health outcomes by identification and selection of proper policies for structural intervention. The health outcome was taken as a

J. Kollárová
Regional Public Health Authority, Ipelska 1, 04011 Kosice, Slovakia
e-mail: kollarova@ruvzke.sk

Á. Molnár
Centre for Research on Inner City Health, Li Ka Shing Knowledge Institute,
St. Michael's Hospital, 209 Victoria St., Rm. 3-26.22, Toronto, ON, M5B 1C6 Canada

University of Debrecen, Kassai 26, 4028 Debrecen, Hungary
e-mail: MolnarAg@smh.ca; molnar.agnes@sph.unideb.hu

B. Ádám
University of Southern Denmark, Niels Bohrsvej 10, 6700 Esbjerg, Denmark

University of Debrecen, Kassai 26, 4028 Debrecen, Hungary
e-mail: badam@health.sdu.dk; adam.balazs@sph.unideb.hu

S.R.J. Kræmer
University of Southern Denmark, Niels Bohrsvej 10, 6700 Esbjerg, Denmark
e-mail: skraemer@health.sdu.dk

M. Geremek • J. Kobza
Medical University of Silesia, 18 Medykow Street, 40-752 Katowice, Poland
e-mail: m.geremek@poczta.onet.pl; koga1@poczta.onet.pl

R. Fehr
University of Bielefeld, Universitätsstraße 25, 33615 Bielefeld, Germany
e-mail: rainer.fehr@uni-bielefeld.de

starting point and assessment through levels of risk factors and determinants of health lead to identification of policies needed to reduce burden of health outcome.

The present chapter illustrates through eight case studies conducted in seven different countries a bottom-up policy risk assessment model aiming to describe casual pathways upstream, from a single health outcome (effect) up through risk factors and health determinants leading to a list of policies. The purpose of this approach is to emphasize that results in health outcomes are related to many different policies at the same time, bringing up the need to adopt proactive inter-sectoral negotiations and putting health in the agenda of non-health sectors. Special interest was put on identifying the type of information needed for the description of the full-chain, possible discrepancies in defining health outcomes, risk factors or health determinants, the availability of data, the designation of possible scenarios related to political options, and the characterization of uncertainties. A strong effort was made to include quantitative risk assessment methods by providing numerical information on how the health status of the population can be improved by a policy. The quantification approach has been suggested to facilitate the decision making process by clarifying the weight of the options, and incorporating the use of economic instruments such as cost-benefit analysis (Joffe and Mindell 2005; Veerman et al. 2005).

The health outcomes proposed as starting point for this full-chain analysis were selected in all case studies by their relevance at European or national level. They include a variety of topics from osteoporosis (Denmark), road traffic fatalities (Spain), road traffic injuries (Germany), chronic liver disease (Hungary), cirrhosis (Slovak Republic), life expectancy (Poland), asthma (Slovak Republic), and chronic obstructive pulmonary disease (Slovenia). The first great challenge was clearly define the selected health outcomes since several stages of a pathogenic process can be considered as outcome. A description of the severity, reversibility and frequency of occurrence of each outcome has been addressed in all cases, with special emphasis on quantification gathering data mostly from publicly available statistics and surveys. The next step was to enlist all possible risk factors that according to the existing scientific evidence can positively (protective factors) or negatively modify the health outcome. Information on the quantitative relation between risk factors and health outcomes, as well as a description of the interrelation among risk factors has been searched for each topic. In the upper level the analysis continued by the qualitative/quantitative characterization of the relation between the previously described risk factors and wider determinants of health. Several models can be used for this purpose, being the model of Lalonde the most frequently applied in the reported case studies. Finally, for each casual pathway that emerged from a health outcome, relevant policies were identified taking the following aspects: the importance of the issue, the need of policy makers for assistance in the decision-making process, and the feasibility of a quantitative assessment. Cross-cutting issues addressed throughout the full chain analysis were the quantification of results in the process when possible and the analysis of uncertainty. The bottom-up approach might be considered useful to put health issues on policy agenda of all sectors which are identified for a single health outcome.

From Road Traffic Fatalities Towards Setting Policy: The Spanish Experience

Introduction

Transport is an essential component of contemporary life. Positive effects of transport result in providing access to education, employment, services, goods, leisure activities, and by contributing to economic development. However, the increase in road transportation has also been accompanied by numerous negative side effects related to health. According to the World Health Organization's data (WHO), road crashes result annually in almost 120,000 fatalities and 2.4 million injuries in the European Region, numbers similar to those caused by many communicable diseases. In economic terms, the direct and indirect costs of road traffic injuries could be as much as 3 % of the European gross domestic product. The problem is especially severe for adolescents and young adults, for whom road traffic injuries are the leading cause of death (WHO-Europe 2004, 2009).

Recognizing that road crashes represent a major preventable public-health burden, increased political attention is being paid by the international community to this topic in last years (European Commission EC 2001; United Nations 2008).

The present case study applies a bottom-up policy risk assessment procedure describing pathways (causal/association-based) from a single health outcome (effect) up through risk factors and health determinants eventually leading to a list of policies. In particular we have focused on "road traffic fatalities" (RTF) given the extensive availability of large public datasets. This study also addresses the prospective quantification of a possible reduction in RTF by assuming different scenarios in which the implementation of a policy (e.g. the "Penalty Point System") could result in decreased exposure to certain risk factors (e.g., "safety belt use"). This approach from health outcomes towards policy–setting is an attempt to provide decision makers outside the health sector with a whole picture of the process and issues that should be addressed and prioritized when proposing new actions that would not only benefit their sectoral political interest, but also improve the health and wellbeing status of citizens.

Important research on trends and data analysis referring to RTF has been undertaken in Spain over the last decade by several research groups, including the Spanish Traffic Authority (in Spanish, *Dirección General de Tráfico*, DGT). However, the main objective of the present study is not to perform a systematic literature review but to illustrate the process and the methodology for policy risk assessment, with special emphasis on differences in the definition of health outcomes, the availability of data for risk exposure characterization, and the quantification process.

Health Outcome Description

The most commonly accepted definition of RTF adopted by European Union (EU)-Member States is the one proposed by the United Nations Economic Commission

Table 4.1 Historical evolution (2001–2009) in EU-27 and Spain of RTF and people injured	Year	RTF		People injured	
		EU-27	Spain	EU-27	Spain
	2001	54,302	5,517	1,986,645	149,600
	2006	43,104	4,104	1,719,076	143,450
	2009	34,500	2,714	1,571,534	124,966

RTF = Motor vehicle crash deaths at 30 days
(Source: EC-CARE 2010; DGT 2006; 2009)

for Europe as: "*any person killed immediately or dying within 30 days as a result of an injury accident*" (WHO 2004a, b). However, this task requires marshalling a considerable amount of resources to monitor the 30-day track episode, and some countries use shorter periods. To adjust for this variation and enable comparative studies to be done across Europe, various correction factors are applied to arrive at a 30-day equivalent (WHO 2004, 2009). Spain endorsed the European definition of RTF in 1993 by applying an appropriate adjustment factor to motor vehicle crash deaths at 24 h based on police records. However, this adjustment often fails to take into account differences in the severity of injuries and mortality by road user type or other relevant variables (e.g. time and place of the crash, kind of vehicle involved, or age of the victim) (WHO 2004a, b; Pérez et al. 2006). Currently other mechanisms are under study to improve data collection and avoid missed cases. In their investigation, (Perez et al. 2006) reported the utility of hospital discharge registers (HDR) as a complementary source of information to police registry.

According to the European Commission (EC), over the time period 2001–2009 the number of RTF for the entire EU was reduced by 36 %, still far from the 45 % proposed target for 2009 under the EU Road Traffic Policy (EC 2001). In the case of Spain this decrease was larger accounting for 51 %. Nonetheless, personal injuries during the same period did not show such a great decline, dropping only by 16 %. In fact, when calculating the ratio of non-fatal injury per fatality, this ratio increases over time, ranging from 27 in 2001 to 42 in 2009 (Table 4.1).

All types of road users are at risk of being killed in a road traffic accident, but there are differences between groups. The so-called "vulnerable road users" are mainly pedestrians, cyclists and riders of motorized two-wheelers (moped and motorcycle) (WHO 2009). In Spain, the proportion of RTF among vulnerable road users became greater over time, increasing from 32 % in 2001 to more than 41 % in 2009. This is very relevant for urban pedestrians who accounted for 46 % of all urban RTF for year 2009 (DGT 2009).

The proportion of fatalities in the category for cars and taxis (modes of transportation categories registering the highest RTF in Europe) trended smoothly downward from 57 % in 2001 to 47 % in 2009 (DGT 2009).

In Spain, RTF by gender was almost four times greater among men than women, regardless of the year (DGT 2006, 2009). This ratio increased up to fivefold in the age range of 25–44 year olds. The distribution curve of RTF in Spain for age groups shows the highest fatality numbers for those between 25 and 44 years, followed by adults between 15 and 24 years of age (DGT 2006, 2009).

According International Classification of Diseases, version 10 (ICD-10) traffic-related injuries and fatalities are coded as V01-V99 (http://apps.who.int/ classifications/icd10/browse/2010/en). However, we have to mention that data is most often based on police statistics not taking in account ICD classification.

Risk Factors and Determinants of Health

According to Haddon's matrix, car crashes can occur as the result of factors related to humans, roads, the environment, and the vehicle itself. All these factors can interact differently depending on the phase of the car crash (Haddon 1968; WHO 2004a, b): pre-crash, crash and post-crash.

Pre-crash risk factors include Spain's *rapid motorization, demographic factors (ageing population)*, the *increased need to travel*, and the *mixture of high-speed motorized traffic with vulnerable road users* (DGT 2009).

The most relevant pre-crash human-related risk factors that influence the probability for a crash to occur are:

- *Speeding* (excessive or inappropriate speed). Speeding was present in 15 and 13 % of all road accidents with casualties in Spain for years 2006 and 2009, respectively. Those percentages were as high as 31 % for accidents with fatal consequences. During 2009 the police performed over 26.5 million radar speed controls and 2.9 % of vehicles were reported (DGT 2009).
- *Drinking and driving*. In most high-income countries about 20 % of fatally injured drivers exceed the legal limit of blood alcohol concentration (BAC). In Spain the percentage of alcohol testing conducted on deceased drivers increased from a 50.7 % in 2003 to 54.6 % in 2009. The percentage of drivers killed in traffic crashes who had BAC levels equal or above the legal limit of 0.3 g/dl decreased from 37.4 % in 2003 to 30 % in 2009 (DGT 2009).
- *Medicinal and recreational drugs*. During 2009 in Spain, about 22 % of deceased drivers with high BAC levels tested positive for simultaneous drug use (DGT 2009).
- *Using earphones or any other hand-held mobile device*. Evidence suggests the risk of suffering a car crash is four times higher for drivers who use mobile phones while driving compared to those who do not use them (WHO 2004a, b). The research undertaken by Gras et al. (2007) found that more than 60 % of drivers (a sample of Spanish university workers) in the Cataluña region (Spain) used a mobile phone while driving. The reported frequency of using a mobile phone to talk on urban roads was significantly correlated with crash involvement.
- Other risk factors are *fatigue*, being a *young male*, being a *vulnerable road user in urban and residential settings* and *poor road user eyesight* (WHO 2004a, b).

The most relevant pre-crash road-related risk factors are (WHO 2004, 2009) *travelling in darkness* or *without daytime running lights* on cars; *defects in road design*; and *inadequate visibility* due to environmental factors.

Finally, the most relevant vehicle-related pre-crash risk factors are *poor conditions of braking, handling and maintenance systems* in vehicles (WHO 2004, 2009).

Once the crash has occurred, human-related factors influencing crash severity and health consequences, include the following:

- *Seat belt and child restraints not used.* While they do not prevent crashes from taking place, they do play a major role in reducing the severity of injury to vehicle occupants. A review on the effectiveness of seat-belts found that their use reduces the probability of being killed by 40–50 % for drivers and front seat passengers, and by about 25 % for passengers in rear seats (Foundation for the Automobile and Society 2009). In non-urban settings in Spain the number of all deceased car occupants who didn't use seat belts decreased by 17 points from February 2006–2009, ranging from 39 % of all deaths in 2006, to 22 % in 2009. However, in urban settings negative effects were recorded, with a net increase of two points in the percentage of total deaths related to the non-use of a seat-belt for this period (32 % in 2006, and 34 % in 2009) (DGT 2009).
- *Not wearing a crash helmet.* Helmet use has proven to be the most successful approach for preventing injury among users of two-wheeled vehicles.
- Other factors are *human tolerance factors* (age, health conditions, etc.), *inappropriate or excess speed* or presence of *drugs or alcohol*.

Other risk factors influencing crash severity and health consequences can be road related, such as "*Roadside objects not crash protective*," or vehicle-related, such as "*Insufficient vehicle crash protection for occupants and for those hit by vehicles*."

Finally, post-crash risk factors related to caring for persons injured in a car crash can be human related, such as *first aid skills* or *access to medics*; vehicle related, for example, *ease of access* or *fire risk*; and road related, such as *rescue facilities* or *congestion*.

All these risk factors could be grouped into determinants according to the following categories: "*Biological factors*," for those related to age, health status or sex; "*Behaviours*," for those influenced by health-related behaviours such as excessive or inappropriate speed, drinking and driving, using mobile while driving, not using helmet, failing to comply the safety distance or improper use of safety seat belts and/or child restraint systems; "*Material circumstances as physical environmental factors*" for defects in road design, inadequate visibility due to environmental factors or roadside objects not crash protective; "*Access to services*" for the access and quality of health services or resources (ambulance, police, etc.); "*Social and economic factors*" such as rapid motorization and need to travel, income and wealth, or education; and "*Public Policies*" for the range of policies linked with determinants and risk-factors (next section).

In terms of information availability, it is crucial to characterize correctly the level of exposure to different risk factors adjusted to specific scenarios (concrete areas and affected populations). Without this information it is impossible to quantify any health gain related to changes in risk factors linked to specific policy measures. Presently this type of information in the field of RTF is not systematically recorded in Spain for all main risk factors.

Relevant Policies

Traffic safety and road traffic injury prevention have strong political support in Spain. National targets have been established and enjoy wide acceptance by society and key agencies. Interim targets are set within a specific time frame of the national road safety strategy. They are ambitious but realistic.

Targets and other safety performance indicators are continuously monitored, establishing the effectiveness of specific road safety measures by carrying out before and after studies. The main strategies and policies developed in Spain on this topic have been: the National Strategic Plan on Road Safety 2005–2008 and the Penalty Point Driving License System (PPS), adopted in 2006. The PPS mostly exerts an influence on individual risk behaviour factors such as discouraging driving after alcohol consumption, or promoting the use of safety belt at all times by all car users.

Quantification of the Reduction of RTF

As stated earlier, any approach that seeks to quantify the health impact of a policy requires the application of an integrated model capable of describing the interactions among all possible risk factors and related health determinants. Some proposals for integrated models are currently under discussion (i.e. DYNAMO-HIA) but they have not been yet properly adapted to the road transport sector. An operative approach would be based on estimating RTF reduction, by assuming scenarios under which potential policies would result in decreased exposure to certain health determinants and related risk factors. Well-based epidemiological evidence on the dose-response function between health outcomes and risk factors is essential for this characterization. To illustrate this approach we have selected the "use of safety belt" as a risk factor (protecting factor), incorporated in the previously mentioned PPS policy.

The data entry used for this exercise were: population data, health data (RTF data by subgroups for year 2006, prior to the implementation of PPS), exposure data (use of safety belt by population subgroups at year 2006 and 2009), and effectiveness (dose response function) of the safety belt in preventing occupant's car from being killed in a road traffic accident (data previously reported). The method used was the one proposed by Chris Schoon, well described by the European Transport Safety Council (ETSC 2010). Two possible scenarios were defined: (1) safety seat belt wearing rate registered in 2006 (pre-PPS policy implementation) for drivers of light vehicles (82 % according to DGT 2009); and (2) the percentage of those wearing seat belts would be improved to the maximum possible rate (99 %). This approach excludes possible interactions with other risk factors and health determinants, so several assumptions were also defined.

According to our calculations, it was estimated that 1,500 (CI: 1,264, 1,770) RTF could have been prevented among drivers of light vehicles in non-urban roads in Spain during 2006 by using properly the safety seat belt (scenario 1). About 333

(CI: 281, 393) more drivers could have survived if 99 % of all drivers would have been wearing a safety seat belt (scenario 2). We have assumed that the accident risk for current non-wearers was the same as for current wearers, and that other risk factors remained equal.

Conclusions

This approach emphasizes that health outcomes can be modified by many different policies at the same time through a variety of health determinants and risk factors. It provides evidence for the policy-making process and encourages the design and introduction of more inter-sectoral and innovative policies, projects or programmes.

A quantitative bottom-up approach is a useful perspective for decision makers to gain deeper insight about the main issues that need to be addressed and prioritized in policy-development.

It is crucial to improve data collection referring to risk factors and social health determinants adjusted to specific scenarios. These data should be publicly available, harmonized and linked within integrated databases, if possible, into information systems.

From Road Traffic Injuries Towards Setting Policy: The German Experience

Introduction

The aim of this analysis is to improve the level of knowledge concerning road traffic injuries (RTI) and crash hotspots in road traffic in order to further develop or improve schemes for reducing traffic accidents and their health implications.

Many different factors influence the volume of traffic, traffic management and road users. The questions of to whom, how, and where traffic crashes happen is important. Furthermore the trends in regional development indicate a strengthening of the suburban settlement structures, which leads to an increasing volume of traffic. Mobility is acquiring an ever higher status both in working life and in leisure activities. The distances travelled between home and the work place are increasing and the proportion of leisure traffic is growing.

Trends in future road traffic volume are dependent on the population development, the settlement structure and mobility behaviour. The shift in age structures indicates a population growth in precisely those groups in which an increase in the traffic volume leads to a rising frequency of traffic crashes. This means particularly young motorists with a newly acquired driving licence and the increasing for a proportion of those in gainful employment (IT.NRW 2010).

Health Outcomes

Road traffic injuries (RTI) refer to road users who are injured or killed in a road crash. These are the health outcomes that we consider in this bottom-up-approach. Road traffic injuries are categorized as fatal (road traffic mortality) and non-fatal injuries (serious and slight injuries). The official statistics provide no deeper categorisation for serious injuries. Such pattern of injuries, e.g. accident trauma or definition of patients, as documented in clinical data provide more details on health consequences of road traffic injuries (RTI).

For this first approach we used road safety statistics which distinguish between crashes, casualties, persons involved and crash causes (DESTATIS 2008). These are basically important for the analysis of the health outcomes and risk factors.

The description of the severity of road traffic injuries and crashes includes three categories:

1. Persons who are injured in a road traffic crash and die within 30 days after the accident are reported as road traffic deaths.
2. Persons who are injured in a road traffic crash and need immediate hospital or inpatient treatment of at least 24 h are classified as seriously injured.
3. Persons who are injured in a road traffic crash but do not need inpatient treatment are classified as slightly injured.

Passengers who are injured or killed in the crash are documented as casualties. The statistics discriminate between casualties with personal injury (seriously, slight and minor injuries) and major crashes with damage to property. According International Classification of Diseases, version 10 (ICD-10) traffic-related injuries and fatalities are coded as V01-V99 (http://apps.who.int/classifications/icd10/browse/2010/en). However, we have to mention that data is most often based on police statistics not taking in account ICD classification.

In Fig. 4.1 the bottom-up risk assessment approach for road traffic injuries is displayed and this is described in detail in the subsequent chapters. The interrelationship between health outcomes (circles), exposure (lozenge shape), risk factors (white), wider health determinants (light grey) and relevant policies, programmes and interventions (grey) is illustrated.

Determinants of Health and Risk Factors

Identification of known risk factors is mostly described within the data relating to the causes of crashes. A distinction is made between general causes, such as road conditions or weather, and person-related incorrect behaviour (such as speeding etc.), which is attributed to the individual driver, passenger or pedestrian, i.e. the road user involved. A total of 89 different cause designations grouped in ten main types of crash causes are listed (DESTATIS 2008). The main causes of all crashes involving personal injury in North Rhein Westfalia (NRW) 2009 were speed with

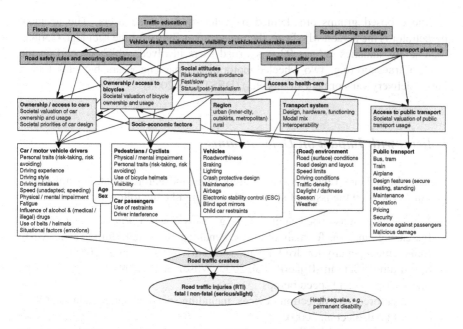

Fig. 4.1 Causal diagram for bottom-up risk assessment of road traffic injuries

22 %, 17 % insufficient safety distance and 15 % failure to give way. In 2009, speeding crashes resulted in 37 % of all road traffic fatalities in NRW (IT.NRW 2010). Another risk factor is the age of road users. Of all age groups, young adults from 18 to 25 years have the highest road traffic crash risk. Alcohol use and failure to adjust speed are the main causes in younger age, while with rising age the failure to yield right of way becomes more important in Germany and NRW.

In the preceding section, risk factors, and proximal determinants of health were discussed. Wider distal determinants of health are introduced in Fig. 4.1 (light grey). Those determinants with impact on risk factors are often interrelated with social status and attitudes in society. These determinants of health are:

– *Ownership or access to cars and bicycles* are influenced by societal valuation of car/bicycles ownership and societal priorities of car/bicycles usage and design.
– *Socioeconomic factors* and social attitudes are determinants that are interrelated to ownership of cars, bicycles as well as the use of public transport.
– *Transport system* with elements such as design, hardware and functioning as well as the modal mix and interoperability between the different modes of transport.
– *Regions* are differentiated into urban and rural regions. Urban regions can be further disaggregated into inner-city, outskirts, and metropolitan area.
– *Access to public transport*: with societal valuation of public transport usage as a key determinant.
– *Access to health-care* may determine the care of persons injured in road traffic crashes and the consequences of the injuries.

The exposed groups are defined by categories of road users. The accident perpetrator is the person who bears the main responsibility for the accident. German road safety statistics defines 93 types road users involved, which depend on the mode of transport (e.g., two-wheeled motor cycles, passenger cars, bicycles, tourist buses, delivery vans or pedestrians etc.) (DESTATIS 2008).

Policies with Impact on Determinants

Among the policies related to road safety rules and enforcement, several policy measures focus on the issue of speed and speeding like the following:

- Nation-wide safety speed campaigns: e.g. "slow down" (*"Runter vom Gas"*).
- Increasing sanctions for main offences: Penalty point system (Pulido et al. 2010).
- Enlargement penalty for drinking and speed driving (Goss et al. 2008).
- Speed limits (Schram-Bijkerk et al. 2009; Wilson et al. 2009).
- Speed displays and speed bumps.
- Speed enforcement detection devices, including speed cameras, radar and laser devices (Wilson et al. 2009).
- Police controls/patrols (Goss et al. 2008).

Speed Limits and Speed Enforcement Detection Devices

Among the multitude of policies to potentially reduce the numbers of injuries due to speeding two policies were selected: speed limits and speed enforcement detection devices (SEDs). The selection was based on following reasoning:

- Speed limits are the core of most speed management policies.
- In road traffic safety, speed enforcement detection devices are rated as an effective speeding control enforcement measure and therefore often implemented.
- It was anticipated that the scientific evidence on the effectiveness of these policies would allow a full-chain modelling of the potential reduction of injuries due to implementation of speed limits and speed enforcement detection devices.

The general speed limit of 50 km/h applies within built-up areas. On arterial roads within urban areas, the speed limit may be raised up to 60 or 70 km/h. According to the location (built-up areas, outside built-up areas and on motorways) the most speeding crashes with personal injury occur on motorways (43 % in NRW 2007) (DESTATIS 2008). In 2006, 57 % of the German motorways were without any speed limit. On motorways and highways outside of towns a recommended speed limit of 130 km/h or 120 km/h applies.

The use of speed enforcement detection devices is essential for the prevention of road injuries and deaths. The aims of speed enforcement detection devices are firstly to reduce all kinds of road traffic injuries and secondly to control speeding. Since 1959 speed cameras are established in Germany. Currently, there are 3,588 fixed speed cameras ("*Starenkästen*") installed in Germany. In North Rhine-Westphalia are 918 fixed speed cameras in use.

Modelling the Reduction of Fatal and Non-Fatal Road Traffic Injuries in NRW Due to Selected Policy Measures

The quantification of the effect of the two policies on road traffic injuries is based on the approach of using "crashes" and "casualties" as dependent variables and "speed" as independent variable. It is predicted that, if the number of speeding drivers is lowered, both the likelihood and severity of a road crash will be reduced (Schram-Bijkerk et al. 2009). Because the higher the speed, the higher the crash risk and the more severe the crash consequences. But the relationship between speed and risk of a crash, of course, is more complex and to quantify this relationship needs different variables.

The reduction of the proportion of speeding vehicles/drivers disregarding the speed limit depends on the speed threshold given and/or on the localisation (settings: urban, rural) and may differ substantially from country to country (WHO 2004a, b). Some studies found that roads with a larger speed variance had a higher crash rate than roads with a smaller speed variance (Aarts and van Schagen 2006).

Speed Limit: Dose-Response Assessment

A review of WHO on the effectiveness of the introduction of speed limits (WHO 2004a, b) shows that only three studies with quantitative "dose-response" relationships are significant for the outcome road traffic injuries. A study in Denmark revealed that the number of traffic fatalities could be reduced by 24 % by an inner-city speed reduction from 60 to 50 km/h (WHO 2004a, b). A lower effectiveness of 6 % was identified in the case of speed limits on country roads in Switzerland (outside built-up areas), compared to urban regions and motorways.

These results were used for a model for the situation in NRW. The road safety statistics provide the number of fatalities which occurred on different type of roads with a speed limit under consideration (Table 4.2). In 2009, nine persons were killed in traffic crashes in built-up areas with speed limit zones of 60 km/h (IT.NRW 2010). The statistics of North Rhine-Westphalia reveal that speeding is the second most frequent crash cause outside built-up areas. These crashes on roads outside built-up areas (country roads) end most frequently in fatalities. For the modelling the focus was on those fatalities which occur within speed limit zones of 130 km/h on motorways. In NRW, three persons were fatally injured despite this speed limit on motorways (Table 4.2).

Table 4.2 Number of fatalities by type of road and speed limit NRW 2009 (IT.NRW 2010, p. 32)

Type of road	Speed limit at crash location (km/h)	Number of fatalities in NRW in 2009
Motorways	130	3
Country roads	100	34
Roads in built-up areas	60	9

Table 4.3 Estimated road traffic mortality avoidable by lowering speed limits

Type of road	Speed limit change from...	Estimated number of prevented fatalities in NRW
Motorways	130–120 km/h	0.3
Country roads	100–80 km/h	2
Roads in built-up areas	60–50 km/h	2

Speed Limit: Estimation of Health Impact

Based on the quantitative relationship between the shift to a lower speed limit, the effect on fatalities and the reported number of fatalities at this speed limit the potential reduction was estimated (Table 4.3).

The lowering of the speed limit from 60 to 50 km/h on roads in built-up areas in NRW would potentially prevent the death of two persons. In 2009, 34 persons died in crashes on country roads in NRW with a prevailing speed limit at crash location of 100 km/h. 6 % of these fatalities might be avoided by lowering the speed limit from 100 to 80 km/h. This would result in two persons less killed due to traffic crashes on these roads per year. In 2009, three persons died in car crashes on NRW motorway-sections with a speed limit of 130 km/h. If this speed limit would be lowered to 120 km/h, according to this model, 12 % of the fatal injuries could be prevented. For the NRW situation this would result on average in 0.3 persons prevented from dying in a car crash on these motorway-sections annually. In other words: the life of one person could be saved every 3 years.

On a large part of NRW motorways, there is no speed limit at all. 47 persons were killed in car crashes on NRW motorway-sections without a speed limit in 2009. Unfortunately, no dose-response function for the situation: no speed limit vs. speed limit could be identified in literature. If the dose-response relationship for lowering the speed limit from 130 to 120 km/h would also be valid for introducing a speed limit of e.g. 130 km/h on motorway sections that had no speed limit before, 12 % of the fatalities could be prevented. For the year 2009 in NRW, this would result in 5–6 lives saved. Only the effects on fatal road traffic injuries could be quantified in this approach. Due to lack on information on the dose-response function of change in speed limit on non-fatal road traffic injuries, the effect of speed limits for these health outcomes are not modelled.

Table 4.4 Potential
effectiveness of speed
enforcement detection
devices (SEDs)
(Wilson et al. 2009)

| | Estimated reduction (%) | |
Outcome	Minimum	Maximum
All road crashes	14	72
Injury crashes	8	46
Fatalities and serious injuries (casualties)	19	31

Speed Control (SEDs): Dose-Response Assessment

A Cochrane systematic review (Wilson et al. 2009) on the effectiveness of speed
control systems shows estimated relative changes (%) in the outcome after intervention. The majority of the studies examined in the Cochrane review consider road
traffic crashes as a target variable, only a few examine the number of those injured
or killed as a target variable. If road traffic crashes are used as a target variable, the
disadvantage is that not all persons involved in a crash are included in the calculations, occupants and passengers are not considered. Since cars are frequently occu-
pied by more than one person, the number of "casualties" in road traffic crashes is
higher than the number of "crashes with personal injury" recorded.

The range of the estimated reduction of all road crashes (also incl. damage to
property) varies between 14 and 72 % (Table 4.4). The effect on crashes with personal injury (those killed and injured) ranges from 8 to 46 % reduction. According
to the review, the number of people seriously injured and killed (fatalities and serious injuries) in road traffic crashes could be reduced by as much as 31 % by deploy-
ing more stationary and mobile speed control systems.

Speed Control (SEDs): Estimation of Health Impact

On NRW roads 561,749 crashes occurred in total in the year 2009. Of those, 63,209
crashes with personal injury are reported, and 14,217 persons died or were seriously
injured. For the calculation of an interval estimate the published minimal and maxi-
mal outcome reduction was used (Table 4.4). In contrast to the health impact quantification of the effect of speed limits, it was not differentiated between various
types of roads, as the evidence on the dose-response relationship is not available for
this differentiation. The wide range of the estimates reflects this situation.

It can be estimated that between 78,645 and 404,459 road crashes on NRW roads
could potentially be avoided by the installation of additional speed control systems
(Table 4.5). As not all road crashes do result in persons injured, this figure is less
informative with regard to the estimation of the health impacts of this measure.
Based on the available evidence on the effect of implementation of speed enforcement devices on fatal and serious injuries, potentially 2,701–4,407 causalities could
be avoided by implementation of these control systems (Table 4.5).

Table 4.5 Estimated impact of implementation of speed enforcement devices in NRW

| | Estimated number of avoidable cases | |
Outcome	Minimum	Maximum
All road crashes	78,645	404,459
Injury crashes	5,057	29,076
Fatalities and serious injuries (casualties)	2,701	4,407

Discussion

In quantifying health impacts the concept of exposure assessment and exposure-response relationship was used. In case of modelling the health impacts of road traffic crashes, the "exposure" concept is harder to apply. Quantitative knowledge of the dose-response relationship of the selected policy measures is rather poor with regard to the considered health outcomes. Most of the studies consider crash with personal injury as target variable. Crashes with personal injury can result in multiple casualties, and no standard default ratio for these casualties can be given. The dose-response relationships based on this target variable are of limited value for quantifying the health impacts. In only a few studies, the number of road traffic injuries is considered. In case of the quantification of the effect of lowering speed limits, only fatal road traffic injuries are investigated in dose-response studies. High quality dose-response study which investigated non-fatal injuries could not be found in literature.

Different findings (WHO 2009; Wilson et al. 2009) show that, if speed cameras are in place, the number of people killed or injured is reduced. Despite the methodological limitations of the studies reviewed, the consistency of reported positive reductions in speed and crash outcomes across all studies suggest that SEDs are a promising intervention (SafetyNet 2009):

- Speed cameras are more effective than physical policing methods (i.e. police spot check on traffic) in reducing speeds and crashes.
- Speed cameras are more effective in reducing crashes within urban areas than on rural roads.
- Fixed speed cameras are more effective in reducing speed and crashes than mobile speed cameras.

The methodological quality of the majority of studies included in the Cochrane review relevant for this analysis was judged as poor by the reviewers. The research outcomes show highly differing results. Varying study designs and variable definitions decrease comparability (SafetyNet 2009; Wilson et al. 2009). Limitations can be summarized as:

- Varying definitions and measures of speed, crashes, injuries and deaths. In some studies, results for "all injury crashes" may include property damage crashes.
- Injury crashes are not always a subset of those which are speed related.

- The type of intervention on speeding varied between studies: overt or covert cameras, fixed or mobile position, or combined; no differentiation of the effects between the different cameras; e.g. no separation of effects of red light versus speed cameras; some studies reviewed the possible difference between the effectiveness of hidden versus visible speed camera different settings: urban, rural, rural or semi-rural, mixed urban-rural, semi-rural.
- Different types of roads: highway, residential road, arterial, trunk.
- Duration of intervention.
- Most studies were conducted some decades ago and may be not appropriate for being applied to the current traffic situation in Europe.

Conclusion

It can be concluded that evidence-based study results on the effect of speed surveillance are rare, although speed control has been in practice for many decades. Modelling has to combine exposure-response relationships and available data. As a result, the quantification of health effects due to the reduction of road traffic injuries and injury crashes range widely.

From COPD Towards Setting Policy: The Slovene Experience

Introduction

Chronic obstructive pulmonary disease (COPD) is one of the largest population health concerns. COPD is common disease affecting 5–10 % of the US population. During the last two decades, death from COPD has continued to increase, especially among women (Eisner et al. 2010). At present it is the third cause of mortality in EU−27 countries (Eurostat 2010a, b) and seventh cause of lost year of life. In review of recent studies, the estimated fraction of COPD mortality attributable to smoking was 54 % for men 30–69 years of age and 52 % for men >70 years of age (Ezzati and Lopez 2003). The corresponding attributable fractions for women were 24 % and 19 %, respectively.

Health Outcome

Chronic obstructive pulmonary disease (COPD) refers to chronic bronchitis and emphysema, a pair of commonly co-existing diseases of the lungs in which the airways become narrowed. This leads to a limitation of the flow of air to and from the lungs causing shortness of breath. In contrast to asthma, the limitation of airflow is poorly reversible and usually gets progressively worse over time. It is a chronic progressive disease leading to complete respiratory and cardiovascular failure. According International Classification of Diseases, version 10 (ICD-10) COPD is classified under code J40-44 and J 47 (http://apps.who.int/classifications/icd10/browse/2010/en).

The treatment at late stages is very difficult (oxygen therapy, removal and transplantation of lungs). The only medical therapy that clearly reduces disease progression and mortality is supplemental oxygen (Nocturnal Oxygen Therapy Trial Group 1980; Anthonisen et al. 1994).

We assume that the numbers in Slovenia are similar to Austria (a doctor diagnosis of COPD was reported by 5.6 % of population), because of traditional and geographical patterns. The prevalence rate is around 5 % among population over 40 years of age (Schirnhofer et al. 2007). 600 (two-thirds were men, one-third women) people died of COPD in 2008, which is equal to 4 % of all deaths that year (Institute of Public Health of the Republic of Slovenia 2008). The number of hospitalizations for COPD was little below 2,100 (1 % out of total hospitalizations) (Institute of Public Health of the Republic of Slovenia 2008); hospitalized patients are mostly population over 15 years of age. Sensitive population groups are smokers, population living in areas with high air pollution and occupationally exposed workers (coal miners, hard-rock miners, tunnel workers, concrete-manufacturing workers) (Eisner et al. 2010). COPD represents enormous financial expense for Europe (38 billion euro in total; 2.7 billion for medication, 2.9 billion for hospital treatment, 28.4 billion for lost working days and 4.7 billion for outpatient services) (EUGLOREH 2007).

COPD continues to be an important cause of morbidity and mortality worldwide (Mannino 2002). In 1990, COPD ranked sixth among all causes of death worldwide, in 2006 ranked already fifth and it is projected to rank third in 2020 (Murray and Lopez 1997).

Determinants of Health and Risk Factors

The fundamental causes of COPD are not completely understood. The strongest risk factors for developing COPD are: exposure to cigarette smoke, exposure to air pollution, exposure to air pollution at work place and genetic risk factors.

Research finds that both the occurrence of the disease and exacerbation of COPD are affected by smoking. The strength of evidence that smoking is a cause of COPD has been growing for more than 40 years and has been extensively reviewed in three US Surgeon General's Reports. There is a consistent exposure-response relationship. Recent evidence confirms that the majority of COPD is attributable to smoking. Smoking is the cause of 85–90 % of all cases of COPD, although some studies report that this number is not higher than 80 %. On average it is estimated that 15–25 % of regular smokers get COPD. Studies of bar and hospitality workers who were heavily exposed to second hand smoking in the workplace indirectly address the issue of second hand smoking as a possible cause of COPD. Other risk factors are exposure to outdoor air pollution, which occurs during the entire lifespan. Strong evidence indicates that daily variation in exposure to outdoor air pollution correlates with acute exacerbations of COPD. Exposure to air pollutants, such as particulate matter, O_3, and NO_2, can produce deleterious effects on the airway: airway oxidative stress, pulmonary and systemic inflammation, reduction in the airway ciliary activity, amplification of viral infections, and increases in bronchial reactivity These mechanisms could produce irreversible loss of pulmonary function over time and COPD. Recent studies show strong dependency on development and exacerbation of COPD. Longitudinal studies of the effects of occupational exposures and COPD have been performed in coal miners, hard-rock miners, tunnel workers and concrete-manufacturing workers. Quantitative pathological assessment of emphysema as an outcome variable has confirmed a relationship between dust exposure and degree of emphysema in several studies of coal and hard-rock miners. Genetic risk factors are also important, but there is limited/suggestive evidence of familial aggregation of pulmonary function among nonsmokers.

In review of recent studies, the estimated fraction of COPD mortality attributable to smoking was 54 % for men 30–69 years of age and 52 % for men >70 years of age (Ezzati and Lopez 2003). The tobacco industry is deliberately targeting women and the youth. The price of tobacco is close to family/partner/friends, with 47 % agreeing that it made them think about quitting. The price of tobacco products is most motivational among 40–54 year olds, those who are self-employed, manual workers and students. Not surprisingly, younger smokers are more influenced by price than older people (15–24 year olds 55 % versus over 55 years 47 %), the unemployed (66 %) more than white collar workers (managers 35 % and other white collar workers 46 %) and those from lower social groups more than those from higher social groups (66 % of groups 1–4 versus 49 % of groups 5–6 and 39 % of groups 7–10) (Eurobarometer 2010). Longitudinal studies of the effects of occupational exposures and COPD have been performed.

The two main identified determinants of health are environment and lifestyle; both of them are closely linked to socioeconomic determinant of health. Price of cigarettes, education, unemployment and income of population are socioeconomic determinants that are having impact on life style (smoking rate). Exposure to air pollution (environmental health determinant) is also influenced by lifestyle and socioeconomic determinants of health. Air pollution exposures may affect people differently depending on education and income—socioeconomic position. The effect of pollution is greater for children of lower socioeconomic status, indicating that pollution is one potential mechanism by which education and income—socioeconomic status affects health (Neidell 2004). Level of air pollution depends on the price of fuel. Urban lower social class households were more likely to be located in areas of poor air quality, mostly because lower property prices and in addition they use cheap fuels (wood, coal) often increasing level of air pollution. Low social class and poor air quality were independently associated with decreased lung function which leads to COPD (Wheeler and Ben-Shlomo 2005).

The main determinant of health that causes exposure to outdoor air pollution is environmental determinant of health. Outdoor air pollution depends on number of reasons such as traffic density, industry, relief, and heating plants. Socioeconomic determinants of health (taxation, price of fuels, income and employment) are influencing environmental determinant of health. Use of cheap fuels—with high polluting potential by people with low income and unemployed has impact on environmental determinant of health-air pollution. There is dependency even within the group of the same determinant (socio—economic determinant); unemployment has impact on income and poor income on use of cheap high polluting fuels. Behavioural and personal determinant is having impact on environmental determinant of health, by different lifestyle. Smoking rate (behavioural determinant) also depends on other determinants of health—socio—economic determinant of health, mostly on price, taxation, education and unemployment. There is also dependency between sub determinants of the group (education has impact on employment and employment on smoking rate).

The main determinant of health that causes exposure to cigarette smoke is behavioural and personal determinant leading to risk of smoking expressed via smoking rate. Smoking rate depends on number of reasons (personal, psychological, lifestyle). Smoking rate also depends on socio—economic determinants of health, mostly on price, taxation and unemployment. From quantification process it was found that price (socio—economic determinant) of cigarettes has impact on smoking rate although very likely not as important one as behavioural and personal determinant do. The determinant—access to goods and public services very likely plays a role in smoking rate, although there was no quantification done. The same goes for environmental determinant of health—indoor air pollution—pollution with second hand cigarette smoke, it is entirely depending on smoking rate. In a case of smoking rate there is connection between determinants, at first sight it looks that the main one is behavioural and personal determinant, the others just having impact on later. Socio—economic determinant and sub determinants of the group are having impact the most obvious is price, but also unemployment and education could have a significant impact. Therefore policies aiming to prevent smoking rate and diseases coming from smoking must be pointed to many directions. The main determinant of health that causes exposure to outdoor air pollution is environmental determinant of health.

Policies Having Impact on Determinants

Many policies having impact on risk factors and determinants of health are leading to protection of population from development of COPD. The most important policies are definitely those that protects people from tobacco smoke such as ban of smoking in public places and policies setting environmental air pollution standards.

There is a number of existing and proposed policies with aim to prevent people from exposure to tobacco smoke and environmental air pollution. Because of comprehensive impact of different determinants of health on risk factors and horizontal interaction between them, there is a need to target all determinants and risk factors what may bring decrease of exposure to tobacco smoke and air pollution.

Conclusions

The aim of study was to see which are the policies, actions, activities and programs that have impact on development of COPD. To identify them a full chain bottom—up assessment was undertaken. COPD represents increased burden of disease in EU, therefore it is important to take any measure on national level to reduce burden of disease. Such aim could be achieved with identification of existing policies and programs, with planned programs and policies and always by implementing them. Usually a lot of policies seem to have no impact on disease occurrence like COPD and people are on general not aware that something completely unrelated at first sight to issue (like tax on gas) is connected with level of air pollution and development of COPD on a long run. COPD is in terms of risk factors quite well defined. There are very clear risk factors (exposure to cigarette smoke and exposure to outdoor air pollution). It looks quite easy what might be done to reduce burden of disease, it is important to reduce exposure to main risk factors. Good identification of health determinants is indeed essential. There are a number of policies, programs, actions and activities that can act on determinants having impact on cigarette smoke exposure and outdoor air pollution exposure. It is important that at the same time we go on with as many measures acting on all relevant determinants. Going just with one (like dramatic rise of price of cigarettes) is not enough and tricky because of some other possible consequences on long run. All the participating stakeholders at meetings and in discussions emphasized education, communication, training and raising public awareness about harmful impact of cigarette smoke and outdoor air pollution.

From Asthma Cases Towards Setting Policy: The Slovak Experience

Introduction

Allergic diseases and asthma are among the most common chronic diseases worldwide. Approximately 300 million people around the world have asthma, and it has become more common in both children and adults globally in recent years. Asthma is still one of the most common causes of absence from school and the workplace (Hruškovič 2004).

Availability of health outcome data for asthma depends on health information systems at national level, which is main source for other higher levels. There is a question, how reliable the data are for public health policies and interventions, because there is still a poor access to data. Global and European level tried to find scientific ways how data could be comparable due different methods of data collection within the countries for the future health impact assessments.

Health Outcome Description

The veritable causes of asthma are still not known. In trying understanding the problem, asthma should be divided into two levels: its initiation and management of asthma (Loddenkemper, 2003).

Asthma is a chronic disease characterized by recurrent attacks of breathlessness and wheezing, which vary in severity and frequency from person to person. Asthma has a relatively low fatality rate compared to other chronic diseases (Hruškovič 2004). According International Classification of Diseases, version 10 (ICD-10) asthma is classified by code J45 (http://apps.who.int/classifications/icd10/browse/2010/en).

Occupational asthma is defined as a disease characterized by variable airflow limitation and/or airway hyper responsiveness due to condition attributable to a particular occupational environment and not to a stimuli encountered outside the workplace (Gergelova, et al. 2008).

In the population of children, the incidence of asthma is greater in boys than in girls, but from puberty girls begin to prevail, what is also typical for the adult population. Studies estimate that 5–18 % of asthma may be attributable to occupational exposure, with one review study suggesting a median value of 15 % for the highest quality studies (WHO, 2002). Around 30 million people in Europe have asthma, and as many as 6 million suffer symptoms which are characterized as severe. Around 1.5 million people in Europe live in fear of dying from an attack (Loddenkemper, 2003). Number of bronchial asthma in Slovakia increased since 2000 in the entire population more than two times, in children almost three times. Asthma morbidity in children up to 18 years recorded in units of clinical immunology and allergology was 5,853 diseases per 100,000 children in 2007 vs. 2,247 per 100,000 children in 2000 (Health statistics year book of the Slovak Republic 2008).

It is necessary to mention financial burden of asthma. The total cost of asthma in Europe is 17.7bn per year, and productivity lost to poor asthma control is estimated at 9.8bn per annum (Loddenkemper, 2003). The cost of asthma treatment is rising annually and in Slovakia this represents up to 68 Mil EUR per year (Košturiak 2008). Asthma is under-diagnosed and under-treated. It creates substantial burden to individuals and families and often restricts individuals' activities for a lifetime.

Estimates have shown that the number of people with asthma could grow to as many as 400–450 million people worldwide by 2025 (Loddenkemper, 2003). Ontario study used population-based personal health data and time series models to describe and forecast the patterns of asthma prevalence and asthma health services use in the province of Ontario, Canada. Based on data from 1996 to 2006, time-series projection estimated the current (2010) prevalence rate of asthma to be 14.10 % and that it would increase to 16.25 % (95 % CI: 16.19, 16.30) by 2020. This translates to a 15.22 % increase from 2010 (To, 2011).

Determinants of Health and Risk Factors

The fundamental causes of asthma are not completely understood. The strongest risk factors for developing asthma are a combination of genetic predisposition with environmental exposure to inhaled substances and particles that may provoke allergic reactions or irritate the airways.

Many environmental risk factors have been associated with asthma development and morbidity, or asthma attacks. Research finds that both the occurrence of the disease and exacerbation of asthma are affected by outdoor air pollutants. The main inhaled substances and particles could be: indoor allergens (for example, house dust mites in bedding, carpets and stuffed furniture, pollution and pet dander), outdoor allergens (such as pollens and molds), tobacco smoke, chemical irritants in the workplace, air pollution. Other triggers can include cold air, extreme emotional arousal such as anger or fear, and physical exercise. Even certain medications can trigger asthma: aspirin and other non-steroid anti-inflammatory drugs, and beta-blockers (which are used to treat high blood pressure, heart conditions and migraine). Urbanization has been associated with an increase in asthma. But the exact nature of this relationship is unclear (Lanea et al. 2006).

Sulphur dioxide, ozone and nitrogen oxides in the external environment are the strongest triggers of asthma; their impact is determined by local climatic and geographical conditions. This is particularly the environment of cities with significant air pollution and with strong car traffic. Diesel particles from the exhaust gases significantly lead to the exacerbation of allergic respiratory diseases and the mechanism of absorption of pollen allergens on its surface with a concomitant increase their allergenic potential (Hruškovič 2004).

When we are talking about exposed groups we should think about two levels—general population and population of employees. Asthma has become more common in both children and adults globally in recent years (Hruškovič 2004). In the population of children, the incidence of asthma is greater in boys than in girls, but from puberty girls begin to prevail, what is also typical for the adult population. The highest reported rates of asthma in occupation were in craft and related occupations, followed by plant and machine operative. The analyses of asthma by industry show rates generally higher in primary and manufacturing industries and much lower in health and social services (Gergelova et al. 2008).

The level of exposure to common risk factors, particularly tobacco smoke, frequent lower respiratory infections during childhood and air pollution (indoor, outdoor, and occupational exposure) are main determinants very often described in literature. There is a need to determine exposure-response functions. In practice, exposure-response functions for air pollution are estimated to be concentration-response functions. These functions specify the risk of a particular health outcome (e.g., asthma attacks, bronchitis, premature mortality) relative to an incremental increase in air pollution exposure, controlling for other known risk factors (Holloway et al. 2005).

The two main identified determinants of health are genetics and environment when we are talking about disease incidence. It is necessary to mention health care as also important determinant of health because of asthma management. Asthma exacerbations and deaths related to asthma could be results of inappropriate asthma management.

Environmental risk factors (indoor, outdoor air pollution) could be also linked with the management of asthma. When the asthma control is optimal, we can expect less sensitivity to the effects of environmental risk factors. Many environmental risk factors have been associated with asthma development and morbidity, or asthma attacks. Research finds that both the occurrence of the disease and exacerbation of asthma are affected by outdoor air pollutants.

Asthma risk factors are very often and significantly described in literature (2,045 findings in PubMed, 7,001 findings in Current Contents Connect, 60,482 findings in Science Direct, 8,680 findings in Web of Science). There are very few publications focused on asthma and risk factors research which has been done in Slovakia (52 findings in PubMed, 10 findings in Current Contents Connect, 12 findings in Web of Science). For the purpose of risk assessment phase in health impact assessment we strongly recommend using review articles. The main affected factors of asthma are genetics potented by outdoor and indoor air pollution. The physical environment is an important determinant of health. In the built environment, factors related to housing, indoor air quality, and the design of communities and transportation systems can significantly influence physical and psychological well-being. Both are very important asthma triggers.

Genetics and physical environment are crucial within the process of initiation of asthma. Asthma as a chronic disease is determined again by environmental determinants, we can observe exacerbations of asthma, worse quality of life, asthma deaths, or asthma hospitalizations. The most important determinants we have identified as environment (air pollution) and health care (management of asthma/asthma control).

Policies Having Impact on Determinants

Karen Lock and Martin McKee have written in 2004: "many new member states are developing more broadly based models of HIA, adopting multisectoral approaches to public health. For example Slovakia has been developing methods for HIA, supported by a range of capacity building activities." In 2010 there are still no visible multisectoral approaches focused on pathways from health outcome to interventions at policy level.

Some environmental groups and community activists have made asthma a key focus, and in several areas, have entered into coalitions with academic research centres, health providers, public health professionals, and even local and state governmental public health agencies. Despite grassroots efforts to highlight environmental factors in asthma, this remains a contentious debate; these disputes are important because they substantially influence public health prevention and government regulation.

The Slovak Government approved the State Health Policy Resolution No. 910 on 8 November 2000. Ministry of Environment has created Environment Strategy for protecting and enhancing the health of citizens SR based on State health Policy. Results are: Strategy documents—Declaration of Ministers and Action Plan for Environment and Health children for Europe (CEHAPE) and updating of Action plan for environment and human health SR for the years 2006–2010 (NEHAP III).

Primary health care policies should be oriented on asthma guidelines implementation in health system. Corticosteroids represent the main therapeutic modality in asthma treatment and their safety has been much more improved during the past decades. Other agents, such as LABA, antileukotrienes, methylxantines or anti-IgE can be combined with corticosteroids. In Slovakia, all of these therapeutic modalities are available, so there are ideal settings for putting guidelines into the clinical practice. Optimal control of asthma is the goal defined in guidelines (Košturiak 2008).

Conclusions

Available data on asthma prevalence in Slovakia are mainly from routine sources of health care data and very few are results of epidemiological studies/surveys focused on asthma. There are no accessible prevalence data. Asthma is a disease, which could be underestimated in the population. Chronicity of this disease could represent problems with health outcome measures. Age specificity and work related specificity could represent problems with data sources (paediatrician's health records vs. physician's health record vs. occupational physician's health records).

Risk assessment is the most important and also most tough part of whole pathway. Assessment should bring evidence as a result of suitable epidemiological approaches, designs. When it is not possible to do own further research within risk assessment, we can use number of publications from electronic information sources allowed assessing risk estimation by using existing epidemiological research.

This writing provides case study on possible risk assessment methodology taking into account whole pathway from health outcome to risk factor, from risk factor to health determinants and from health determinants to policy. It could be the starting point to processes of "healthier" policy choices. It was told by local decision makers in Sydney (Lock and McKee 2005) that it may be helpful for them to provide some of the evidence from health literature as "healthy design" principles that could be incorporated into planning instruments.

In general we can conclude there is not too much available data of asthma disease in Slovakia. There is chance that situation will improve in the future after implementation of the E-health project coordinated by the Ministry of health in the Slovak republic.

This writing describes the findings of the review and outlines options for the future risk appraisal methodology, which must be further discussed and improved. It would be helpful if the writing could leads to the development of planning instruments such as Local Environment Plans, or to the implementation of already developed guidelines for asthma management at national level in the future.

From Liver Cirrhosis Towards Setting a Policy: The Slovak and Hungarian Experience

Introduction

Chronic liver disease and cirrhosis are one of the leading causes of morbidity and mortality in Europe, with especially high burden of disease in Central and Eastern European countries. Liver cirrhosis, an end-result of a wide variety of the liver diseases, is a worldwide health problem and is a complication of many liver diseases that is characterized by abnormal structure and function of the liver. The diseases that lead to cirrhosis do so because they injure and kill liver cells and the inflammation and repair that is associated with the dying liver cells causes scar tissue to form. The main risk factors of liver cirrhosis are preventable, such as chronic hepatitis and excessive alcohol consumption. Its rates have closely followed alcohol consumption level in European countries.

At a global level, alcohol consumption is among the top risk factors for disease and disability. In developed countries, it has been ranked third among the main risk factors, following tobacco use and high blood pressure (International Centre for Alcohol Policies, 2008).

European level policies and strategies, as well as the activity targets of international bodies give a broad framework of alcohol policy development. The need for concerted action at supranational level is, among others, presented by the European Union's Alcohol Harm Reduction Strategy, the Alcohol Policy Framework in the WHO European Region of 2006 or the WHO Global Alcohol Strategy. Several policy interventions directed at the population as a whole have been proven to be effective in reducing the harm done by alcohol consumption. Considering patterns and trends observed in Mediterranean countries, alcohol control in Central and Eastern Europe can lead to an appreciable reduction of premature mortality from cirrhosis (Rehm et al. 2007).

Applicability of different policy options and interventions should be investigated, potential alternatives prioritized and adjusted to national/regional/local health needs and targets, in which health impact and risk assessment methods can play an important role. This case study details a bottom-up (health outcome, risk factors, determinants of health, policy) risk assessment aiming to decrease the burden of chronic liver disease and cirrhosis through adequate policy development.

Health Outcome Description

Liver cirrhosis (K 74 according to the *International Classification of Diseases, 10th Revision* (ICD-10) http://apps.who.int/classifications/icd10/browse/2010/en) is defined as a degenerative disease of the liver in which hepatic tissue is replaced with connective tissue, commonly a result of chronic alcoholism.

Cirrhosis and chronic liver disease are among the leading causes of morbidity and mortality in Europe. Though, the EU as a whole experienced decrease in mortality in the past decades, disease burden due to chronic liver disease and cirrhosis differs widely among countries. Mortality from cirrhosis has been steadily declining in most countries worldwide since the mid or late 1970s. In southern Europe, rates in the early 2000s were less than halved compared to earlier decades. In contrast, since the 1980s a band of countries in south and central Europe from Slovenia and Croatia through Hungary, Romania to the Baltic states have reported a considerable increase in mortality, typically peaking in the mid-1990s (Boseti et al. 2007; Szűcs et al. 2005). While some of these countries returned to pre-transition rates, others such as Hungary remain in unfavourable position. In all countries men experience much higher rates of death than women. In Hungary 85 % of premature deaths from gastrointestinal disease is caused by liver diseases in men. Mortality was peaking in 1994, when death rates from chronic liver disease and cirrhosis in men were more than seven times, while in women six times higher than the EU15 average. Morbidity shows significant differences between regions of Hungary with higher prevalence in rural areas among males. In addition, morbidity monitoring based on a sentinel station program revealed considerable unknown morbidity from chronic liver disease and cirrhosis (Széles et al. 2005).

Premature mortality rates due to liver cirrhosis increased in both genders in Slovakia until 1990 (67/100,000 in men and 16/100,000 in women). After 1990 a dramatic decrease was observed, but after 1996 (33/100,000 in men and 9/100,000 in women) the rates began to increase again. In 2002 the rates averaged 44/100,000 in men and 14/100,000 in women. In both genders the rate was comparable to average of the EU10 countries (42/100,000 and 14/100,000 respectively), but was more than twice the rate in the EU15 countries (17/100,000 and 7/100,000 respectively). In 2002 the ratio of the Slovak and EU15 rates was 2.6 for men and 2.4 for women (Zatoński et al. 2008).

Risk Factors and Determinants of Health

Single or multifactorial insults to the liver ultimately lead to cirrhosis, with the majority of preventable cases attributed to excessive alcohol consumption (60–70 %), chronic hepatitis B and C infection (10 %), and obesity with concomitant non-alcoholic fatty liver disease (steatohepatitis, 10 %) (Heidelbaugh and Bruderly 2006). Other risk factors of chronic liver disease and cirrhosis (aside from hereditary conditions, biliary system and other disorders) include viruses and parasites and chemical exposures including use of certain drugs. Many people with cirrhosis have more than one cause of liver damage. Cirrhosis is not caused by trauma to the liver or other acute, or short-term, causes of damage. Usually years of chronic injury are required to cause cirrhosis (NIDDK 2000).

Risk factors and related health determinants were investigated according to the following categories. For the sake of complexity we review most of risk factors but our case study for bottom-up risk assessment aims to investigate alcohol consumption as the main, modifiable risk factor of chronic liver disease and cirrhosis in detail.

Excessive Alcohol Consumption

Alcohol abuse and dependence continue to be a major health problem all around the world. Although moderate alcohol consumption has some health benefits (WHO 2004a, b) the WHO identified the consumption of alcohol as one of the top-10 risks for worldwide burden of disease. In 2002, more than 1.9 billion adults ($\geq$15 years of age) around the world were estimated to be regular consumers of alcoholic beverages, with an average daily consumption of 13 g of ethanol (about one drink). Most authors agree that an upper limit of 80 g of ethanol per day should not be exceeded. A moderate drinker is considered as one who consumes 5–25 g of ethanol per day and a light drinker as one who consumes 0.2–5 g per day.

Alcohol consumption increases the risk of liver cirrhosis that is the most frequently used indicator of alcohol related harm at the individual level. The dose-response relationship follows an exponential curve, with relatively little risk increase in the low range, and steep rise at large amounts of consumption. At any given level of alcohol intake, women have a higher relative risk of developing liver cirrhosis than men. Women appear to be more vulnerable than men to many adverse consequences of alcohol use. Women achieve higher concentrations of alcohol in the blood and become more impaired than men after drinking equivalent amounts of alcohol. Research also suggests that women are more susceptible than men to alcohol-related organ damage. Compared with men, women develop alcohol-induced liver disease over a shorter period of time and after consuming less alcohol. In addition women are more likely than men to develop alcoholic hepatitis and to die from cirrhosis.

The relationship between alcohol intake and chronic consequences such as liver cirrhosis seems to depend mainly on volume of drinking, though; some evidence also indicates a potential effect of drinking pattern. Average volume of consumption as a risk factor has long-term health effects mainly through biochemical mechanisms or through dependence. Drinking patterns such as intake of alcohol outside mealtimes, consumption of spirits and multiple different beverages are indicated to increase the risk of developing alcohol-induced liver damage. Episodes of clinical intoxication and binge drinking can also facilitate chronic health consequences. Some studies indicated that even moderate drinking may affect the progression of cirrhosis in some individuals, especially in those with underlying liver failure caused by hepatitis infections. Individual sensitivity may also be determined by genetic variances.

Mortality rates from cirrhosis correlate with the level of drinking, often with a time lag. A 1-1 increase in per capita consumption at population level was on average estimated to cause three to four additional cirrhosis deaths per 100,000 for men and one additional death for women (Ramstedt 2007). Higher proportion in total mortality is experienced in young adulthood than is in any other age groups.

The European Union has the highest volume of alcohol consumption in the world with the average level of 11 1 of pure alcohol per adult per year. Within the EU there are significant variations in alcohol consumption levels. Considering also unrecorded consumption — accounting for smuggling, home production and cross border shopping — the highest levels of consumption relate to CEE countries. Regarding the patterns of alcohol consumption, Hungary belongs to Euro C region of the WHO, characterized by high per capita alcohol consumption, dominance of spirits within the total consumption and high percent of heavy drinkers and alcohol-dependent persons. The consumption of unregistered or illegally produced alcohol counts for a considerable part of total consumption in Hungary; estimates vary from 9 to 20–22 % (WHO), latter being more likely (National Addictology Centre 2009). Recorded adult per capita consumption is around 12.3 1 of pure alcohol and has remained stable according to recent trends. Some unrecorded alcohol production is also estimated in the country, adding around 4.0 1 to recorded volumes that puts annual total adult per capita consumption of pure alcohol around 16.3 1 in Hungary (WHO 2009).

Studies suggest that the consumption of unrecorded alcohol means additional risk for the development of alcohol-induced cirrhosis. Increased hepatotoxicity can be due to higher ethanol content and contamination with methanol and other short and branched chain aliphatic alcohols, like isoamyl alcohol. Despite concern about the potential harm to health from drinking unrecorded alcohol, there are only few reliable data about this phenomenon in Europe. Low quality of homemade spirits may explain the rise in mortality from liver disease in Hungary as well as in other CEE countries in the previous decades, which was accompanied by a decreasing tendency in per capita legal alcohol consumption in the same period (Szűcs et al. 2005). Besides chemical contamination, illegally traded alcohol can also pose a health risk due to its lower cost leading to higher consumption volumes.

Alcohol consumption can be influenced by several determinants of health in direct or indirect ways. The volume and pattern of alcohol consumption is associated with *age and gender*. In older age groups, both men and women drank smaller quantities of alcohol and were more likely to stop drinking altogether, but drinking frequencies did not change consistently with age (NIAAA 1998). Men are more likely to drink and drink more than women, though this gender gap is decreasing in many aspects, such as in drunkenness in young adults. Patterns of drinking are influenced by the social context. Research on social determinants of alcohol drinking patterns has emphasized several factors, among them social class and culture of drinking. Alcohol dependency and binge drinking are more characteristic for those with lower SES for both genders (Anderson and Baumberg 2006). Due to the different cultural backgrounds and levels of social development, considerable variations can be experienced in drinking patterns among countries of the EU.

People with low *socioeconomic status* (SES) may exhibit higher alcohol consumption, and as a consequence suffer from worse health in comparison with high SES people. High SES (father's occupation, mother's education, mother's employment status) of a family was connected with healthy habits (concerning smoking, drinking, physical exercise) among Finnish male adolescents (Pietili et al. 1995). The highest occupational group of parents, family type, and type of the adolescent's school were strongly related to smoking, alcohol use, and (lack of) physical exercise among Finnish adolescents (Karvonen and Rimpeli 1996). In the case of drinking, however, the adolescents whose fathers had higher SES used alcohol to a somewhat greater extent than the others did. Prevalence of smoking, episodic heavy drinking, lack of physical exercise and also clustering of health risk behaviour were inversely related to SES based on parent's education and family income among adolescents in the USA (Lowry et al. 1996). Scottish adolescents from lower (non-manual) social class households were most likely to smoke and drink (Green et al. 1991). It has also been consistently found that those with lower socioeconomic status are more likely to abstain from alcohol. Men with less *education* are more likely to be heavy drinkers, in contrast to women. The type of school itself appeared to have a strong effect on the occurrence of smoking, drinking, and drug use among Hungarian adolescents (Piko 2000). The school, its setting, organizational structures, activities and atmosphere may influence health risk behaviour in adolescents. Considerable influence may also be attributed to classrooms, which are important arenas for peer group formation and friendship relations.

Several studies have shown that heavy consumption has a negative impact on *earnings, incomes and wages*, because it reduces individual productivity and may create problems with working arrangements for the employer (Mullahy 1991; Cercone 1994). Using a panel probit model and controlling for gender, age, education, work experience, wage rate and the ownership type of the employing organization, it was found that alcohol has a positive and statistically significant effect on the probability of being fired (Suhrcke et al. 2007).

Chronic Liver Infections (Hepatitis B, Hepatitis C)

Chronic liver infections, such as hepatitis B and particularly hepatitis C, are commonly linked to cirrhosis. People at high risk of contracting hepatitis B include those exposed to the virus through contact with blood and body fluids. This includes healthcare workers and intravenous (IV) drug users.

Recent reports have documented high but heterogeneous HCV prevalence rates among injection drug users (IDU) and other non-IDU groups (Abdala et al 2003; Reshetnikov et al. 2001) suggesting the presence of an ongoing HCV epidemic.

People with lower *educational* attainment have poorer self-reported health, higher rates of infectious disease and shorter life expectancy than the better educated (Feldman et al. 1989; Guralnik et al. 1993).

Corrao et al. (1995) performed a case-control study assessing the interactions between alcohol intake, chronic hepatitis C virus (HCV) infection and *nutrient intake* on the risk of liver cirrhosis. The analysis of principal components showed that a pattern of higher lipid but lower protein and carbohydrate intakes was significantly associated with the risk of cirrhosis and it modifies multiplicatively the risk of cirrhosis associated with alcohol intake and/or chronic HCV infection.

Literature shows that viral hepatitis is still one of the main complications in haemodialysis (HD) patients, with hepatitis C being the most common one (Sun et al 2009).

Obesity with Concomitant Non-Alcoholic Fatty Liver Disease

Obesity is a risk factor in non-alcoholic fatty liver disease (NAFLD) and non-alcoholic steatohepatitis (NASH). NAFLD is now the most common cause of chronic liver disease in the world. 2–3 % of adults in the US have NASH and 20 % of these will develop liver cirrhosis (Metabolic Syndrome Rounds, 2006).

Inverse associations were found between childhood socioeconomic position (SEP) and adulthood obesity in 70 % (14 of 20) of studies in females and 27 % (4 of 15) in males. Childhood socioeconomic disadvantage in developed countries may be important in the development of adulthood obesity, particularly in females. Early childhood is a critical period for the development of food and flavour preferences, as well as the ability to self-regulate food consumption (Ventura et al. 2005).

A recent systematic review demonstrated that positive associations between *adulthood SEP and obesity* typically exist in developed countries, while in developing countries, the associations are generally negative (McLaren 2007). Unhealthy behaviours including unhealthy diets (Kawachi and Berkman 2003; Drewnowski and Specter 2004; Braddon et al. 1988) tend to be higher in adults with low SEP compared with high SEP. These behaviours can be modelled as normative behaviours to offspring (Hanson and Chen 2007).

Exposure to Toxic Substances (Drugs, Toxins, Infections)

Other causes of cirrhosis include drug reactions, prolonged exposure to toxic chemicals, parasitic infections, and repeated bouts of heart failure with liver congestion.

Drug-induced hepatotoxicity is a frequent cause of liver injury (Kaplowitz 2004). The predominant clinical presentation is acute hepatitis and/or cholestasis, although almost any clinical pathological pattern of acute or chronic liver disease can occur. The pathogenesis of drug-induced liver disease usually involves the participation of the parent drug or metabolites that either directly affect the cell biochemistry or elicit an immune response. Each hepatotoxin is associated with a characteristic signature regarding the pattern of injury and latency. However, some drugs may exhibit >1 signature. Susceptibility to drug-induced hepatotoxicity is also influenced by genetic and environmental risk factors.

Inherited Liver Diseases

Liver cirrhosis can also be a result of diseases that run in families (inherited diseases). Cystic fibrosis, Alpha-1 antitrypsin deficiency, Hemochromatosis, Wilson disease, Galactosemia, and Glycogen storage diseases are inherited diseases that interfere with how the liver produces, processes, and stores enzymes, proteins, metals, and other substances the body needs to function properly (Kamath and Piccoli 2003). Especially health workers (doctors, nurses) have a key role in increasing public awareness and educating patients and their families about these condition to enable early detection and effective management in inherited liver diseases. It is important that these patients receive information regarding appropriate dietary management and especially the risks of alcohol misuse.

Quantitative Assessment

The Hungarian case study modelled the exposure change required to achieve the arbitrary target of 20 % reduction in the mortality of chronic liver disease and cirrhosis attributable to alcohol consumption. Frequency measures of the condition were taken from the most reliable sources accessible in Hungary. As all required data were available for 2006, this year was chosen to determine baseline values. Association measures for morbidity and mortality by gender and exposure categories (daily pure alcohol consumption in grams) were acquired from the literature (Rehm et al. 2010). The assessment was based on the calculation of gender specific disease burden measured in attributable death (AD) and disability adjusted life years (DALY). The quantification followed the methodology of the WHO Global burden of disease study, 2004. 3 % discount rate was applied without age-weighting.

Among those consuming alcohol in the Hungarian population, the majority drinks large volumes falling into the highest exposure category used by Rehm et al. (>60 g/day). The modelling found that if these heavy drinkers reduced their consumption to fit the next exposure category (48–60 g/day), the number of cirrhotic death attributable to alcohol consumption would decrease by around 20 %, fulfilling the set target. The same reduction was found in the potential years of life lost, while the number years of life lived with disability almost halved and DALY fell by more than 23 %. In conclusion, in the hypothetic situation if all the drinkers falling into the highest exposure category reduced their consumption volume under 60 g/day, 1,439 lives and over 28,500 DALYs could be saved annually in the Hungarian population of 10 million inhabitants.

Horizontal Interactions

Interactions between alcohol consumption and hepatitis C may be studied at several levels, including epidemiology, virology (including viral load), histology (effect on the severity of liver lesions), carcinogenesis (the role of alcohol in the occurrence of hepatocellular carcinoma), and the effect on the extrahepatic manifestations or severity of HCV infection. At the epidemiological level, a high prevalence of HCV infection was noted in patients with alcoholic liver diseases (14–37 %), also characterized by a high rate of viral replication as detected by PCR, which was present in over 90 % of patients tested (Degos 1999). The effect of moderate (<80 g/day) and heavy (>80 g/day) alcohol intake on the histological and clinical progression of HCV infection and their associated risk of hepatic cancer was investigated in a group of Japanese patients (Khan, 2000). There was no difference in the age, length of exposure to HCV infection and HCV RNA serum levels in the alcohol and alcohol-free groups. Kruskal-Wallis analysis among four groups (based on alcohol consumption pattern) demonstrated a significant transition to fibrosis ($P < 0.05$) for alcoholics with HCV infection. In this study alcohol consumption was considered to be an important risk factor in the histological and clinical progression of HCV infection.

Policies Having Impact on Determinants

Healthy public policies have just recently become a mainstream policy approach for tackling alcohol-related public health problems. Over the past three decades significant efforts have been taken to clarify the relationship between alcohol policies, alcohol consumption and alcohol-related problems and the evidence base on the effectiveness and cost effectiveness of interventions aimed at reducing alcohol-related problems has widened. Effectiveness of alcohol policy interventions can be examined according to the following main categories of interventions.

Policies that Regulate the Alcohol Market

Price and tax policies are regarded among the most effective measures to reduce total alcohol consumption and hence alcohol-related harm, indicating that a rise in price will lead to drop in demand and consumption. Policies that increase prices are especially effective in dropping alcohol consumption among youth, since they are more sensitive to price changes due to their smaller disposable income. Increased prices delay the time when young people start to drink, slow their progression towards drinking larger amounts, and reduce binge drinking. Evidences from economic models have shown that setting a minimum price per gram of alcohol can be as effective as an across-the-board tax increase, with both options increasing the cost to heavy consumers far in excess of the cost to light consumers.

Price and tax policy can only be effective if applying severe regulation methods and sale monopolies. Tax policies should be complemented by different interventions such as limiting unregistered alcohol consumption, measures against illegal alcohol production and sale, directing consumers to lower risk beverages, or by actions against discount pricing practices (happy hours) and minimum price regulations at the on-premise trade (e.g. Apple Juice law) (Koós, 2009).

Addressing the Availability of Alcohol

Substantial evidence is available on the correlation between alcohol availability and consumption. Restricting access to alcohol is one of the oldest measures in response to the harms caused by alcohol. Availability of alcohol can be regulated by limiting the hours and days of sales, and by controlling the density and type of sales locations. Limitations can be extended to different social groups as juveniles. State monopoly and restrictions on retail are considered as effective measures to reduce alcohol consumption and alcohol-related problems.

Limiting Marketing of Alcoholic Beverages

The impact of alcohol advertising on alcohol consumption has been debated for long. Three major categories of alcohol promotion control policies can be distinguished: industry self-regulation, restriction of alcohol advertisements, and social responsibility messaging. The alcohol industry and interest groups usually claim that advertising has an effect only on the proportion of purchase between specific products. In contrast, studies published in recent years indicate an increase in consumption and initiation of consumption at an earlier age due to advertisements. It is therefore not surprising that an effective alcohol policy includes the restriction of the marketing of alcohol as an essential element.

Targeting Illegal Production and Sale

Policies aiming to address unrecorded alcohol consumption include several intersectoral action areas, such as clear definition and control of illicit alcohol, prevention of cross-border traffic, and enforcement of quality and purity standards for non-commercial licit beverages (International Centre for Alcohol Policies 2008).

Besides its direct adverse health effects, illegal alcohol production and the availability of these products undermine the effectiveness of alcohol policy interventions such as taxation, pricing and restriction of availability. For these reasons, regulatory, fiscal and trade measures against illegal production and distribution are among the most efficient alcohol policy intervention instruments and the prerequisites for other policy instruments e.g. pricing and tax policies, as well.

Policies that Support the Reduction of Harm in Drinking and Surrounding Environments

There is growing evidence for the impact of strategies that alter the drinking environment in order to reduce the harm done by alcohol. These strategies are primarily applied to drinking in bars and restaurants, and their effectiveness relies on adequate enforcement (Anderson and Baumberg 2006).

Interventions may include the training of bar personnel for dealing with drunk persons and managing conflicts; active enforcement of alcohol sales laws; enforcement of on-premise regulations; improving public transport, operating party driving services; and providing safer bar environment (Babor et al. 2003).

These interventions can reduce or prevent acute consequences of drinking (violence, injuries and traffic accidents); however, have little effectiveness in tackling the damages related to excessive alcohol consumption. Passing a minimum drinking age law, for instance, will have little effect if it is not backed up with a credible threat to remove the licenses of outlets that repeatedly sell to the under-aged. Such strategies are also more effective when backed up by community-based prevention programs.

Policies that Reduce Drinking and Driving

It is well known that alcohol consumption can reduce driving ability even in small quantities. Legislation along with enforcement can influence the chance of getting caught, the expected severity of punishment and the promptness of the consequences. Policy measures include the reduction of blood alcohol concentration (BAC) limits, setting up sobriety checkpoints, and increased penalties for drink-driving.

The combination of these factors is detectable in the Hungarian drunk-driving legislation. Zero blood alcohol level was specified by law in 2008, focusing on the promptness of consequences. At the same time the n umber of road traffic controls increased, followed by enlarged media attention. The police is entitled to demand the closure of the vehicle and to take the driving licence. The campaign was credited with a significant reduction in the number of accidents and fatalities due to drink-driving.

Policies that Support Education, Communication, Training and Public Awareness

These interventions are, in the traditional sense, integrated into health education and community health promotion program frameworks. Evidence for the effectiveness of direct health education altering alcohol-related behaviours is unclear. However, these programs can be particularly effective if they seek to enforce or complement existing rules and provisions. In this sense, effective community—e.g. workplace— alcohol prevention programs can function in combination with other types of policy measures.

Isolated mass media campaigns may play an essential role in: raising awareness about alcohol-related issues, reinforcing health-related messages or changing social norms regarding alcohol consumption and drink driving (McQueen and Jones 2007). Although there is limited evidence for the impact of warning labels on alcoholic products in reducing the harm done by alcohol, European consumers should receive accurate and consistent information on the potential of the harms done by alcohol (Anderson and Baumberg 2006).

Policies that Support Interventions for Individuals with Hazardous and Harmful Alcohol Consumption and Alcohol Dependence

Health sector's response to the alcohol misuse and problem drinking includes, in particular, short intervention and early treatment of alcohol-related problems and harm reduction interventions that decrease the negative consequences of intoxication. Brief intervention is considered as a highly effective intervention that favourably influences the prevalence of hazardous and harmful drinking and reduces alcohol consumption, mortality, morbidity, alcohol-related injuries, alcohol-related social consequences and the use of health care resources (Kaner et al. 2007).

There is a substantial research literature on policies that are effective in reducing or holding down rates of alcohol-attributable problems. However, relatively few interventions are designed to target social inequities within societies or between societies, and there remains plenty of unexploited terrain for applying existing and evolving evidence-based approaches to groups of low socioeconomic status and the developing world (Schmidt et al. 2010).

In terms of policy responses, evaluations of cost effectiveness of different interventions suggest that taxation, restricted access, and advertising bans are among the most cost-effective policy options. In populations with moderate or high levels of drinking, population-wide measures, such as taxation, represent the most cost-effective interventions, whereas more targeted strategies, such as brief physician advice, roadside breath testing and advertising bans are indicated in case of a lower level of alcohol consumption (Chisholm et al. 2004). National alcohol strategies are recommended to include the combination of the above policy measures.

In Hungary the last two decades of alcohol policy were characterized by several political declarations, and by a lack of implementation, consensus and concerted action at the policy level (Koós 2010). The elaboration of a comprehensive alcohol strategy is still on the way, to which international recommendations and available national examples can offer evidence base.

In Slovakia the focus was on policies within health sector. Slovakia is a country with a plenty of laws, directives, regulations, policies and programs. The following policies in the health sector were identified regarding to selected health outcome, related risk factors and determinants of health:

- National Action Plan on Alcohol Problems.
- Vaccination Program of the Slovak Republic.
- State Health Policy Concept of the Slovak Republic.
- National Program on Health Promotion.
- National Program for Prevention of Cardiovascular Diseases.
- Recovery Nutrition Program of Slovak population.
- National Program on Obesity Prevention.
- National Program on Sport Development.
- National Program of Care for Children and Adolescence.
- Act No 355/2007 on Protection, Support and Development of Public Health (and related regulations and directives and).
- Drug policy of the Slovak Republic.
- Act No 576/2004 on Health Care and Services related to Health care.
- Health Insurance Act No 580/2004.

Conclusions

Relations among determinants of health, risk factors and liver cirrhosis are apparently complex and multilevel. The most important factor is alcohol consumption which is determined by lifestyle. Lifestyle leading to excessive alcohol consumption is also influenced by socioeconomic determinants of health. SES plays an important role in affecting lifestyle. Infection with Hepatitis B and C has also origin partly in life style (sexual behaviour, drug injection) and is again partially influenced by socioeconomic status.

High burden of disease due to chronic liver disease and cirrhosis necessitates public health actions at the level of risk factors. Given that approximately 60–70 % of liver disease is caused by excessive alcohol consumption, the reduction of exposure levels by adequate interventions can significantly reduce the burden of disease.

Prioritization of impact pathways was challenged in several terms in our case. Selection of risk factors and influenced health determinants were limited by our intention to examine potential responses to alcohol-related harm, as well as on the availability of evidence for casualty and feasibility of assessment. Mechanistic models of these associations, toxicological studies and evidence on the impacts and effectiveness of policy measures were needed to quantify necessary changes in exposure levels and determinants. The existence of valid frequency data of chronic liver disease and association measures for the risk assessment were critical. The estimation of potential harm associated with unrecorded alcohol consumption was hampered by the lack of information on the size and composition of the market of illicit alcohol, the demographics of the drinkers, as well as the trends in the consumption. Since applicable numerical results of studies investigating the association between quality of consumed alcoholic drinks and health outcomes are not available, our risk assessment was restricted to the analysis of how reduction of quantity consumed can reach the above aim. Quantification was limited in terms of stratifying data by socioeconomic status, ethnicity or other categories linked to upstream determinants of health, therefore, was not able to provide information on inequalities to support the planning of targeted actions.

Planning and implementation of targeted interventions, however, depends on the availability of a reliable monitoring system and exact data on the alcohol-related harm. This can make it possible to assess the magnitude of the problem, and predict and optimize the impacts of policy alternatives so as to support policy development at different level and sectors of government.

From Osteoporosis Towards Setting Policy: The Danish Experience

Introduction

Osteoporosis is a disease that affects more than 75 million people in Europe, Japan and the USA, and causes more than 2.3 million bone fractures annually in Europe and the USA alone. These fractures typically occur at the hip, vertebral and forearm and the lifetime risk for these fractures have been estimated to be approximately 40 %, similar to that of coronary heart disease. Osteoporosis-related fractures can cause disability, deformity and chronic pain, and influence social activities and the perception of being healthy (Pongchaiyakul et al. 2008). It is estimated that more than 50 % of hip fracture patients over 60 years of age, need more assistance with activities of daily living after fracture, than before. It is further estimated that osteoporosis-related fractures will cause 6.7 % of women to become dependent in basic activities of daily living during their lifetimes (WHO 2003). Prevention of osteoporosis is expected to improve health, quality of life and independence among a growing population of elderly (WHO 2003). The consequences of osteoporosis represent a major public health and financial burden to individuals, societies, and healthcare systems globally. As life expectancy seems to continue to increase, the prevalence of osteoporosis is predicted to increase and thereby also cause an increase in the health and financial burden over the next 50 years. In order to reduce this burden it is necessary to develop effective strategies and interventions, targeting those most at risk for osteoporotic fracture as well as population-based public health interventions to improve bone health in general (WHO 2003).

Health Outcome Description

Osteoporosis is a major public health issue, because of the associated fragility fractures (Winsloe et al. 2009).

Osteoporosis is a disease with the codes M80 (Osteoporosis with pathological fracture), M81 (Osteoporosis without pathological fracture) and M82 (Osteoporosis in diseases classified elsewhere), according to the International Classification of Diseases, 10th Revision (ICD-10, http://apps.who.int/classifications/icd10/browse/2010/en). The definition for osteoporosis is:

[...] A systemic skeletal disease characterized by low bone density and micro architectural deterioration of bone tissue with a consequent increase in bone fragility (Consensus development conference 1991).

Bones consists primarily of four types of cells: Osteoblasts, osteoclasts, osteocytes and lining cells. Osteoblasts are primarily responsibility for bone formation and are more active than osteoclasts in infancy and childhood. Later they can either be incorporated into bone as osteocytes or remain on the surface as lining cells. The process of osteoblasts in shaping the skeleton during growth is called modelling, and slows down during adolescence and comes to a stop at the mid-twenties. Osteoclasts are primarily responsible for bone resorption. The process of resorption combined with the continuous formation of new bone, is called re-modelling. Re-modelling increases at the mid-twenties and can either contribute to maintenance of bone mass or cause a loss of bone mass. Any reduction in the rate of re-modelling can increase the risk of spontaneous fractures. When re-modelling results in bone loss, osteoporosis occurs. More precisely there are three scenarios where this may happen:

1. Osteoclasts may create an excessively deep cavity, which cannot be filled by the action of the osteoblasts.
2. The function of the osteoblasts may be diminished, such that even a normal sized lacuna is not filled.
3. An increased number of osteoclasts can be activated which, when in combination with either of the above mentioned two processes, may result in increased bone loss.

(Pongchaiyakul et al. 2008).

In the adult skeleton, approximately 5–10 % of the existing bone is replaced every year through re-modelling (WHO 2003).

Prevention and treatment can be difficult to separate (Prentice 2004), and there are numerous confirmed and suspected risk factors, which will be further explored later in this text. However, common to all of them is that the frequently assessed health outcome is in fact fracture or BMD, rather than the diagnosis of osteoporosis.

Osteoporosis can be divided into two main categories, primary osteoporosis and secondary osteoporosis. Primary osteoporosis primarily affects postmenopausal women and older men where a secondary cause of osteoporosis cannot be identified. Secondary osteoporosis occurs when an underlying disease, deficiency or drug causes osteoporosis (Kok and Sambrook 2009). For patients with osteoporosis quality life is often assessed by the ability to perform the tasks of daily life, engage in social activities, and function without pain.

In general osteoporosis is three times more common in women than in men (WHO 2003), but osteoporosis in men is an increasing problem. It is expected that one in five men over the age of 50 years will suffer an osteoporotic fracture during their lifetime, and men who sustain fractures have an increased mortality risk. The original World Health Organization criteria for diagnosing osteoporosis is based on women, therefore it has been debated whether these criteria were appropriate for men. It seems that the relationship between BMD and fracture risk is stronger among younger men versus that of older men, compared to women (Khosla 2010).

The onset of substantial bone loss is usually around age 65 years in men and 50 years in women. At age 50 years the lifetime risk of hip fracture in Scandinavian women exceeds 20 %. Based on current mortality in Swedish men and women, the lifetime risk of hip fracture are 8.1 % and 19.5 %, respectively, but is anticipated to rise to 11.1 % and 22.7 %, respectively, if life expectancy does increase as expected. For women aged 65–69 the odds of having osteoporosis seems to be 5.9 fold higher than that of women aged 50–54, and the odds for women aged 75–79 having osteoporosis also compared to women aged 50–54 is 14.3 fold. Early osteoporosis is not usually diagnosed and remains asymptomatic; it does not become clinically evident until fractures occur (WHO 2003).

The Danish population aged 65 or older accounted for 15.9 % of the collective population of Denmark 2009 and is expected to increase to 25.0 % by 2,035. More than half of this population (56.1 %) is women. 6.4 % of the elders in Denmark have at this point in time been diagnosed with osteoporosis (Sundhedsstyrelsen 2010). Within the Danish population of 5,534.738 (assumed unchanged from current population) inhabitants that would indicate an increase of elders aged 65 or older from approximately 880.023–1,383.684, and if the rate of diagnosed cases of osteoporosis remains the same that would further indicate that the number of inhabitants with diagnosed osteoporosis would increase from approximately 56.321–88.555.

Determinants of Health and Risk Factors

Risk factors can be grouped in different ways, but collectively they are mainly either lifestyle related, biological or other.

Lifestyle

Lifestyle risk factors include diet, cigarette smoking, alcohol abuse, physical inactivity and certain medications (Prentice 2004; Pongchaiyakul et al. 2008).

Diet

Among nutritional factors that can cause bone loss there is deficiencies in calcium, vitamin D (Pongchaiyakul et al. 2008; WHO 2003), caffeine intake (Pongchaiyakul et al. 2008), phosphorus, magnesium, flouride (Prentice 2004) and low protein intake (Meunier 1999; Bonjour et al. 1997). The skeleton acts as a reservoir of alkaline salts for maintenance of adequate acid–base homeostasis, and foods such as fruits and vegetables may diminish the demand for skeletal salts to balance acid generated from foods such as meat (Prentice 2004).

Low body weight, particular in connection with anorexia and frailty of old age, is associated with an increased risk of fractures, whereas being overweight is associated with a reduced risk. Lean young people and older men and post-menopausal women who have a lower lean-to-fat ratio are positively related to bone mineral. Interpretations of these data include the osteogenic effects of muscle in younger people, the shock-absorbing effects of adipose tissue in older people, and the possible endogenous production of oestrogens by adipose tissue, which may be important in particular for women after the menopause (Prentice 2004).

Further suspected diet related risk factors include: lactovegetarian-, vegan—or macrobiotic diets, lactose intolerance, body weight and composition, and vegetarianism, but there are no significant evidence that justifies they should be included in a risk assessment (Prentice 2004).

Vitamin D

Vitamin D is associated with a reduction of vertebral fractures and possible also for non-vertebral fractures (Rizer 2006). Vitamin D can be obtained either through diet or through the skin when exposed to sunlight. The efficiency of the conversion of sunlight (UV radiation?) on the skin to vitamin D is reduced with age, skin pigmentation, and potentially with the extensive use of sunscreens applied on the skin. Recently it has been increasingly recognized that vitamin D insufficiency is common in the elderly, and particularly those who are no longer fully independent and therefore less exposed to sunlight. This problem is greater at higher latitudes. In addition, vitamin D insufficiency leads to secondary hyperparathyroidism and consequently to greater bone loss. It also impairs muscle metabolism and may increase the likelihood of falls. Therefore it is important to ensure either that foods are fortified or that foods containing vitamin D3 is consumed (WHO 2003; Compston 2009).

The relative risk of vertebral fractures when adhering to the recommended doses of vitamin D is 0.63 (CI 95 %: 0.45–0.88; $P < 0.01$) (Royal College of Physicians. Fractured Neck of Femur. London: Royal College of Physicians, 1989), but there is no evidence that higher intake further decreases this risk (Prentice 2004).

Calcium

99 % of the body's calcium is located in bone and teeth. The calcium residing in the extracellular compartment (0.1 %) is regulated by a dynamic equilibrium between the levels calcium in the intestine, kidney and bone (WHO 2003). One of the reasons that calcium is considered important is that the intake of calcium has a significant positive impact on BMD, albeit it is a small effect (Prentice 2004). As an

example hip-fractures are strongly associated with BMD, and this type of fractures are further very costly and cause more disability that other types of fractures (Rizer 2006). Calcium intake cannot explain variation in fracture risk on a world-wide basis. Interestingly, those countries with a low calcium intake have the lowest hip fracture incidence, while the highest rates of fracture occur in those populations with a high calcium intake (Prentice 2004). When supplementing with calcium citrate maleate rather than with calcium carbonate there seems to be a more effective change in risk of fracture (Rizer 2006).

Other Nutrients (Protein, Caffeine, Phosphorus, Magnesium, Fluorine)

The recommended dietary allowance of protein in young adults is 0.8 g/kg of body weight, studies in the elderly have shown that, even when healthy, their requirement for protein is modestly increased, and a daily intake of 1 g/kg is recommended. Protein intake is therefore often inadequate in the elderly and protein restriction may be inappropriate (WHO 2003). The long term effect of protein in bone health is debated. Some are concerned that high intake of protein is harmful for long-term bone health, but there is no evidence to that effect (Sebastian et al. 2001; Heaney 2001; Mowe et al. 1994; Larsson et al. 1990). On the other hand elderly patients with osteoporosis admitted to hospital in western countries, are also mainly diagnosed with clinical protein-energy malnutrition and these patients are more likely to fall. Patients admitted to hospital due to hip-fractures, who are given protein supplements, have lower bone loss and shorter hospitalisations. There are no current guidelines on protein intake related to osteoporosis (Prentice 2004).

Caffeine intake has been associated with increased risk of osteoporosis (Pongchaiyakul et al. 2008) but more recent population-based studies do not confirm this (Prentice 2004). Caffeine intake is associated inconsistently with low bone density and fractures (Rizer 2006). Phosphorus is like calcium an essential bone-forming element, and intake according to guidelines is appropriate throughout all life stages. If there is depletion of phosphate bone mineralisation is impaired and it will compromise the osteoblastic function. Regardless there are no studies that use osteoporotic fractures as outcome, and there is no evidence that intake of phosphorus affects the risk of osteoporosis with the exception of very-low-birth weight infants. Conversing there has been raised concerns of an adverse effect in relation to high intake of phosphorus in western-style diets (Prentice 2004). Magnesium is also involved in bone growth and stabilization, but it is unknown, how it affects osteoporotic fractures (Prentice 2004). Fluoride can stimulate osteoblastic activity and inhibit bone crystal dissolution and thereby increase BMD, however high intake of fluoride is known to cause fluorosis that further cause joint stiffness, limb deformities and staining of the teeth (Prentice 2004). Further vitamins and minerals that may be important for bone health are: zinc, copper, manganese, boron, vitamin A, vitamin C, vitamin K, the B-vitamins, potassium and sodium. However there, evidence is mostly lacking (Prentice 2004).

Smoking and Alcohol

Smoking and excessive drinking has been associated with osteoporosis (Pongchaiyakul et al. 2008). Studies of smoking and bone density indicate that postmenopausal bone loss is greater in current smokers than in nonsmokers and that the risk for hip fracture was higher for thinner smokers than for normal or overweight smokers (Rizer 2006).

Excessive alcohol consumption is associated with decreased BMD and moderately increased fracture risk, and alcoholism is a major risk factor for osteoporosis (Prentice 2004). There is no consistent evidence, however, that moderate alcohol consumption is detrimental and there are some studies that suggest that it may be protective in post-menopausal women. Alcohol use is thereby an inconsistent predictor of bone mass and fractures (Rizer 2006).

Physical Activity

Low levels of physical activity is also associated with risk of fractures (Pongchaiyakul et al. 2008) and moderate physical activity should be encouraged throughout life, but should be particularly emphasized during childhood and adolescence (WHO 2003). Improvements in muscle strength or balance may decrease fracture risk but that is not attributed with change in BMC or BMD (Prentice 2004).

Biological Risk Factors

Gender and age are two major risk factors for osteoporosis and risk of fracture as is family history or genetics (Prentice 2004; Pongchaiyakul et al. 2008).

Major determinants of osteoporotic fracture risk in later life also include peak bone mass, reached in adulthood (Winsloe et al. 2009; Prentice 2004) and the rate of subsequent bone loss (Prentice 2004) Skeletal factors not associated with BMD include skeletal geometry, turnover, trabecular connectedness, osteocyte viability and osteonal distribution. These factors are due to family history and genetics and may be influencing risk of fracture (Prentice 2004). Genetic or inherited factors are suggested to account op to 50 % or more of the variance in BMD and BMC values in the population (WHO 2003). However the severity of bone loss due to immobilization is much greater than that for postmenopausal osteoporosis. Fracture rates are substantially higher. Several studies have reported incidence rates from 4 to −34 % (Kok and Sambrook 2009).

Race has also been identified as a risk factor however it is not fully understood yet how it is related. Caucasian women living in temperate climates have higher hip-fracture rates than women from Mediterranean and Asian countries and women from Africa have the lowest hip-fracture rates. Some countries like Hong Kong however seem to be facing a significant increases in age-adjusted fracture rates in recent decades whereas the same fracture rates in Western countries seems to be more stable (Prentice 2004). The significant geographical variation in fracture incidence is largely unknown, but theories including effects at the genetic, anatomical, biochemical, nutritional and lifestyle level. The only element that seems to be sure is that the variation is not due to differences in the deterioration of bone mineral mass, and that bone loss at the menopause and low bone mineral status in old age, seem to be a universal phenomenon (Prentice 2004).

The outcome of gender, age, family history/gender, and race as risk factors is fairly certain but it can be predicted and the effects can be moderated. BMD is accepted as a risk factor for fractures, however in contrast to gender, age, family history and race it is possible to affect directly.

Other Risk Factors

Aromatase inhibitors and Gonadotropin-releasing hormone (GnRH) agonists are commonly used to treat hormone-dependent cancers, for example, prostate and breast cancers are associated with negative effects on BMD and risk of fractures (Kok and Sambrook 2009).

Rheumatic diseases are amongst the most common causes of secondary osteoporosis and rheumatoid arthritis and ankylosing spondylitis, are associated with excess fracture risk. The most common drugs causing secondary osteoporosis are glucocorticoids, AIs and GnRH agonists (Kok and Sambrook 2009).

Depression is a common problem in older people, is more likely to manifest as reduced appetite and weight loss in the elderly than in younger adults and is an important cause of weight loss and under nutrition in this group, accounting for up to 30–36 % of the total in medical outpatients and nursing home residents. Under nutrition may worsen depression. Treatment of depression is effective in producing weight gain and improving other nutritional indices (McPhee and Chapman 2007). In Denmark 56.3 % of the elder reports to being psychologically well (Sundhedsstyrelsen 2010).

Apparently all major determinants of health categories according to Lalonde model of health are involved and above enlisted risk factors could well be regrouped according to interest of a policy or risk assessors. Environmental determinants are crucial and do influence physical activity, nutrition, smoking, vitamin D intake as well as pre-condition of falls (if we consider osteoporosis together with falls as health effect). Social and economic determinants via education do influence ability of people to get and understand lifestyle oriented messages, improve health literacy and moreover, they do influence access to health education and health services. Behavioural determinants are a key group for individual behaviour and lifestyle habits; what do we eat, how we move, smoking and alcohol-related choices although influenced by social and environmental conditions but they are still largely individual choices. The individual biological determinants consisting of age and sex are very relevant for case of osteoporosis as well, yet likely not that relevant for risk policy risk assessment as they are not subject of policies mostly. As last group among determinants according Lalonde, by intention we discuss health care as a determinant of health. Apparently, the issue of definition of osteoporosis the issue of osteoporosis and fractures as health effect, many risk factors linked to health education and literacy, screening-related issues compliance with diet, physical activity, vitamin and calcium subsidization preventive therapies and recommendations makes health care as the most important determinants to a full chain risk assessment.

Policies Having Impact on Determinants

A variety of strategies to encourage better adherence to osteoporosis therapies have been proposed, and some have been researched (Gold and Silverman 2006).

To impact adherence, physicians must form a partnership with their patients. Communication and trust between the physician and patient are crucial. The patient must understand the problems presented by impending bone loss and appreciate his or her personal involvement in the solution. Information exchange should occur at the point of service. The physician must interact effectively with patients and make accommodations for their life styles and needs as part of choosing the optimal osteoporosis therapy (Gold and Silverman 2006; Compston 2009).

There is a need, therefore, to develop effective strategies and interventions that will reduce the fracture risk associated with this condition, particularly among the elderly, who are at increased risk for both developing osteoporosis and falling. These strategies include better systems to identify individuals at risk, as well as therapeutic interventions to prevent or treat the progressive loss of bone mass and the accompanying alteration of bone microarchitecture, thereby reducing the incidence of fracture, the accompanying negative effects on individuals, and the rising healthcare burden (Siris et al. 2009). The daily intake of 400–800 IU of vitamin D is a straightforward, safe and inexpensive means of prevention (WHO 2003).

No study has evaluated the effect of screening in reducing fractures in this younger population. Although several studies have tested screening tools, the Osteoporosis Society of Canada recommends targeted case finding strategies for those at increased risk, using at least one major or two minor risk factors (Box 1), along with BMD measurement with central dual-energy x-ray absorptiometry (DEXA) at age 65 years [13] (Rizer 2006).

To reduce risk of fall accidents it is recommended to develop a fall preventive policy and action plan with clear procedures for the municipalities. Furthermore it is recommended that procedures are drawn up for early tracing of elderly at risk (Sund By Netværket 2010).

According to the Danish National Prevention Committee 72 % of the Danish population wants the public sector to claim responsibility for health, and is willing to accept measures including bans, and punishments when it comes to changing the habits among children and adolescents (Det Nationale Forebyggelesråd 2010).

Conclusions

Osteoporosis is a global problem with several individual, societal and financial adverse effects. Several determinants of health are linked to the changeable risk factors and further there are policy options that can affect these determinants. However osteoporosis is an asymptomatic disease (WHO 2003) and therefore often diagnosed to late leaving the primary options for intervention treatment and fall prevention of which compliance is a major problem.

Life Expectancy in Aspect of Main Health Risks and Policies; Experience of Poland

Introduction

Life expectancy at birth in Poland has been changing constantly, through '1950–1980s there were also episodes of small decrease in the life expectancy what was different from high developed countries. In the beginning of 1990's.life expectancy for newborns in Poland was on low rate comparing to Western European countries. The political transformation in 1989, the brand new challenge for the Polish society, brought health and socioeconomic threats, what in the beginning resulted in decrease of life expectancy at birth. In 1990 it was: 66.24 years for men and 75.24 years for women, in 1991: 65.88 for men and 75.06 for women (MSO 2010). The level for EU-15 in 1990 was 72.8 years for men and 79.4 years for women, so it was longer: 6.56 years for men and 4.34 for women (Eurostat 2010a, b).

Availability of health outcome data for life expectancy depends on health information systems at national level, which is main source for other higher levels. There is a question, how reliable the data are for public health policies and interventions, because there is still knowledge and methodology gap.

Health Outcome

Life expectancy is defined as the average number of years a person can expect to live if in future if current age-specific mortality rates in the population persists. Life expectancy at birth takes into account the complete mortality level of population; it sums up the mortality pattern that prevails across all age groups (WHO 2010). Life expectancy at birth is considered the best mortality-based summary indicator of the health status of the population (Murray et al. 2002). It is also useful for measuring long-term health changes (Zatoński et al. 2008).

Newborn mortality and cardiovascular diseases mortality are the most frequent causes of mortality which determine life-expectancy. In 1990 Poland had one of the highest newborn mortality rates in Europe (19.3/1,000) comparing to other post-communist countries: Czech Republic 10.8/1,000, Hungary 14.8/1,000 and Western European countries: France 7.3/1,000, Germany 7.0/1,000, Great Britain 7.9/1,000. In 2005 infant mortality rate in Poland was 6.4/1,000; comparing to Czech Republic 3.4/1,000, Hungary 6.2/1,000, France 3.8/1,000, Germany 3.9/1,000, United Kingdom 5.1/1,000 (Eurostat 2010a, b). There has been a constant decrease of infant mortality rate over past decade due to better effectiveness of health care system (particularly by introducing more newborn intensive care units), prenatal care (especially for women from households with lower incomes) and better equipped paediatric hospitals.

Another important factor which influences life expectancy is cardiovascular disease mortality. In majority of high developed countries cardiovascular death rate has been decreasing since '1970s. At the same period CVD mortality had a dramatic steady increase in Poland until 1991. In the beginning of 1990s CVD mortality in Poland was among the highest in Europe, both for men and women. Since 1991 there has been observed significant decline in cardiovascular mortality and during next 10 years it decreased in the young and middle aged population (aged 20–64) by 40 %. The decline was three times bigger in Polish women than in the EU15 and two times bigger in Polish men than in the EU15 in this period (Zatoński et al. 2008). In this case study authors concentrate their attention on the reasons of CVD mortality decrease as a main factor connected with life expectancy prolongation.

Life expectancy value in Poland has started to increase constantly since 1993 and after the almost last two decades it was estimated on level of 71.53 years for men and 80.05 years for women in 2010 (MSO 2010). Various recent researches show that increases in life expectancy were mainly achieved by reductions in cardiovascular diseases mortality and in infant mortality (Yang et al 2010).

Determinants of Health and Risk Factors

People's health is influenced and determined by the surrounding environment both, in place of living and working area. Lalonde describes human life and health as related with lifestyle in 50 %, genetics in 20 %, and environmental factors in 20 % and health care activity in 10 %. Dahlgren and Whitehead model includes the following factors: general socioeconomic, cultural and environmental, living and working conditions, social and community factors and individual lifestyle factors.

Life expectancy indicator in Poland was different regarding rural and urban population. For instance in 2007 females in urban areas lived 8.2 years longer than males (in 1990 it was—8.75) while in rural areas the difference was 9.7 years (in 1990–9.5) (Wojtyniak and Goryński 2008).

According to the WHO Global Health Risk report, eight risk factors: alcohol and tobacco use, hypertension, high BMI, high level of cholesterol, high blood glucose level, low fruit and vegetable consumption, and lack of physical activity account for 61 % of cardiovascular deaths reasons and WHO estimated that reducing exposure to these eight risk factors would increase global life expectancy by almost 5 years (WHO 2009). People's lifestyle strongly influences health, quality of life and longevity. Among basic lifestyle factors there are: diet, physical activity, and tobacco and alcohol consumption.

Diet

Economic conditions result in a different diet quality which contributes to health status. The economic transformation changed diet of Polish population, what especially concerned: sugar products, fruits and its products, meat and fish products, fats. There was a significant change in access to these products comparing to the decade of '1990s. Fruits consumption and vegetables has increased since 1991. Poultry became more popular than red meat. Plant fat consumption doubled in the period of 1989–2004, animal fat consumption level decreased about 50 % in this period of time. Additionally there was an increase in vegetable oil consumption in the same period, in particular in rapeseed and soybean oils which became the most common oils in the beginning of '1920 (Czapiński and Panek 2009).

Physical Activity

Physical activity positively influences health conditions. Physical activity of Polish citizens has also changed and now is close to European Union average, although 2/3 of adult men and women don't achieve adequate, recommended by experts level of physical activity (Drygas et al. 2005).

Smoking

In the beginning of 1980s Poland belonged to the group of countries with the highest tobacco consumption in the world. In 1982, at the peak of smoking prevalence, about 68 % of men and 34 % of women aged 20–64 years smoked, and for that time tobacco consumption has been constantly decreasing, this favourable change has improved health indices such as infant mortality and life expectancy and now tobacco consumption for the entire Polish population remains now on level 27.8 % (2009) comparing to 37.9 % (1995), 32.3 % (2000), 30.7 % (2003), 29.3 % (2005), 29.6 % (2007) (Zatoński et al. 2008).

Alcohol Consumption

As regards alcohol consumption historically Poland was a spirits drinking country. At the beginning of the '1980s vodka constituted 70 % of the alcohol consumed.

Since the beginning of '1990s a decreasing share of spirits and an increasing share of beer were observed. In the beginning of twenty-first century beer constituted 55 % of total alcohol consumption, spirits 26 % and wine 19 % (Zatoński et al. 2008).

Socioeconomic Background

The temporal decrease of life expectancy value in Poland in period of 1990–1992 could have been influenced by rapid economic, social, cultural and other changes, which affected the majority of Polish population. Unemployment, high-increasing inflation rate, inadequate salaries were brand new phenomena. *Unemployment rate grew up from 6.5 % in 1990 to 14.9 % in 1995* (*Szczapa* 2009). During last decade the unemployment rate in Poland decreased significantly and majority of the socio-economic factors in Poland have become closer to European average.

Health Care System: Access to Public Services

Strong primary care was one of the main aims of health care changes and reforms after 1989 to eliminate the existing differences in health status between Poland and Western Europe. Introduction of Universal Health Insurance Act in 1999 (Ministry of Health 2010) finally changed the health care financing model, from budget system to insurance one. Non-integrated primary care based on four specialists: paediatrician, gynaecologist, dentist, internist was replaced by general practitioners. Introducing medical specialization in the field of family medicine finished historical undervaluation of primary care in Poland. General practitioners became active in the area of health promotion.

Invasive Cardiology in Poland

It was observed stable increase in access to modern treatment procedures in Poland. The invasive cardiology significantly developed in Poland during last decades. Angioplasty in Polish cardiologic centres was introduced at the beginning of '1980s. The number of 1,000 angioplasties per year was achieved in 1989 and in 1997 it reached 5,000. The vital moment for invasive cardiology in Poland was 1999 (after introducing Universal Health Insurance Act). In 1999 total number of coronarographic procedures grew up for 31.8 % and angioplastic procedures for 32.8 % comparing to 1998 (Gil et al. 2003). There is still a significant progress in increasing number of new cardiologic centres and invasive procedures in Poland.

Exposed Group

The case is looking the total population, with emphasize on population being subjects for risk factors for cardiovascular diseases which are the most important cause of mortality. There are other causes of mortality as well which could be looked (e.g. cancer).

Determinants of Health Having Impact on Risk Factors

The two main identified determinants of health are socioeconomic and lifestyle. The first one having impact on employment rate and the second one is connected to most important risk factors such as smoking, alcohol consumption and unhealthy diet. It is important to consider also the possibility of access to health services, which can prevent worsening of diseases and prolong life-expectancy. Cardiovascular death is also result of inappropriate and late management of diseases.

Horizontal Interaction

Socioeconomic determinant of health, such as unemployment is having impact on lifestyle and also on access to health services. Well-being of nation, good education and employment which are the main socioeconomic determinants of health are having practically the most important impact on other determinants.

Policies Having Impact on Determinants

Health care, including public health and social care, is organized and financed on central, regional and local level. Ministry of Health is the main institution responsible for health policy. Some aspects of health care system are also coordinated by Ministry of Labour and Social Policy, Ministry of National Defence and Ministry of Interior and Administration. Other institutions playing key role in health care policy on central level are: National Institute of Public Health-National Institute of Hygiene, National Food and Nutrition Institute, Institute of Occupational Medicine, Chief Sanitary Inspectorate and others. National Health Fund is the only public provider of health care procedures in Poland and plays a significant role in health care financing and administration. Regional government offices manage health policy on regional level. Municipalities are also responsible for health policy and social care.

Health Promotion Programs

Poor health outcomes of Polish population at the beginning of '1990s provoked implementation of various health promotion programmes and increased public health activity in Poland. In 1995, National Health Programme 1996–2005 was approved. It consisted of multiple national and regional range sub-programmes, which constantly and permanently were to enhance the health status of Polish population. Among the main targets the following two were mentioned:

- Increasing the physical activity of Polish society, as lack of physical activity combined with negative food patterns and unawareness of nutrition value of products resulted in the higher mortality rate for both cardiovascular and digestive system diseases.

- Reducing the tobacco and alcohol consumption, thus the high tobacco consumption and negative structure of alcohol consumption were characteristic for the majority of post-communist societies at the beginning of '1990s (Ministry of Health 2010). The second National Health Programme was established on years: 2007–2015. The first strategic goal concerns decreasing incidence proportion and premature death from cardiovascular diseases (cerebro-vascular accidents included). Operational targets concern health determinants such as: low tobacco and alcohol consumption combined with reducing negative health effects of alcohol, fighting obesity, increasing nutrition of the population and food quality, physical activity, reducing psychoactive substances consumption and number of risk factors in living and working environment and their health effects (Ministry of Health 2010).

Summary of Polices

The main goal of National Programme for Cardiovascular Diseases Treatment and Prophylaxis (Polkard—the first edition) 2003–2005 was to keep on cardiovascular death rate reduction in Poland (observed in the period of '1990s and later). According to specialists this reduction was achieved by actions started by National Programme of Heart Protection (1993–2001) and positive lifestyle and nutrition changes of Polish society. The main goal of the second edition of Polkard programme 2006–2008 was to maintain the cardiovascular diseases death rate achieved in period 1990–2004, to achieve 3 % decrease of this death rate every year for the 10 years period 2003–2012. Among main POLKARD targets the following were mentioned: cholesterol level reduction below 5 mmol/l, blood tension level of population above 65 years old—below 140/90 mmHg, reducing tobacco consumption level 1 % per year, social access to health promotion activities and health prevention activities (based on EBM) with special focus on such health problems like: obesity, type 2 diabetes, heart inefficiency. The above mentioned goals were supported with needs of health education (particularly among children and adolescents), better equipped cardiologic and cardiosurgery centres, access to cardiovascular procedures in Poland similar to European standards, introduction of modern and safe medical technologies with prophylaxis interventions, diagnostics and treatment. As to next targets of programme the following were mentioned: necessity of integrated and complex database collection and frequent epidemiological monitoring, increase of the efforts for identifying new health risk factors and identifying social risk factors affecting cardiovascular diseases. Development of the cardiovascular indicators had to be combined with similar development of neurological medical centres, especially to decrease number of cerebro-vascular accidents and better reconvalescence (POLKARD 2010).

There were two vital programmes financed by National Health Fund concerning cardiovascular diseases prevention (NHF 2010):

- National Programme for Preventing Overweight, Obesity and Chronic Non-communicable Diseases by Increasing Nutrition Quality and Physical Activity 2007–2011 (Ministry of Health 2010) was introduced to establish early prevention of overweight and obesity in order to reduce incidence proportion on chronic diseases and to reduce health care expenditures and premature death.

- National Programme for Prophylaxis and Solving Alcohol Problems 2006–2010, established by Ministry of Health was the response to the increasing role of social degradation as an effect of alcohol abuse. It consisted of three administrative levels: local programmes for alcohol prophylaxis and solution for alcohol problems (implemented by municipalities and local governments followed by the local decision makers), regional programmes for alcohol prophylaxis and solution for alcohol problems (implemented on the regional levels), national programmes for alcohol prophylaxis and solution for alcohol problems (implemented by governmental institutions and central agendas) (Ministry of Health 2010).

Legal Acts

Physical Activity

The Act on Physical Culture of 18 January 1996 described physical culture and physical activity as a part of national culture and underlines its law protection. The Act defined activity of Central and Local governments, non-public associations and other organizations in aspect of physical culture, sport and rehabilitation (Ministry of Health 2010). The Act on Physical Culture was amended by The Act on Sport of 25 June 2010 (Ministry of Health 2010).

Alcohol Consumption

Due to Act on Upbringing in Abstinence and Prevention of Alcoholism of 26 October 1982, amended in 2002, life in abstinence was acknowledged as necessary factor to achieve moral and material wellness of the nation. Local authorities were obliged to take actions which effect in reducing alcohol consumption and changing alcohol consumption patterns. Supporting of NGOs activity and employing establishments was underlined as the one of the main duties of central and local authorities (Ministry of Health 2010).

Smoking

Poland was the first Eastern European country which introduced a comprehensive tobacco control program in 1995. According to new anti-tobacco law (accepted on 8 April 2010 as amendment of The Act on Health Protection Against Tobacco Products of 9 November 1995 r.) it is forbidden to smoke in public indoor spaces. Advertisement and tobacco companies sponsoring are also limited (Ministry of Health 2010).

Conclusion

Our findings suggest tremendous impact of the policy on chosen risk factors reduction, like tobacco and alcohol consumption or diet in CVD mortality decrease, what directly provide to the life expectancy prolongation. The bottom–up policy risk assessment approach seems to be a useful methodology to identify challenges involved in analyze of risk factors reduction policies and in assessing how the related health indicators have changed over time.

Since 1990 almost all health indicators in Poland have improved. The most important change in health status was a significant and steady decline of mortality from cardiovascular diseases. Effective public health policy needs translating scientific research into policy and practice. Bottom-up case study template can be one of the focal tools in this process.

Methodological Guidelines Bottom-Up Guidance

Guidance for the bottom-up approach of identifying policies having impact on health outcome in an integrated manner was elaborated based on presented national case studies. The process of identification of policies requires analysis of the health outcome, to identification and description of relevant risk factors and identification and description of relevant determinants of health linked to risk factors. Finally, policies related to selected determinants of health are identified and assessed.

At each level published scientific evidence needs to be used to identify links and epidemiological information to assess the relations. A strong focus needs to be on use of quantitative risk assessment techniques at various stages (Ádám et al. 2013), integration of quantitative and qualitative assessment elements in specified pathways, evaluation of horizontal interactions between elements of the same impact level, and characterization of uncertainties.

The consensual recommendations are presented as guidance by the levels of the full impact chain, followed by common, cross-cutting issues. The tool is intended to be used for the identification of policies having impact on various health outcomes and by doing so helping public health experts and advocates to place concrete health issue on agenda of all sectors of the society.

Health Outcomes

Health outcomes are the starting point of the impact chain to the identification of policies having impact on them via causally related risk factors and associated determinants of health.

They must be clearly defined, since various stages of a pathomechanism can be considered as outcomes, like a disease or health stages and events related to a disease. A definite solution for clarification is the application of ICD codes. When characterizing health outcomes according to their importance in the assessment, strength of evidence for causality, as well as the condition's severity (related morbidity, disability and mortality), reversibility and frequency of its occurrence in the population—in short, its public health importance—should be taken into consideration.

Health outcomes can be assessed in a qualitative or, if feasible, in a quantitative way. Qualitatively the direction of effect can be stated or the size of effect can be categorically described. However, a critical issue in the assessment of health outcomes is the possibility of quantification. Quantification needs a decision on what kind of health measures (i.e. epidemiological frequency measures), to use as input and output data of the calculation process. In addition, consideration of availability of valid baseline frequency data of the health condition, as well as that of dose/exposure-response functions applying dose-response coefficients or relative risks is indispensable for the success. Values of frequency measures of health conditions and of exposures must be available for the affected population. They usually derive from routine statistics, population-based registries or from surveys. Availability and validity of data is crucial in the process and therefore should be clearly described. The result of quantification can be a frequency measure, like frequency of occurrence, morbidity, hospitalization, mortality, or favourably a complex measure of disease burden, like attributable deaths, potential years of life lost or disability adjusted life years. The latter is an advantageous choice for expressing results of a risk assessment in a quantitative way, since it is a complex measure of disease burden combining effect on both morbidity and mortality.

Risk Factors

This level of assessment process aims to enlist known risk factors and if feasible describe quantified relation of risk factors and level of established causality for population of interest. Risk factors are those factors of the impact chain that directly affect health. Risk factors are defined according to the Health Promotion Glossary of WHO as "social, economic or biological status, behaviours or environments which are associated with or cause increased susceptibility to a specific disease, ill health, or injury" (WHO 1988). However, one has to be aware that a risk factor could also be a protective factor having a positive effect on health.

The prevalence or level of their contact with individuals is referred to as exposure. It is imperative to make a distinction between the risk factors acting in the impact chain and the risk factors modifying individual susceptibility. The latter is to be considered when identifying susceptible subgroups of the affected population. To be able to assess the possible health outcomes of the selected causal pathways, thorough review and enlistment of all influenced risk factors is indispensable. The exposed population, the routes of exposure and the exposure pattern in different population groups should be described.

Because of their possible high number risk factors should be prioritized with aim to tackle the most important ones. The process of prioritization should take into account strength of evidence for causality considering reliability of literature source and biological plausibility as well as significance of induced health effects that is determined by the size of exposure change influenced by the policy, size of population affected and severity of related health outcomes.

Since the extent of being exposed to risk factors may be characterized not only qualitatively but measured in a quantitative way, an important consideration of selection for detailed analysis is the feasibility of numerical explanation. The quantification of exposure change due to policy implementation is based on the availability of applicable exposure measures and numerical information on the baseline level/prevalence of exposure, as well as on the expected change of exposure related to policy implementation (exposure assessment).

The demand for quantification depends on the interest of policy-makers and other stakeholders. Since the quantitative assessment of health outcome is the final goal, it is worth to consider the availability of valid data and dose/exposure-response coefficients for health outcome assessment already in the selection process of risk factors, making internal loops of consideration between any levels of the causal chain.

Health Determinants

This level aims to systematize knowledge on the relation between wider determinants of health and risk factors that are likely to be influenced by the policy level. In some cases, determinants of health might overlap with risk factors. Determinants of health are defined by the Health promotion glossary of WHO as "the range of personal, social, economic and environmental factors which determine the health status of individuals or populations" (WHO 1988). Determinants of health are factors which influence occurrence of risk factors.

Those factors that are considered as the determinants—or wider determinants, upstream determinants, causes of causes—of health have typically rather qualitative nature in the assessment process.

As for non-public health researchers it might be hard to identify and describe groups of determinants of health use of a model with a pre-set list of determinants of health is recommended to overcome this problem. There are various models to describe the structure of health determinants; those presenting the holistic model of health are preferable. The model of Lalonde is frequently used (Lalonde 1974), another option could be the Dahlgren and Whitehead model (Dahlgren and Whitehead 1991) further developed by Barton and Grant (Barton and Grant 2006).

The ways for identifying important health determinants having impact on risk factors can vary, therefore a transparent determination of the used methods for selection should be applied. Extensive literature review, expert opinion or involvements of stakeholders in form of interview process are the most often recommended

Table 4.6 Tool for horizontal prioritization

Determinants of health	Risk factors	Number of people affected	Quality of life affected	Related national expenses	Strength of literature evidence	Sum
Determinant of health I						
	Risk factor I.1					
	Risk factor I.2					
Determinant of health II						
	Risk factor II.1					
	Risk factor II.2					

Remarks
Add as many lines (determinants of health or risk factors) as necessary
Scoring is from 1 (no or minimal effect) to 5 (maximum effect expected)

methods to identify determinants of health. The key issue in the selection of influenced health determinants is availability of evidence for causality.

Two approaches for selection can be distinguished: the broad consideration (not to lose any) and the strict one that prioritizes health determinants. The selection process also depends on the primary intention of the assessment, that is, what public health practitioners (experts) want to use the assessment for, as well as on the scale of resources available.

To conclude, a clear strategy for choosing health determinants for assessment is necessary. If selection is to be narrowed down, the way of prioritizing among the various pathways should consider the strength of available evidence for causality, as well as the size/importance of the effect (size of population affected, severity of health effects, costs involved etc.). The formalization of the prioritization process by using a scoring system can further increase transparency (Table 4.6).

Policy

The policy (strategy, program or regulation) is of great importance from a population health point of view, regardless of the level and sector of its initiation that can be either central, regional or local government, industry or other organizations.

All in all while enlisting policies relevant to influence the health determinant linked to risk factors and to health outcome of interest the following issues should be taken into consideration; the importance of topic, the need of policy makers for assistance in the decision making process and the possibility of a quantitative assessment.

Usually, there is a number of policies having impact on health determinants linked to risk factors and finally to health outcome. In principle any policy that has impact should be considered and enlisted. To be sure that all the policies are listed a multidisciplinary assessing team should perform the task.

After the policies are defined, a good understanding of the policy context is of crucial importance in order to be able to link the policies to impacts on health determinants: map the impact structure, prioritize impact pathways and identify where the challenges come from. A comprehensive collection of policies must be presented to policy makers and importance of each stressed.

Placing the policies into an international context helps to identify the driving forces of policies making, meanwhile allows finding similar policies implemented in other countries whose experiences can be fruitfully applied in the assessment process. A list of information sources for the description is of help. It is worth understanding the history of the policies, how they developed with time. The understanding of the legal environment and the relationship between the suggested and other related policies allows their interactions to be considered.

Cross-Cutting Issues

A key issue in policy health impact assessment is the quantification of results. Quantitative assessment can be perceived as the quantitative expression of expected changes in health outcome measures by using numerical information on how a policy affects health outcomes directly or through induced changes in exposure levels of risk factors. Quantitative expression of results has advantages to qualitative description. It is favoured in the decision making process, since it helps in prioritizing issues and considering cost-benefit relations, therefore it can effectively assist the bargain process.

Constructing a mathematical model from the health outcome up to determination of policies reducing health outcome is essential for possibility to compare different policy options of different sectors. Quantification needs to be done for individual causal pathways to avoid double counting; *horizontal interrelation* between various causal pathways at different levels should be assessed, too.

Transparency is important prerequisite for the description of any assessment processes. Assessors should provide a clear explanation on the method of information search, evidence evaluation, prioritization of health determinants, risk factors and health outcomes, selection of applied measures and functions, data collection and validity assessment. An important factor of transparency is the description of uncertainties in the assessment process.

An important issue is the acknowledgement of limitations in the use of methodology. The admission of inability to assess health outcomes due to lack of data, functions, expert skills, etc., is a prerequisite of a transparent process description and relates to the phenomenon of uncertainty.

Uncertainty is a natural attendant of predictions. The assessment of the impact of a policy, especially when it is prospective making projection for the future, always involves uncertainty. It derives, among others, from the questionable strength of evidence and validity of data and functions applied. Numerical information is usually an estimate with inherited uncertainty due to random error of sampling, and it can be further enlarged by the presence of bias and by the extrapolation of information from one situation/population to another. Therefore the repeated statement that uncertainty exists has not much added value; rather its extent should be described in a qualitative or quantitative way. In the latter case, a range can be specified functioning as an interval estimate of the result. More about uncertainties and the way to communicate them could be found in the WHO-IPCS guidance document on characterizing and communicating uncertainty (WHO 2008).

Realization of impact may need time. The description of probable *latency* of effects is important information to be considered in the decision-making process. There is a latency period between the planning and implementation of a policy, as well as a lag phase between policy implementation and development of health effects. The consideration of health outcomes dependent on time, i.e. differentiation between short and long term effects is a favorable product of an assessment.

To describe and assess *strength of evidence* on different levels of the full chain assessment, users are recommended to use guidance on levels of evidence developed by the National Institute for Health and Clinical Excellence of the United Kingdom (National Institute for Health and Clinical Excellence 2005; Weightman et al. 2005).

Bottom: Up Checklist

The methodological guidance is summarized as a checklist that can be used as a tool for the determination of policies related to health outcome (Table 4.7).

Usability of the Combined Tool

One of the main goals of the RAPID project was to provide a methodological tool for those who want to carry out the comprehensive selection of policies having impact on health outcome. The structure of the bottom—up assessment of policies having impact on health outcome suits the process of putting public health issues on agenda of any sectors of a government.

It starts with the selection of health outcome, determines risk factors and health determinants and finally makes a selection of policies having impact on determinants of health.

The developed combined tool includes a guidance and a checklist. The guidance provides detailed description of the assessment process and explains critical theoretical and practical issues; it helps to understand and use the checklist in practice. The checklist offers a logical framework of assessment. It enlists the required steps and highlights the important issues that must be considered during the assessment process. The checklist addresses not only what to do but also how to do that by giving advice on practicalities of the assessment process.

Table 4.7

	Content of analyses	How to do
Health outcome	Identify the health outcome, briefly describe its nature and driving forces of the assessment	Literature search including medical, epidemiological and health outcome literature
	Provide a definition of selected health outcome, ICD code	
	Identify population groups affected by outcome	
	Provide available/accessible epidemiological/population health data (incidence, prevalence, hospitalization,…) and describe the source of data and its validity	International, national, local statistics
	Provide information on overall burden of disease with area of interest (international, country, region, local), time trends and international comparison	
	Forecast how the problem is expected to develop	
	Set objectives and define what kind of change(natural and size of it) would be desirable in occurrence of health outcome	
	Provide information upon cost related to health outcome	
Risk factors	Enlist the known risk factors	Literature search with focus on epidemio-logical literature
	Provide quantitative expressions of risk using available epidemiological association measures such as risk ratios, hazards, coefficients, odds ratios, relative risk, attributable risk fractions, etc…	Database search
		Prioritize among enlisted risk factors aiming to identify the most important ones to reach the expected change in occurrence of health outcome defined in previous level
	Provide information upon strength of evidence (level of causality), source and method of reaching the enlisted expressions of risk	
	Define and specify exposure based on available epidemiological association measures, enlist exposure measures if not available use proxy measures (and describe the proxy measure in terms of strength of evidence, source and method)	
	Identify and describe dose-response, dose (exposure)-effect relations	Epidemiological scientific literature and exposure database are likely to be the main source of informa-tion on this level

(continued)

Table 4.7 (continued)

	Content of analyses	How to do
Determinants of health	Define which model of determinants is use (Lalonde, Dahlgren &Whitehead, others...) Group the risk factors according wider determinants of health user either categories of determinants of health according selected model (e.g. biological, environmental health system and lifestyle if Lalonde model is use) Describe how does the determinant affect prevalence of risk factors(causality/association) and provide information upon strength of evidence; if no direst measures available please use proxy measures Link wider determinants to sectors (branches of the government, ministries, etc.) which could act Prioritize horizontally among determinants of health if necessary taking into account relevance of enlisted determinants, culture of cross-sectoral collaboration, existing infrastructure and governance rules	Literature search with focus broader public health literature Most likely qualitative research methods such as documentation analysis, focus group of key informant interviews are the most relevant methods to get information
Policy	Describe baseline policy and legislative environment Identify alternative policy options-enlist policies with likely influence on selected determinants of health Enlist interventional opportunities at relevant policy level (International/national/regional/local Discuss costs related to policies Enlist and discuss implementation processes link to the policies Specify policy options/interventions (level, sector stakeholders, policy instrument, scope, target group, time scale) compare policy options Indicate efficiency and effectiveness based on available scientific evidence Consider consistency with existing legislation, infrastructure, culture of cross-sectoral collaboration and other constraints Create a shortlist of preferred options, explain reasons of discarding Establish mechanisms for monitoring and evaluation (indicators, methods, time scale)	Qualitative research methods such as documentation analysis, interview processes Policy analyses Implementation research

(continued)

Table 4.7 (continued)

	Content of analyses	How to do
Cross-cutting issues	The assessment process should be transparent and replicable data collection methods and forms of analysis should be identified and be scientifically sound; references should be provided where necessary	
	At any relevant level role of time as important variable needs to be discussed! There are two levels of latency: first from when a policy is planned until implemented and second from implementation time to development of health effect (the epidemiological lag time)	
	Uncertainties, errors, biases should be enlisted at relevant points and an overall discussion of uncertainties related to full chain should be given in report	
	Data gaps should be indicated and recommendation for elimination should be discussed	

The combined tool is expected to be used by public health professionals to determine policies and actions to positively influence trends of a health outcome. The tool can be effectively used by professionals having practice with HIA and risk assessment; however, the tool can also provide assistance for those who have limited previous experience but would like to gain an insight in the process of determination of policies having impact on health outcome. Health promoters, health advocates, health policy developers, public health practitioners are very important potential users of the bottom-up guidance.

References

Aarts, L., & van Schagen, I. (2006). Driving speed and the risk of road crashes: A review. *Accident Analysis and Prevention, 38*, 215–224.

Abdala, N., Carney, J. M., Durante, A. J., et al. (2003). Estimating the prevalence of syringe-borne and sexually transmitted diseases among infection drug users in St Petersburg, Russia. *International Journal of STD and AIDS, 14*, 697–703.

Ádám, B., Molnár, Á., Gulis, G., & Ádány, R. (2013). Integrating quantitative risk appraisal in health impact assessment: Analysis of the novel smoke-free policy in Hungary. *European Journal of Public Health, 23*(2), 211–217.

Ældrebefolkningens sundhedstilstand i Danmark - analyser baseret på Sundheds- og sygelighed-sundersøgelsen 2005 og udvalgte registre. Sundhedsstyrelsen (2010). Retrieved August 29, 2013, from http://www.si-folkesundhed.dk/upload/aeldrebefolkn_sundhedstilst.pdf

Anderson, P., & Baumberg, B. (2006). *Alcohol in Europe A public health perspective. A report for the European Commission*. UK: Institute of Alcohol Studies. Retrieved March 1, 2013, http://www.ec.europa.eu/health-eu/doc/alcoholineu_content_en.pdf

Anthonisen, N. R., et al. (1994). Effects of smoking intervention and the use of an inhaled anticho-linergic bronchodilator on the rate of decline of FEV1, the Lung Health Study. *Journal of the American Medical Association, 272*, 1497–1505.

Babor, T., Caetano, R., Casswell, S., Edwards, G., Giesbrecht, N., Graham, K., et al. (2003). *Research and public policy. Alcohol: No ordinary commodity.* London: Oxford University Press.

Bambra, C., Gibson, M., Sowden, A., Wright, K., Whitehead, M., & Petticrew, M. (2010). Tackling the wider social determinants of health and health inequalities: Evidence from systematic reviews. *Journal of Epidemiology and Community Health, 64*, 284–291.

Barton, H., & Grant, M. (2006). A health map for the local human habitat. *Journal of the Royal Society for the Promotion of Public Health, 126*(6), 252–261.

Bonjour, J. P., et al. (1997). Protein intake, IGF-1 and osteoporosis. *Osteoporosis International, 7*(suppl. 3), S36–S42.

Boseti, C., Levi, F., Lucchini, F., Zatonski, W. A., Negri, E., & La Vechia, C. (2007). Worldwide mortality from cirrhosis: An update to 2002. *Journal of Hepatology, 46*(5), 827–839.

Braddon, F. E., Wadsworth, M. E., Davies, J. M., et al. (1988). Social and regional differences in food and alcohol consumption and their measurement in a national birth cohort. *Journal of Epidemiology and Community Health, 42*(4), 341–349.

Busse, R., Blümel, M., Scheller-Kreinsen, D., & Zentner, A. (2010). *Tackling chronic disease in Europe: Strategies, interventions and challenges.* Copenhagen: WHO, European Observatory on Health Systems and Policies.

Cercone, J.A. (1994). *Alcohol related problems as an obstacle to the development of human capital.* World Bank Technical Paper No. 219. Washington, DC: World Bank.

Chapman, M. I. (2007). The anorexia of aging. *Clinics in Geriatric Medicine, 23*, 735–756.

Chisholm, D., Rehm, J., Van Ommeren, M., & Monteiro, M. (2004). Reducing the global burden of hazardous alcohol use: A comparative cost-effectiveness analysis. *Journal of Studies on Alcohol, 65*(6), 782–793.

Compston, J. (2009). Recent advances in the management of osteoporosis. *Clinical Medicine, 9*(6), 565–569.

Consensus Development Conference. (1991). Diagnosis, prophylaxis and treatment of osteoporosis. *American Journal of Medicine, 90*, 107–110.

Corrao, G., Ferrari, P. A., & Galatola, G. (1995). Exploring the role of diet in modifying the effect of known disease determinants: Application to risk factors of liver cirrhosis. *American Journal of Epidemiology, 142*(11), 1136–1146.

Czapiński, J., & Panek, T. (2009). *Social Diagnosis 2009, the subjective quality and objective conditions of life in Poland.* Warszawa: The Council for Social Monitoring. Retrieved December 10, 2010, http://www.diagnoza.com/pliki/raporty/Diagnoza_raport_2009.pdf

Dahlgren, G., & Whitehead, M. (1991). *Policies and strategies to promote social equity in health.* Stockholm, Sweden: Institute for Future Studies.

Degos, F. (1999). Hepatitis C and alcohol. *Journal of Hepatology, 31*(1), 113–118.

DESTATIS, Statistisches Bundesamt. (2008). *Verkehr. Verkehrsunfälle 2007. Fachserie 8 Reihe 7* (p. 316). Wiesbaden: Statistisches Bundesamt. http://www.destatis.de

Det Nationale Forebyggelsesråd. (2010). *Det er tid til handling—forebyggelse er en politisk vindersag.* København, Denmark: Det Nationale Forebyggelsesråd.

Dirección General de Tráfico (DGT). (2006). *Anuario estadístico de accidentes 2006.* Retrieved December 15, 2010, from http://www.dgt.es/was6/portal/contenidos/es/seguridad_vial/estadistica/publicaciones/anuario_estadistico/anuario_estadistico001.pdf

Dirección General de Tráfico (DGT). (2009). *Anuario estadístico de accidentes 2009.* Retrieved December 15, 2010, from http://www.dgt.es/was6/portal/contenidos/es/seguridad_vial/estadistica/publicaciones/anuario_estadistico/anuario_estadistico013.pdf

Drewnowski, A., & Specter, S. E. (2004). Poverty and obesity: The role of energy density and energy costs. *American Journal of Clinical Nutrition, 79*(1), 6–16.

Drygas, W., Kwaśniewska, M., Szcześniewska, D., Kozakiewicz, K., Głuszek, J., Wiercińska, E., Wyrzykowski, B., & Kurjata, P. (2005). Ocena poziomu aktywności fizycznej dorosłej populacji Polski. Wyniki programu WOBASZ. *Kardiologia Polska, 63*(6 supl. 4), 632–635.

Eisner, M., Anthonisen, N., Coultas, D., et al. (2010). An official American Thoracic Society Public Policy Statement: Novel risk factors and the global burden of chronic obstructive pulmonary disease. *American Journal of Respiratory and Critical Care Medicine, 182*, 693–718.

EUGLOREH. (2007). Retrieved November 8, 2010, from http://www.eugloreh.it/default.do
Eurobarometer. (2010). *Tobacco. European Commission.* Retrieved November 8, 2010, from http://ec.europa.eu/public_opinion/archives/ebs/ebs_332_en.pdf
European Commission (EC). (2001). *White Paper. European transport policy for 2010: Time to decide.* Luxembourg [on line]. Retrieved December 17, 2010, from http://ec.europa.eu/transport/strategies/doc/2001_white_paper/lb_texte_complet_en.pdf
European Commission: Road Traffic-Community Database on Accidents on the Roads in Europe (EC CARE). (2010). *Road safety evolution in EU [on line].* Retrieved December 17, 2010, http://ec.europa.eu/transport/road_safety/pdf/observatory/historical_evol.pdf
European Transport Safety Council (ETSC). (2010). *PIN Flash n16. Methodological notes on behavioral indicators [on line].* Retrieved December 27, 2010, from http://www.etsc.eu/documents/Methodological%20note_PIN%20Flash16.pdf
Eurostat. (2010). *Infant mortality rate in Europe,* Luxembourg. Retrieved December 1, 2010, from http://www.epp.eurostat.ec.europa.eu/portal/page/portal/eurostat/home
Eurostat. (2010). http://epp.eurostat.ec.europa.eu/portal/page/portal/eurostat/home/
Ezzati, M., & Lopez, A. D. (2003). Estimates of global mortality attributable to smoking in 2000. *The Lancet, 365,* 847–852.
Feldman, J. J., Makuc, D. M., Kleinman, J. C., & Cornoni-Huntley, J. (1989). National trends in educational differences in mortality. *American Journal of Epidemiology, 129,* 919–1033.
Foundation for the Automobile and Society (FIA). (2009). *Seat-belts and child restraints: A road safety manual for decision-makers and practitioners.* London [on line]. Retrieved December 22, 2010, from http://www.who.int/roadsafety/projects/manuals/seatbelt/en/index.html
Gergelova, P., Corradi, M., Acampa, O., et al. (2008). New techniques for assessment of occupational respiratory diseases. *Bratislavské Lekárske Listy, 109*(10), 445–452.
Gil, R., Witkowski, A., & Różyłło, W. (2003). Przezskórna angioplastyka wieńcowa w Polsce. *Historia i teraźniejszość.* Retrieved November 20, 2010, from http://www.kardiologiainwazyjna.pl/mod/archiwum/2407,przezsk%C3%B3rna,angioplastyka,wie%C5%84cowa.html
Gold, D. T., & Silverman, S. (2006). Review of adherence to medications for the treatment of osteoporosis. *Current Osteoporosis Reports, 4,* 21–27.
Goss, C. W., Van Bramer, L. D., Gliner, J. A., Porter, T. R., Roberts, I. G, DiGuiseppi C. (2008). Increased police patrols for preventing alcohol-impaired driving. *Cochrane Database of Systematic Reviews,* Issue 4. Art. No.: CD005242. DOI:10.1002/14651858.CD005242.pub2
Gras, M. E., Cunill, M., Sullman, M. J., Planes, M., Aymerich, M., & Font-Mayolas, S. (2007). Mobile phone use while driving in a sample of Spanish university workers. *Accident Analyses and Prevention, 39*(2), 347–355.
Green, G., Macintyre, S., West, P., & Ecob, R. (1991). Like parent like child? Associations between drinking and smoking behaviour of parents and their children. *British Journal of Addiction, 86*(6), 745–758.
Guralnik, J., Land, K., Blazer, D., Fillenbaum, G., & Branch, L. (1993). Educational status and active life expectancy among older blacks and whites. *The New England Journal of Medicine, 329,* 110–116.
Haddon, W., Jr. (1968). The changing approach to the epidemiology, prevention, and amelioration of trauma: The transition to approaches etiologically rather than descriptively. *American Journal of Public Health, 58,* 1431–1438.
Hanson, M. D., & Chen, E. (2007). Socioeconomic status and health behaviors in adolescence: A review of the literature. *Journal of Behavioral Medicine, 30*(3), 263–285.
Health statistics yearbook of the Slovak Republic 2007. (2008). *[pdf] Národné centrum zdravotníckych informácií,* Bratislava. ISBN 978-80-89292-13-4. Retrieved December 15, 2011, from http://www.nczisk.sk/Documents/rocenky/rocenka_2007.pdf
Health Statistics Yearbook (2008). Retrieved August 29, 2013, from http://www.ivz.si/Mp.aspx?ni=202&pi=18&_18_view=item&_18_newsid=407&pl=202-18.0
Heaney, R. P. (2001). Reply to a Sebastian et al. (letter). *American Journal of Clinical Nutrition, 74,* 412.

Heidelbaugh, J. J., & Bruderly, M. (2006). Cirrhosis and Chronic Liver Failure. *American Family Physician, 74*(5), 756–762.

Holloway, T., et al. (2005). *Application of air quality models to public health analysis.* [pdf] Energy for Sustainable Development l Volume IX No. 3 l. Retrieved December 6, 2011, from http://www.aseanenvironment.info/Abstract/41013076.pdf

Hruškovič, B. (2004). *Alergia a astma v Európe.* Bratislava: [pdf] Alergologická a imunologická ambulancia. Retrieved December 6, 2011, from http://www.solen.sk/index. php?page=pdf_view&pdf_id=540&magazine_id=1

Institute of Public Health of the Republic of Slovenia (NIPH). (2008).

International Center for Alcohol Policies (ICAP). (2008). *Quick reference guide to the ICAP Blue Book: Implementing alcohol policy and targeted interventions.* Washington, DC: ICAP. Retrieved March 1, 2013, from http://www.icap.org/PolicyTools/ICAPBlueBook/BlueBookM odules/21NoncommercialAlcohol/tabid/180/Default.aspx#3

IT.NRW, Information und Technik Nordrhein-Westfalen. (2010). *Statistische Berichte. Straßenverkehrsunfälle in Nordrhein-Westfalen 2009* (p. 199). Düsseldorf: IT.NRW. http://www.it.nrw.de

Joffe, M., & Mindell, J. (2002). A framework for the evidence base to support health impact assessment. *Journal of Epidemiology and Community Health, 56,* 132–138.

Joffe, M., & Mindell, J. (2005). Health impact assessment. *Occupational and Environmental Medicine, 62,* 907–912.

Joffe, M., & Mindell, J. (2006). Complex causal process diagrams for analyzing the health impacts of policy interventions. *American Journal of Public Health, 96,* 473–479.

Kamath, B., & Piccoli, D. (2003). Heritable disorders of the bile ducts. *Gastroenterology Clinics of North America, 32,* 857–875.

Kaner, E. F., Dickinson, H. O., Beyer, F. R., Campbell, F., Schlesinger, C., Heather, N., Saunders, J. B., Burnand, B., Pienaar, E. D. (2007). Effectiveness of brief alcohol interventions in primary care populations. *Cochrane Database of Systematic Reviews* 2007, Issue 2. Art. No.: CD004148. DOI: 10.1002/14651858.CD004148.pub3.

Kaplowitz, N. (2004). Drug-induced liver injury. *Clinical Infectious Diseases, 38*(Suppl 2), S44–S48.

Karvonen, S., & Rimpeli, A. (1996). Socio-regional context as a determinant of adolescents' health behaviour in Finland. *Social Science & Medicine (1982), 43,* 1467–1474.

Kawachi, I., & Berkman, L. F. (2003). *Neighborhoods and health.* New York, NY: Oxford University Press.

Kemm, J. (2001). Health impact assessment: A tool for healthy public policy. *Health Promotion International, 16*(1), 79–85.

Khan, K. N., & Yatsuhashi, H. (2000). Effect of alcohol consumption on the progression of hepatitis C virus infection and risk of hepatocellular carcinoma in Japanese patients. *Alcohol and Alcoholism, 35*(3), 286–295.

Khosla, S. (2010). Update in male osteoporosis. *Journal of Clinical Endocrinology and Metabolism, 95*(1), 3–10.

Kok, C., Sambrook, P.N. (2009). *Secondary osteoporosis in patients with an osteoporotic fracture, Best Practice & Research Clinical Rheumatology* 23, 769–779.

Koós, T. (2010). Healthy public policy: Alcohol policy in Hungary. *Népegészségügy, 88*(1), 23–28 [in Hungarian].

Košturiak, R. (2008). Moderný manažment bronchiálnej astmy, *Via pract., roč.* 5(2), 58–62 [online]. Retrieved December 10, 2011, from http://www.solen.sk/index.php?page=pdf_ view&pdf_id=2947&magazine_id=1

Lalonde, M. (1974). *A new perspective on the health of Canadians.* Ottawa, Canada: Government of Canada.

Lanea, S., et al. (2006). An international observational prospective study to determine the cost of asthma exacerbations (COAX). *Respiratory Medicine, 100,* 434–450.

Larsson, J., Unosson, M., Ek, A.-C., Nilsson, L., Thorslund, S., & Bjurulf, P. (1990). Effect of dietary supplement on nutritional status and clinical outcome in 501 geriatric patients—a randomised study. *Clinical Nutrition, 9,* 179–184.

Narodowy Program Profilaktyki i Leczenia Chorób Układu Sercowo-Naczyniowego 2006-2008 POLKARD. (2010). Warszawa. Retrieved December 1, 2010, from http://www.polkard.org/polkard.html

Lock, K., & McKee, M. (2005). Health impact assessment: Assessing opportunities and barriers to intersectoral health improvement in an expanded European Union. *Journal of Epidemiology and Community Health, 59*(5), 356–360.

Lowry, R., Kann, L., Collins, O. R., & Kolbe, L. J. (1996). The effect of socio-economic status on chronic disease risk behaviors among US adolescents. *Journal of the American Medical Association, 276*, 792–797.

Main Statistical Office, (MSO), (in Polish Główny Urząd Statystyczny). (2010). *Life expectancy in Poland.* Warszawa. Retrieved December 1, 2010, from http://www.stat.gov.pl/gus/5840_894_ENG_HTML.htm

Mannino, D. M., Homa, D. M., Akinbami, L. J., Ford, E. S., & Redd, S. C. (2002). Chronic obstructive pulmonary disease surveillance—United States, 1971-2000. *MMWR Surveillance Summaries, 6*(51), 1–16.

McQueen, D., & Jones, C. (2007). *Global perspectives on health promotion effectiveness.* New York: Springer.

McLaren, L. (2007). Socioeconomic status and obesity. *Epidemiologic Reviews, 29*(1), 29–48.

Metabolic Syndrome Rounds, St. Michael's Hospital, Toronto/ON, Canada; March 2006, Vol. 4, Issue 3.

Metcalfe, O., & Higgins, C. (2009). Healthy public policy—is health impact assessment the cornerstone? *Public Health, 123*, 296–301.

Meunier, P. J. (1999). Calcium, vitamin D and vitamin K in the prevention of fractures due to osteoporosis. *Osteoporosis International, 9*(suppl. 2), S48–S52.

Ministry of Health. (2010). *Ministry of health official web page.* Warszawa. Retrieved December 1, 2010, from http://www.mz.gov.pl/

Mowe, M., Bohmer, T., & Kindt, E. (1994). Reduced nutritional status in an elderly population (70 year) is probable before disease and possibly contributes to the development of disease. *American Journal of Clinical Nutrition, 59*, 317–324.

Mullahy, J. (1991). Gender differences in labor market effects of alcoholism. *American Economic Review* (Papers and Proceedings), *81*(2), 161–165.

Murray, C. J. L., & Lopez, A. D. (1997). Alternative projections of mortality and disability by cause 1990-2020: Global Burden of Disease Study. *The Lancet, 349*, 1498–1504.

Murray, C., Salomon, J., Mathers, C., & Lopez, A. (2002). *Editors summary measures of population health: Concepts, ethics, measurements and applications.* Geneva: World Health Organization.

National Addictology Centre. (2009). *National alcohol policy and strategy draft.* Budapest: National Addictology Centre.

National Health Fund (NHF), (in Polish Narodowy Fundusz Zdrowia). (2010). *Profilaktyczne programy zdrowotne realizowane przez Narodowy Fundusz Zdrowia.* Warszawa. Retrieved December 1, 2010, from http://www.nfz.gov.pl/profilaktyka/programy.php

National Institute for Health and Clinical Excellence. (2005). *Guideline development methods. Chapter 7 Reviewing and grading the evidence.* London, UK: NIHCE. Retrieved on December 09, 2012, from http://www.nice.org.uk/niceMedia/pdf/GDM_Chapter7_0305.pdf

National Institute of Diabetes and Digestive and Kidney Diseases (NIDDK). (2000). *Cirrhosis of the Liver.* April http://www.niddk.nih.gov/health/digest/pubs/cirrhosi/cirrhosi.htm

National institute on Alcohol Abuse and Alcoholism (NIAAA). (1998). *Drinking in the United States: Main findings from the 1992 National Longitudinal Alcohol Epidemiologic Survey (NLAES).* US Alcohol Epidemiologic Data Reference Manual (Vol. 6, 1st ed.). NIH Pub. No. 99-3519. Bethesda, MD: Niaaa.

Neidell, M. J. (2004). Air pollution, health, and socio-economic status: The effect of outdoor air quality on childhood asthma. *Journal of Health Economics, 23*(6), 1209–1236.

Nocturnal Oxygen Therapy Trial Group. (1980). Continuous or nocturnal oxygen therapy in hypoxemic chronic obstructive lung disease: A clinical trial. *Annals of Internal Medicine, 93*, 391–398.

Pérez, C., Cirera, C., Plasencia, A., & On behalf of the work of the Spanish Society of Epidemiology for Measuring of the Impact of Road Traffic Accidents in Spain. (2006). Motor vehicle crash fatalities at 30 days in Spain. *Gaceta Sanitaria, 20*(2), 108–115.

Pietili, A. M., Hentinen, M., & Myhrman, A. (1995). The health behavior of Northern Finnish men in adolescence and adulthood. *International Journal of Nursing Studies, 32*, 325–338.

Piko, B. (2000). Perceived social support from parents and peers: Which is the stronger predictor of adolescent substance use? *Substance Use & Misuse, 35*, 617–630.

Pongchaiyakul, C. H., Songpattanasilp, T., & Taechakraichana, N. (2008). Osteoporosis: Overview in disease, epidemiology, treatment and health economy. *Journal of the Medical Association of Thialand, 91*(4), 581–594.

Prentice, A. (2004). Diet, nutrition and the prevention of osteoporosis. *Public Health Nutrition, 7*(1A), 227–243.

Prevention and management of osteoporosis: Report of a WHO scientific group. (2003). *WHO* (Tech. Rep. Series); p. 921.

Pulido, J., Lardelli, P., de la Fuente, L., Flores, V. M., Vallejo, F., & Regidor, E. (2010). Impact of the demerit point system on road traffic accident mortality in Spain. *Journal of Epidemiology and Community Health, 64*(10), 274–276.

Ramstedt, M. (2007). Population drinking and liver cirrhosis mortality: Is there a link in Eastern Europe? *Addiction, 102*(8), 1212–1223.

Rehm, J., Klotsche, J., & Patra, J. (2007). Comparative quantification of alcohol exposure as risk factor for global burden of disease. *International Journal of Methods in Psychiatric Research, 16*(2), 66–76.

Rehm, J., Taylor, B., Mohapatra, S., Irving, H., Baliunas, D., Patra, J., & Roerecke, M. (2010). Alcohol as a risk factor for liver cirrhosis: A systematic review and meta-analysis. *Drug and Alcohol Review, 29*, 437–445.

Reshetnikov, O. V., Khryanin, A. A., Teinina, T. R., Krivenchuk, N. A., & Zimina, I. Y. (2001). Hepatitis B and C seroprevalence in Novosibirsk, western Siberia. *Sexually Transmitted Infections, 77*, 463.

Rizer, M. K. (2006). Osteoporosis. *Primary Care Clinics in Office Practice, 33*, 943–951.

SafetyNet. (2009). *Speed Enforcement.* Web-text. 31. Retrieved date Novermber 23, 2010, from http://ec.europa.eu/transport/road_safety/index_en.htm

Schirnhofer, L., Lamprecht, B., Vollmer, W. M., Allison, M. J., Studnicka, M., Jensen, R. L., & Buist, A. S. (2007). COPD prevalence in Salzburg, Austria: Results from the burden of obstructive lung disease (BOLD) study. *Chest, 131*, 29–36.

Schmidt, L.A., Mäkelä, P., Rehm, J., & Room, R. (2010). Alcohol: Equity and social determinants. In Blas E, Kurup AS: *Equity, social determinants and public health programs.* Chapter 2 (pp. 11–31). ISBN 978 924 156 3 970 Geneva, Switzerland: WHO Press.

Schram-Bijkerk, D., Kempen, V. E., Knol, A. B., Kruize, H., Staatsen, B., & Kamp, V. I. (2009). Quantitative health impact assessment of transport policies: Two simulations related to speed limit reduction and traffic re-allocation in the Netherlands. *Occupational and Environmental Medicine, 66*(10), 691–698.

Sebastian, A., Sellmeyer, D. E., Stone, K. L., & Cummings, S. R. (2001). Dietary ratio of animal to vegetable protein and rate of bone loss and risk of fracture in postmenopausal women (letter). *American Journal of Clinical Nutrition, 74*, 411–412.

Siris, E. S., Selby, P. L., Saag, K. G., Borgström, F., Herings, R. M., & Silverman, S. L. (2009). Impact of osteoporosis treatment adherence on fracture rates in North America and Europe. *American Journal of Medicine, 122*, S3–S13.

Solar, O., & Irwin, A. (2010). *A conceptual framework for action on the social determinants of health. Social Determinants of Health Discussion.* Paper 2 (Policy and Practice). Geneva: World Health Organization.

Suhrcke, M., Nugent, R. A., Stukler, D., & Rocco, L. (2006). *Chronic disease: An economic perspective.* London: Oxford Health Alliance.

Suhrcke, M., Rocco, L., McKee, M., Mazzuco, S., Urban, D., & Steinher, A. (2007). *Economic consequences of noncommunicable diseases and injuries in the Russian federation. United Kingdom* (p. 27). Trowbridge, Wilts: The Cromwell Press.

Sun, J., Yu, R., Zhu, B., Wu, J., Larsen, S., & Zhao, W. (2009). Hepatitis C infection and related factors in hemodialysis patients in china: Systematic review and meta-analysis. *Renal Failure, 31*(7), 610–620.

Sund By Netværket. (2010). *8 anbefalinger til forebyggelse af ældres faldulykker—den gode kommunale model. Anbefalinger, strategier og redskaber til kommunens faldforebyggende indsats.* København, Denmark: Sund By Netværket.

Szczapa J. (2009). *Bezrobocie w Polsce w latach 1990-2007.* Katowice: University of Economics in Katowice. Retrieved December 1, 2010, from http://www.ue.katowice.pl/images/user/File/katedra_ekonomii/J.Szczapa_Bezrobocie_w_Polsce_w_latach_1990_-_2007.pdf

Széles, G., Vokó, Z., Jenei, T., Kardos, L., Pocsai, Z., Bajtay, A., Papp, E., Pásti, G., Kósa, Z., Molnár, I., Lun, K., & Adány, R. (2005). A preliminary evaluation of a health monitoring programme in Hungary. *European Journal of Public Health, 15*(1), 26–32.

Szűcs, S., Sárváry, A., McKee, M., & Ádány, R. (2005). Could the high level of cirrhosis in central and eastern Europe be due partly to the quality of alcohol consumed? An exploratory investigation. *Addiction, 100,* 536–542.

To, T., Moineddin, R., Atenafu, E., Guan, J., McLimont, S., Gershon, A. S. (2011). Forecasting Asthma Prevalence and Health Care Use To 2020, Ontario, Canada Retrieved August 29, 2013, http://www.atsjournals.org/doi/abs/10.1164/arjccm-conference.2011.183.1_MeetignAbstracts. A2933

United Nations. (2012, June 20–22). *Report of the United Nations Conference on Sustainable Development.* Brazil: Rio de Janeiro

United Nations (UN). (2008). *Improving global road safety, United Nations General Assembly Resolution A/RES62/244.* Geneva [on line]. Retrieved December 15, 2010, from http://www.who.int/roadsafety/about/resolutions/A-RES-62-L-43.pdf

Veerman, J. L., Barendregt, J. J., & Mackenbach, J. P. (2005). Quantitative health impact assessment: Current practice and future directions. *Journal of Epidemiology and Community Health, 59,* 361–370.

Ventura, A., Savage, J., May, A., et al. (2005). Early behavioral, familial and psychosocial predictors of overweight and obesity. In R. Tremblay, R. Barr, R. Peters (Eds.), *Encyclopedia on early childhood development* (pp. 1–10). Montreal, Canada: Center of Excellence for Early Childhood Development. Retrieved October 31, 2010, from http://www.child-encyclopedia.com/documents/Ventura-Savage-May-BirchANGxp.pdf

Weightman, A., Ellis, S., Cullum, A., Sander, L., & Turley, R. (2005). *Grading evidence and recommendations for public health interventions: Developing and piloting a framework.* London, UK: Health Development Agency. Retrieved on December 9, 2012, from http://www.nice.org.uk/niceMedia/docs/grading_evidence.pdf

Wheeler, B. W., & Ben-Shlomo, Y. (2005). Environmental equity, air quality, socioeconomic status, and respiratory health: A linkage analysis of routine data from the Health Survey for England. *Journal of Epidemiology and Community Health, 59*(11), 948–954.

WHO Strategy for Prevention and Control of Chronic Respiratory Diseases, Geneva (2002). Retrieved August 28, 2013, from http://www.who.int/respiratory/publications/crd_strategy/en/index.html

WHO. (2004a). *WHO global status report on alcohol 2004.* Geneva: World Health Organization, Department of Mental Health and Substance Abuse.

WHO. (2004b). *Preventing road traffic injury: A public health perspective for Europe* (p. 100). Copenhagen: WHO Regional Office for Europe.

WHO. (2009). *European status report on road safety. Towards safer roads and healthier transport choices* (p. 161). Copenhagen: WHO Regional Office for Europe.

Wilson, C., Willis, C., Hendrikz, J. K., Bellamy, N. (2006). Speed enforcement detection devices for preventing road traffic injuries. *Cochrane Database of Systematic Reviews,* Issue 2. Art.

No.: CD004607. DOI: 10.1002/14651858.CD004607.pub2. Retrieved August 29, 2013, from http://www.hem.waw.pl/index.php?idm=87,139&cmd=1

Wilson, C., Willis, C., Hendrikz, J., Bellamy, N. (2009). Speed enforcement detection devices for preventing road traffic injuries (review). The Cochrane Library. *The Cochrane Collaboration 57*

Winsloe, C., Earl, S., Dennison, E. M., Cooper, C., & Harvey, N. C. (2009). Early life factors in the pathogenesis of osteoporosis. *Current Osteoporosis Reports, 7,* 140–144.

Wojtyniak, B., & Goryński, P. (2008). *Sytuacja zdrowotna ludności Polski.* Warszawa: Narodowy Instytut Zdrowia Publicznego-Państwowy Zakład Higieny.

World Health Organization. (1988). *Health promotion glossary.* Geneva, Switzerland: WHO.

World Health Organization. (2010). *Life expectancy health topic,* Geneva. Retrieved December 1, 2010, from http://www.who.int/topics/life_expectancy/en/

World Health Organization (WHO). (2004). *World Report on road traffic injury prevention.* Geneva. Retrieved December 15, 2010, from http://whqlibdoc.who.int/publications/2004/9241562609.pdf

World Health Organization (WHO). (2009). *Global status report on road safety: Time for action.* Geneva. Retrieved December 15, 2010, from http://www.who.int/violence_injury_prevention/road_safety_status/2009/en/

World Health Organization Regional Office for Europe. (2009). *Country profiles on EU Member States Overview of Member States policies aimed at reducing alcohol-related harm.* Retrieved March 1, 2013, from http://ec.europa.eu/health/alcohol/policy/country_profiles/hungary_country_profile.pdf

World Health Organization-International Programme on Chemical Safety. (2008). *Guidance document on characterizing and communicating uncertainty in exposure assessment. Harmonization Project Document No. 6 (Part 1).* Geneva, Switzerland: WHO.

Yang, S., Ho, K. Y., Harper, S., Smith, G. D., Leon, D. A., & Lynch, J. (2010). Understanding the rapid increase in life expectancy in South Korea. *American Journal of Public Health, 100*(5), 896–903.

Zatoński, W., et al. (2008). Closing the health gap in European Union. *Cancer Epidemiology and Prevention Division. The final publication of the project HEM—Closing the gap.* ISBN 9788388681493

Chapter 5
Quantification of Health Risks

Odile Mekel, Piedad Martin-Olmedo, Balázs Ádám, and Rainer Fehr

Introduction

Health, health determinants, and also the consequences of (ill) health, all these items imply considerable complexity. When trying to define and operationalize these concepts, especially in quantitative terms, difficulties emerge. Within the field of public health, correspondingly, both qualitative and quantitative approaches are established, and they are often used to complement each other.

This chapter concerns quantitative approaches in risk and impact assessment. In risk assessment, quantification (i.e., counting or measuring) is the "standard" approach, and the focus on quantification is taken for granted. In health impact assessment (HIA), however, there is a debate on the usefulness and feasibility of quantification. The chapter therefore is not only concerned with "how" to quantify but also with the "pros" and "cons" of impact quantification.

We start with an outline of the topic. The chapter identifies key approaches to quantification. As for quantified modeling, the focus is on risk assessment and HIA. Both bottom-up and top-down modeling are discussed, and examples of

O. Mekel (✉)
Unit Innovation in Health, NRW Centre for Health (LZG.NRW), Bielefeld 33611, Germany
e-mail: odile.mekel@lzg.gc.nrw.de

P. Martin-Olmedo
Escuela Andaluza de Salud Pública, Cuesta del Observatorio 4, 18080 Granada, Spain
e-mail: piedad.martin.easp@juntadeandalucia.es

B. Ádám
University of Southern Denmark, Niels Bohrsvej 9-10, 6700 Esbjerg, Denmark

University of Debrecen, Kassai 26, 4028 Debrecen, Hungary
e-mail: badam@health.sdu.dk; adam.balazs@sph.unideb.hu

R. Fehr
University of Bielefeld, Universitätsstraße 25, 33615 Bielefeld, Germany
e-mail: rainer.fehr@uni-bielefeld.de

G. Guliš et al. (eds.), *Assessment of Population Health Risks of Policies*,
DOI 10.1007/978-1-4614-8597-1_5, © Springer Science+Business Media New York 2014

quantification, especially from the RAPID project, are given. Finally, "pros" and "cons" of quantification in this field are discussed, and conclusions are drawn.

Quantification Basics

As a foundation for the subsequent contents, we distinguish between individual health (and disease), population health, health determinants forming a causal web, health potentials, and health impacts.

Individual Health and Disease

Individual health and disease is often assessed in qualitative terms. In the most condensed form, we distinguish "good health" from "ill health." The International Classification of Diseases and Related Health Problems (ICD) enumerates thousands of different health impairments and provides code numbers which are labels (nominal scale) but do not constitute quantification.

Both medicine and public health often work with quantitative approaches to characterize individual health, e.g., blood pressure, body weight, concentrations of chemical compounds in body fluids, and optical lens refraction. Such measurements help to establish medical diagnoses. In this process, the information is transformed into categorical scale, e.g., "hypertension yes/no."

Over the years, quantitative measurement of individual health has evolved as a diversified field (e.g., McDowell 2006). A vast array of quantifying tools is now available. The scales and indices are often based on (self-administered) questionnaires. Measurements may refer to physical handicap, mental health, functional status, or overall quality of life. There are dedicated scales for assessing pain, anxiety, depression, etc.

Population Health

Population health is nearly always expressed in numbers. A straightforward way to assess the health status of a population is to count frequencies, especially the prevalence of health-related conditions or the occurrence of health-related events. In this way epidemiology, the methodological core discipline of public health, arrives at frequency measures of morbidity (disease prevalence and incidence, hospitalization, etc.) and mortality (mortality rate, life expectancy, etc.).

Nearly all established population health indicators are quantitative. While few professionals of public health would be fundamentally opposed to quantification, there are strong tendencies to keep it "simple." Compared to other sciences such as psychology or sociology (let alone, say, physics or engineering), the level of sophistication for both measurement and analysis will often be found lower.

A need is felt, however, to go beyond these traditional measures, especially to integrate population experience concerning morbidity and mortality and to express, as it were, the overall "burden of disease" (BoD), experienced by a population over a specified time period. In this sense, the so-called summary measures of population health intend to condense large amounts of detailed information in a transparent and authoritative way. Examples include disability-adjusted life years (DALYs) and health-adjusted life expectancy (HLE).

The need for, and feasibility of, these "population health metrics" as well as their merits and limitations are still subject to intensive debate, and no general consensus has emerged yet. At any rate, to define and apply summary measures is not merely a technical procedure. At least the assignment of weights to various states of health impairment inevitably implies value judgments.

Undisputed is the need to check, for each given context, what population subgroups may need to be considered. Standard criteria include age, gender, and social status, but ethnicity, migration status, location, comorbidity and disability, susceptibility, and many others may also need to be taken into account.

Quantitative information on "baseline" population health can often be found in (local, regional, national, etc.) health reports.

Health Determinants and Risk Factors

Obviously, health and disease of both individuals and populations depend at least partially on the presence or the absence of numerous factors which collectively are often called the "determinants" of health. One possible typology would classify the determinants into biological, behavioral, environmental (both social and physical), and healthcare-related factors.

Some factors more or less directly influence human health, e.g., pollutants contained in the air we inhale, or physical violence we may encounter. But obviously, many such factors do not occur at random but can be traced back along a causal chain or web.

More proximal (or "downstream") causes of health and disease, if they imply negative effects on health, are often called "risk factors" (e.g., tobacco smoke exposure), or "protective" factors if the opposite is the case (e.g., physical exercise).

Risk factors and protective factors do not occur at random. They can, more or less rigorously, be traced back to more distal (or "upstream") factors, e.g., living environments, which themselves are being shaped and developed by many factors, including a multitude of policies, plans, programs, and related activities.

No agent (be it risk factor or protective factor) can influence an individual's health unless there is contact between the agent and the individual. Relevant aspects of "exposure," especially intensity and duration, are captured by various exposure metrics, e.g., average exposure, peak exposure, or aggregated exposure (cf. Sect.

"Exposure and Risk Assessment"). The concept of exposure is well established for physical, chemical, and biological agents, but can likewise be applied to other health determinants.

Closely related with exposure is the concept of "dose" which can be described as the amount of agent that enters an individual (target) after crossing a contact boundary (e.g., lung).

When quantifying exposures and/or doses, variations between different subpopulations as well as specific exposure patterns (by space, time, activity, etc.) need to be taken into account.

Determinants further "upstream" (including policies, programs) more often remain unquantified or are quantified in dimensions (e.g., financial) which do not easily translate into quantitative estimates of "downstream" effects. Again, variations need to be taken into account, e.g., different target groups, populations affected, or susceptible subgroups.

Similar to "baseline" population health, quantitative information also on health determinants can often be found in health reports.

Causal Web

The sequence from policy to distal (upstream) factor, from there to proximal (downstream) factor, and from there to health forms a "causal chain." However, rarely would such chain exist in isolation. In the typical case, each element of the "chain" will depend on a number of other items further "upstream," and will influence several items further "downstream." Policies, health determinants, and health effects are therefore said to form "causal webs." For a given topic, such web can be presented in the form of a causal diagram.

A prototype of causal chain or web is the "DPSEEA" model, representing driving forces, pressures (on the environment), state of environment, exposures, health effects, and any actions taken to influence this chain (Corvalán et al. 1996).

For further analysis, information and evidence are needed concerning the relationship between elements of the causal web. Relevant questions are the following: How do policies influence distant determinants? How do distant determinants influence proximal determinants? And how do proximal determinants influence health outcomes?

Information is needed, indicating the change in dependent items at least in a qualitative manner (same direction or opposite direction, compared to the change in "upstream" item) (Joffe and Mindell 2006). In many cases, more comprehensive information may be obtainable, incl. type of function describing the relationship (e.g., linear) and parameters such as slope (in case of linear function).

Exposure–response curves or dose–response curves describe the relationship between determinants of health on one side and health outcomes on the other. Input information originates either from epidemiological (human) or from toxicological (animal) studies. Such functions are more established in environmental health, especially for chemical and physical (noise, radiation) agents, but the approach can be extended beyond this field.

It should be stressed that for utilizing exposure (or dose)–response relationships in a meaningful way, they need to be based on causal relationships, not merely on statistical associations. For distinguishing one from the other, a set of criteria is commonly used in epidemiology (Bradford Hill criteria – Hill 1965).

Causal Attribution, Health Potentials

If there is sufficient information concerning a causal web, then this can be used to work in either "bottom-up" or "top-down" direction. In the former approach, we can estimate prevention potentials, and in the latter approach, population health impacts.

First we look at the "bottom-up" direction. For this purpose, the causal web or chain is used "against the causal flow," starting from health effects and analytically moving towards proximal (downstream) and then distal (upstream) health determinants, possibly even including policies. In this approach, quantified knowledge about health status and health determinants contained in the causal web provides the opportunity to attribute fractions of morbidity, mortality, or BoD to certain factors.

In a closer look, the bottom-up analysis includes the following steps: (1) analysis of how health outcome is influenced by proximal factors, allowing for the attribution of health effects to proximal cause(s), (2) analysis of how proximal factors are influenced by distal factors, allowing for the attribution of proximal factors to distal factors, and (3) analysis of how distal factors are influenced by policies, allowing for the attribution of distal factors to policies. This is basic idea; in real life, it is often not possible to trace back subsections of the full causal chain.

Fractions of disease burden which are attributable to certain policies can be used to identify (and quantify) policy "potentials", i.e., potential health gains which can be assumed to occur if certain policies would (successfully) be implemented.

An example of well-known "attributions" analysis is the BoD estimates of the World Health Organization (WHO 2009a) (Fig. 5.1).

Health Impacts

Now we look at the "top-down" direction. If we work along the causal web from policies, plans, or programs to distal and then proximal determinants and finally to health effects, i.e., "*with* the causal flow," then the opportunity arises to identify and quantify the overall effects on health, often called health impacts.

In the typical case, the interest is in *prospectively* estimating the likely impacts. In this situation, a strictly empirical approach is not possible since the evidence "is not there yet." However, existing evidence can be used to establish rational estimates of future impacts.

Fig. 5.1 Concept of
attribution: Proportion of
lung cancer deaths attributed
to the risk factors smoking
and air pollution (adapted
from WHO 2009a)

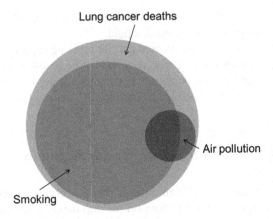

Zooming in on the top-down perspective, the following steps emerge:

- Analysis of how a policy influences determinants of health (distal factors)
- Analysis of how determinants of health (distal factors) influence risk factors (proximal factors)
- Analysis of how risk factors (proximal factors) influence health

Ideally, the top-down analysis allows for comprehensive estimates of the impact of a policy. Such a full description of impacts would cover (Kemm 2013) the nature of the impacts (incl. death, illness, discomfort); the direction of change (increase or decrease); the magnitude of change (number of persons, severity); and the distribution across different groups.

Quantitative Modeling

The preceding section outlined the basic notion of the causal web or chain, i.e., changes in policy(ies) causing change(s) in distal determinants; these changes in turn causing change(s) in proximal determinants; and these changes then causing health change(s).

It has long been recognized that if this causal web from policy(ies) to health outcomes is sufficiently understood, then this knowledge can to some extent be utilized to inform policy-making, for the benefit of population health. In this context, it is often assumed that the usage of quantitative data and the conduction of quantitative analysis will be useful. As indicated, such analysis can either work "bottom-up" or "top-down" through the cascades of causes and effects.

A successful quantitative analysis requires a set of "ingredients." Analysts need at least a basic understanding of the topical domain in question, including the web of causes and effects; access to data of sufficient detail and quality; a notion of substantive variation (e.g., between subgroups and/or over time); strength of evidence; and levels of (un)certainty.

This section starts with presenting key approaches of quantitative risk assessment, including the area of exposure assessment which, under the headline of "exposure science," currently evolves into a discipline of its own. It proceeds to discuss bottom-up (Sect. "Quantification in Top-Down RAPID Case Studies") and top-down (Sect. "Quantification in Bottom-Up RAPID Case Studies") analyses, in both cases utilizing examples from the RAPID project. Over recent years, a suite of software tools supporting quantitative modeling has emerged which is assumed to harbor considerable potential for quantified health analyses.

Exposure and Risk Assessment

Risk assessment and risk management have been activities of banking, insurance, and business operations in industrialized economies for more than 100 years now. Application in human health and safety emerged in the first half of the twentieth century. In the USA, already for more than 30 years, this is a basic element of health, safety, and environmental policy. In other areas of the world incl. the EU, risk assessment is increasingly used, too. Risk assessment evolved in the field of environmental health, closely related with toxicology, epidemiology, and industrial hygiene. Risk assessment, primarily developed for chemical hazards, can be applied to all hazards, whether they are chemical, physical, biological, or psychosocial in nature (ACS 1998; DoH WA—Department of Health and Western Australia 2006; Goldstein 2009).

As described in Chap. 2, one of the pioneers in developing the framework of health risk assessment is the National Research Council in the USA, which was the first to define the risk assessment process as a four-step procedure. The US Environmental Protection Agency (US EPA) uses this framework as a major tool for regulation and risk management. The US EPA developed a vast amount of risk assessment guidance and tools (http://epa.gov/riskassessment) and is a world leading authority in this area. Key elements of the risk assessment methodology are also used in the so-called Public Health Assessments conducted by the US Agency of Toxic Substances and Disease Registry (ATSDR 2005). Such assessments provide an additional public health perspective by integrating more site-specific exposure conditions combined with health effects data and specific community health concerns. Where originally the scope of EPA's risk assessment was on characterizing options for risk control, e.g., at contaminated sites, it was widened to be used for priority setting. In the 1990s the so-called comparative risk analysis (CRA) approach emerged for application in EPA's risk-based priority setting and program planning. This programmatic comparative risk analysis seeks to make comparisons among numerous and widely differing hazards. Besides the quantification of the health risks, qualitative elements especially value judgments are a major component giving participation of experts and stakeholders an important role in the CRA process (Schütz et al. 2006).

A similar term "comparative risk assessment" (CRA) denotes a different approach which evolved in the epidemiological based risk assessment work of the

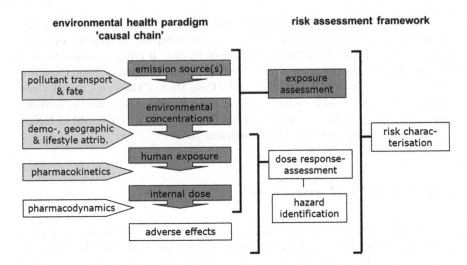

Fig. 5.2 Relationship between an environmental health paradigm and the risk assessment framework (modified after Sexton et al. 1995)

global burden of disease (GBD) studies (WHO 2002; Ezzati et al. 2004). It refers to the "systematic evaluation of the changes in population health which would result from modifying the population distribution of exposure to a risk factor or a group of risk factors" (Murray et al. 2003). It has a strong focus on population health outcomes and the attribution of risk factors to it—with environmental risk factors representing a small share of all risk factors considered.

Health risk assessment aims to provide the best and most objective scientific information about the risks of a specific situation by making empirically based predictions, and explaining observations. It characterizes options for risk control and is used for priority setting.

Risk assessment, at least in the field of environmental health and related disciplines, has evolved into a routine methodology. Today, it is nearly always understood as being quantitative at the core, but incorporating important qualitative features.

Risk assessment implies (see Fig. 5.2):

- Hazard identification (scientific group review, advisory committee process; qualitative in nature)
- Exposure assessment or evaluation (quantitative in nature)
- Dose–response assessment or evaluation (crucial role of assumptions about the shape of the dose–response curve, in particular on the existence or the absence of threshold; quantitative in nature)
- Risk characterization (quantitative and qualitative in nature)

In Chap. 2 these steps were already introduced. In this section, we go into more detail related to quantification issues.

Hazard Identification

This initial step is directed at identifying if an agent (risk factor) could cause particular adverse health effects in a population. In this stage the intrinsic properties of the particular agent are described. For example, will exposure to the agent cause cancer, or will it affect the liver or the nervous system? This qualitative task considers review of animal toxicity data, human data, and/or chemical structure information. Hazard identification is often conducted by scientific group review in advisory committee processes. An example is the classification of agents towards their carcinogenetic potential evaluated by the WHO International Agency for Research on Cancer (IARC). Other examples can be found in the so-called WHO toolkit for health risk assessment (IPCS 2010).

Exposure Assessment

Exposure assessment is the process by which (1) potentially exposed populations are identified, (2) potential pathways of exposure and exposure conditions are identified, and (3) chemical intakes or potential doses are quantified (US EPA 2004). In this process the magnitude, frequency, and duration of exposure to an agent are estimated or measured, along with the number and characteristics of the population exposed. Ideally, it describes the sources, pathways, routes, and uncertainties in the assessment (IPCS 2004). Traditionally seen as part of the risk assessment process, it now evolves into an own specialized field of exposure science (Lioy 2010).

Exposure can in short be described as "contact between an agent and a target" (IPCS 2004). The concepts of exposure and dose are closely related and are often used interchangeably. To distinguish between both, dose can be defined as the amount of an agent that enters the target in a specified time period after crossing a human contact boundary (skin, nose, or mouth). Exposure may occur by ingestion, inhalation, or dermal absorption routes (Fig. 5.3).

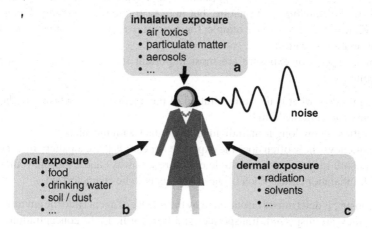

Fig. 5.3 Exposure routes

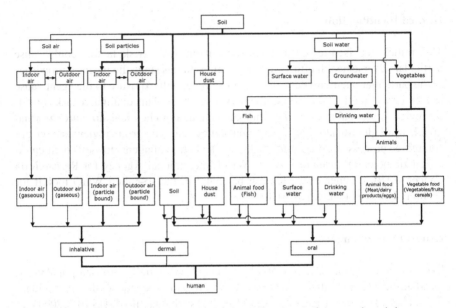

Fig. 5.4 Potential exposure pathways for an exposure assessment of a contaminated site

In order to determine the exposure, conceptual exposure models are instrumental in identifying potential source–pathway–receptor linkages. For example if the source of a chemical is an industrial plant, then several possible exposure pathways are (a) direct occupational exposure for workers, (b) inhalation from outdoor air exposure of the population living near the plant, and (c) deposition of airborne pollutants on local home-grown produce near the plant which could affect allotment gardeners who eat their own produce. Exposure pathways describe how a contaminant travels through the environment from its source to humans. Aspects to consider include the following: source of contamination, environmental media, point of exposure, receptor person or population, and route of exposure. All these elements are still qualitative in nature, but help to frame the exposure characterization. Figure 5.4 shows an example for potential exposure pathways in a land contamination situation.

Three aspects of exposure are most important for determining related health consequences:

- Magnitude—what is the concentration of the agent and the intake into the body of any carrying medium?
- Duration—how long is an individual in contact with the agent?
- Frequency—how often does the exposure appear? Is there a pattern of exposure? Exposure may occur via multiple exposure pathways and exposure routes (dermal, inhalation, oral). Each of these aspects is to be characterized.

Exposure is determined on one hand by the release of agents into the environments, where they are dispersed, transported, and transformed into concentrations in the environmental media, and on the other hand by exposure factors, which characterize the ways those persons come into contact with these agents (mobility, time–activity, consumption patterns, etc.).

Measurements

Techniques for measuring exposure can be indirect or direct. The most common techniques are indirect, which include sampling locations, where contact may occur with an agent, and/or application of survey instruments like (time or activity) questionnaires. Direct techniques comprise personal monitors worn by individuals, or samples of bodily fluids (e.g., urine, blood), which allow measurements of the exposure or the dose for individuals.

The indirect technique implies measuring the concentration of an agent found in an environmental medium at a single sampling site for a specific sampling period—in many cases, this is the only data available for an exposure assessment. Especially concentration measurements taken for regulatory purposes, e.g., air quality measurements conducted at fixed-site ambient air monitoring stations, are typical examples. Use of such measurements in risk assessment might result in high levels of uncertainty (Lioy 2009). Making use of concentration levels in the so-called microenvironments (typically a room, car, back yard, etc.) coupled with activity pattern data (e.g., the time spent in each microenvironment or activity) yields more accurate exposure information and is increasingly used for estimating population exposure distributions (Kruize et al. 2003).

Human exposure occurs in different places, in different settings, at different times, and for different durations. To address these aspects, exposure scenarios can help to develop estimates of exposure. An exposure scenario generally includes facts, data, assumptions, inferences, and—to some extent—professional judgment about how the exposure takes place. An exposure scenario provides the basis for building a mathematical exposure model for calculating population exposure estimates.

A generic equation for characterizing the integrated exposure is shown below. This equation is an exact expression of an individual's exposure, over the course of time, and the integration provides an approximate representation of exposure:

$$E_j = \int_{t1}^{t2} C_{j(t)} \, dt$$

where E_j is the integrated exposure of the jth individual to a concentration C of an agent for time period t_1 to t_2 associated with a biological response.

In practice, simpler equations are used like the generic equation describing a linear relationship between concentration in contact medium, contact frequency and duration, and adjustment for body weight. For each of the exposure pathways the exposure is calculated and summed up for the exposure routes (inhalation, ingestion, and dermal route) to obtain the aggregated exposure over all pathways and routes.

Table 5.1 Sources for exposure factor compendia

Location	Organization	Compendium name	Reference (url)
USA	The US Environmental Protection Agency (US EPA)	Exposure factors handbook (2011) Child specific exposure factors handbook (2008)	www.cfpub.epa.gov/ncea/cfm/ recordisplay. cfm?deid=20563
Europe	EC—Joint Research Centre (JRC)	ExpoFacts (2007) European exposure factor database	www.expofacts.jrc.ec.europa.eu
Germany	Federal Environment Agency (UBA)	RefXP (2011) German exposure factors database	www.uba.de/refxp

General linear equation:

$$E = \frac{C \times IR \times EF \times ED}{BW \times AT} \ mg/kg/day$$

where E is the exposure, C is the agent concentration (e.g., in drinking water: mg/ kg), IR is the ingestion rate (e.g., drinking water consumption: L/day), EF is the exposure frequency (days/year), ED is the exposure duration (years), BW is the body weight (kg), and AT is the averaging time (period over which the exposure is averaged) (days).

The exposure scenario is meant to describe all relevant exposure pathways. For each of these exposure pathways abovementioned linear equations are used. For each of the variables in the equation numerical input is necessary. Concerning the concentration variable, measurement or modeled values are used as input. The other nonchemical variables in the equation are referred to as "exposure factors." Exposure factors are generic or default values that describe contact rates with media, including inhalation rate, drinking-water consumption, food consumption, and soil ingestion. Exposure factors also include anthropometric features of persons, such as body weight and body surface area. These variables are often not available for the population under study, but can be taken from specific compendia (Table 5.1).

Depending on the purpose of the exposure assessment, exposure estimates may reflect the average exposure, peak exposure, or high-end exposures experienced by a small sample of the population. In chemical risk assessment, "conservative" exposure estimates which overestimate the exposure are often used in order to secure health protection.

Traditionally, point values for each of the exposure variables in the model are used: central tendency estimates like mean or median values for estimation of the average exposure for the population under study. For estimating high-end exposures, unfavorable values (e.g., >90th percentile, maximum value) for the exposure variables might be used as input. Here, a difficulty arises: the multiple use of such conservative input values might result in an unrealistic overestimation of the exposure.

To overcome this problem, the employment of distributions for exposure variables in the so-called probabilistic exposure assessments or distribution-based assessments may be used. Instead of a single point value, the statistical distribution for the variables are used in the model and by means of, e.g., Monte Carlo techniques, the exposure is calculated as a final output distribution, too. Distributional or probabilistic exposure assessment is nowadays more easy as several computer programs which can perform such simulations are available. Such assessments are, however, more time-consuming and not easy to evaluate by other assessors. The advantage is that they take into account all available (statistical) information, and deliver detailed information about the variability of the exposure estimate.

A key prerequisite for this kind of analysis is the provision of distributional information for the exposure factors. These and other issues concerning probabilistic exposure assessment were studied in the Xprob-project. Within this project, a database system "Reference values for exposure factors for the German population (RefXP)" was created, including highly detailed data on distributions for exposure factors (Mekel et al. 2007). Further guidance on distributional exposure assessment is compiled by IPCS (2008).

In the past, quantitative information from exposure measurements in epidemiological studies, e.g., concerning occupational pollutant exposure, was often reduced to categorical scale: "exposed yes/no." For exposure to the proximal factors, quantitative measurement devices are increasingly available. Exposure science now clearly moves towards higher levels of quantification. This includes the measurement of chemical and physical agents as well as other relevant parameters, e.g., time spent in various settings, food consumed, and a host of details concerning living area, occupation, and leisure time (Lioy 2009).

Exposure–Response or Dose–Response Assessment

This risk assessment component relates to the determination of the quantitative relation between the magnitude of exposure and the probability of occurrence of the specific endpoint of concern. The three laws of toxicology apply and are specified in this component in detail for the particular agent and induced health effect: (1) the dose makes the poison, (2) chemicals have specific effects, and (3) humans are animals. Two main types of exposure/dose–response curves are distinguished (Goldstein 2009):

- S-shaped curve, with threshold level; assumed to fit all toxic effects *except* those that are produced by direct reaction with genetic material.
- Linear line, no threshold level; covers endpoints caused by persistent changes in the gene (cancer, and inherited mutations).

These curves are normally identified in animal test studies for specific endpoints (e.g., nephrotoxic or cancer in a particular organ). For agents having toxic effects, the threshold level (the so-called no observed adverse effect level—NOAEL) is determined and then translated to effects in human populations. The usual approach is to apply one or more extrapolation factors (interspecies factor, intraspecies factor, and other factors; collectively also known as uncertainty or safety factors). Examples for such human dose specifications are acceptable daily intake (ADI), tolerable daily intake (TDI), reference dose (RfD), or reference concentration (RfC). Negative health effects are not expected to occur below these guidance levels or are assumed to be extremely unlikely in an exposed population.

In case of carcinogenic substances it is assumed that any single molecule of such a substance brings along the possibility of changing a normal cell into a cancerous cell. This implies that there is no safe dose (no threshold), i.e., the dose–response curve starts at zero dose. To extrapolate from observed animal data at high exposure levels to low exposure levels that are relevant for human exposure, multiple mathematical extrapolation models are available. A linearization towards zero is still the current working definition for these substances. Typical examples for human guidance estimates for carcinogenic compounds are unit risk, or unit dose or measures derived from these (e.g., TDI).

Risk Characterization

In the final stage of health risk assessment, the results from the first three components of the risk assessment framework are compiled in order to give an integrated, understandable, and comprehensive description of the predicted potential health effects and the strengths and limitations of the assessment. With regard to quantification, in this step the health effects are quantified by combining the exposure assessment results and the exposure–response results.

The estimated exposure to agents or substances having toxic effects is compared to the guidance values derived from the exposure–response assessment indicating the level of no concern. If the estimated exposure is higher than the guidance value, a health risk is seen to exist. If the estimated exposure is lower, no health risk is to be expected. So in case of toxic agents, the prediction will result in a yes/no answer with regard to the likelihood of a potential health risk.

For carcinogenic agents the combination of exposure and exposure–response assessment results in a different way of expressing health effects. The effects are expressed as the excess cancer mortality (number of people dying of cancer) assuming estimated exposure levels during the lifetime of the population. These risk estimates may be interpreted as more precise than for toxic agents, but in reality, this is not the case. The quantitative estimation of the health effects is only one aspect of the risk characterization component. Considerations about the quality of data, the amount of available evidence, the level of uncertainty in the assessment, as well as other strengths and limitations of the assessment are key elements of this risk assessment component (US EPA 2000; DoH WA—Department of Health and Western Australia 2006; NRC 2009).

In summary, risk assessment faces at least the following major challenges:

- Choosing the appropriate exposure metric.
- Estimating (levels of) future exposures.

- Decision on existence of a threshold below which there is no change in risk.
- Decision on shape of dose–response function: linear? exponential?
- Adequate extrapolation, decision on "safety factors."
- Handling of potential synergism, antagonism.
- Handling of multiple sources of uncertainty.

Uncertainty is a key feature of several of these items.

As pointed out by Schwartz et al. (2011), typical risk assessments for chemical contaminants often make implicit assumptions that simplify the risk assessment, but sometimes fail. These assumptions include the following: risk independence, risk averaging, risk non-transferability, risk synchrony, and risk accumulation.

As mentioned before, in parallel to the risk assessment for chemical contaminants, CRA emerged in the framework of the GBD study (WHO 2002; Ezzati et al. 2004). This framework also uses the risk assessment components of exposure assessment and exposure–response assessments. The starting points of these assessments, however, are not the chemicals or the respective exposures but the health outcomes. Determining what proportion of the BoD (health outcomes) is attributable to a specific risk factor (be it chemicals or other proximal factors) is at the core of this assessment. Epidemiological information and evidence are key in this type of assessment.

Originally the BoD studies focused on describing the mortality and morbidity adequately in a comparable way for all countries around the world. This requires the compilation of health information mainly based on health statistics in a harmonized and intelligent way. In subsequent steps, the attribution of the exposure towards particular risk factors resulting in specific BoD was added. This comparative risk assessment approach is increasingly explored also for use in different contexts of health assessments, e.g., health reporting and HIA.

In BoD, estimates of the years of life lost (YLL), years lived with disability (YLD), as well as DALY as well as number of attributable cases are typical quantitative estimates. Central in estimating the attributable fraction of the BoD related to one risk factor is the calculation of the population attributable fraction (PAF) resulting from information about the dose–response assessment and the exposure assessment.

The attributable burden is estimated by the PAF: The proportional reduction in population disease or mortality that would occur if exposed to a risk factor was reduced to an alternative ideal exposure scenario. The BoD (expressed, e.g., as number of deaths or as DALYs) attributed to a risk factor is quantified by applying the PAF to the total number of deaths or the total BoD (WHO 2009a). The equation for calculating PAF is shown here:

$$PAF = \frac{\int_{x=0}^{m} RR(x)P(x)dx - \int_{x=0}^{m} RR(x)P'(x)dx}{\int_{x=0}^{m} RR(x)P(x)dx}$$

where $RR(x)$ = relative risk at each exposure level, $P(x)$ = proportion of population at each exposure level, $P'(x)$ = counterfactual proportion of population at each exposure level, and m = maximum exposure level.

Estimation of Future Impacts

This section looks at top-down analysis (cf. above), i.e., moving "forward" through the causal chain, starting with policies and moving towards health effects.

Epidemiology is usually concerned with describing and analyzing past experiences. For a prospective assessment of future impacts, the situation is inherently different. To anticipate such future impacts of policies, existing knowledge needs to be utilized in a specific way. Direct observation and analysis are obviously not feasible. In some cases, it may be possible to apply existing knowledge by straightforward analogy or extrapolation. Often, however, this is not possible. In these cases, a detailed understanding of the "mechanics" involved is required to come up with reasonable (conditional) projections or predictions.

There are established ways in science to utilize existing knowledge for such conditional statements and/or predictions. One way is the reliance on expert assessment, e.g., panel of experts issuing statements. Another way is reliance on explicit models.

Throughout the development of HIA, both qualitative and quantitative evidence has been valued as a relevant contribution (Mindell et al. 2001; Joffe and Mindell 2002; McCarthy and Utley 2004; Mindell and Barrowcliffe 2005; Mindell and Joffe 2005; Veerman et al. 2005, 2007; Briggs 2008; Bronnum-Hansen 2009; O'Connell and Hurley 2009; Lhachimi et al. 2010; Bhatia and Seto 2011; Committee on Health Impact Assessment, National Research Council of the National Academies 2011; Kemm 2013). Obviously, to span the full range from policy to health outcome is not a trivial task. Success or failure, to a large extent, depends on the availability of both valid data and appropriate methods.

Veerman et al. (2005) defined quantification, for this context, as the expression in numerical terms of the change in health status of a specific population that can be attributed to a specific policy decision. In a study based on published literature they identified ten (categories of) determinants for which quantified health outcomes were presented, including carcinogens, particulate matter, road transport (vehicle kilometers), employment, income, alcohol, smoking, physical activity, housing, and infectious diseases. It was found that in most studies, the risk measures were derived from epidemiological research, while in three studies toxicological risk measures (derived from animal experiments) were used.

Given the scope of issues encountered on the way from policies to health outcome, the authors divided it into two steps, labeled "exposure impact assessment" and "outcome assessment," respectively. The methods used to estimate effects of policies on determinants of health, not surprisingly, were found to be quite diverse. This was seen to reflect the diversity in factors that influence health. For physical and chemical factors methods seemed well developed, and also for traffic flows and accident rates models were found available. However, few socioeconomic and behavioral determinants were seen quantified up to the level of health outcomes, probably due to the lack of a stable evidence base. Since socioeconomic and behavioral determinants—unlike physical and chemical substances—are context dependent, the evidence is only to a limited extent generalizable across time and space. Therefore, the degree of standardization achieved in environmental HIA was seen as hard to match in HIA that focuses on other policy areas (Veerman et al. 2005).

The appropriate combination of quantitative and qualitative evidence can be seen as a characteristic feature of HIA (O'Connell and Hurley 2009). In particular, the deployment of different scenarios contributes to the usefulness. As Veerman et al. (2005) point out, for "policies that are broadly formulated, or where there is much uncertainty over trends and future developments, the analysis of a number of scenarios might be more informative than a single estimate of the most probable impact. This permits various assumptions to be made without losing scientific credibility, and may convey to decision makers an understanding of the dynamics of the mechanics described by the model."

Quantification may lead end users in the wrong direction. O'Connell and Hurley (2009) underline that "the production of a single estimate, or range of estimates, for the likely health impacts of decisions or actions can obscure the complexities and uncertainties that underlie these figures." Nevertheless, the authors assume that "the development of evidence and methods can and will extend the legitimate range of quantified HIA."

Quantification in Top-Down RAPID Guidance

Quantification aspects are addressed at multiple stages in the RAPID guidance (see Chaps. 3 and 4). Table 5.2 summarizes key items with regard to quantification extracted from the checklist of the RAPID guidance for top-down analysis.

Quantification in Top-Down RAPID Case Studies

Within the RAPID project, several top-down case studies applied various methods of quantification. As shown in Table 5.3, these were case studies from Hungary, Germany, and Romania.

In the *Hungarian* case study the disease burden of active and passive smoking was calculated for a baseline situation (year 2006) and for a future scenario after the health impact of the proposed tightening of the anti-smoking policy realizes. The exposure assessment was based on observed reduction in active smoking and in environmental tobacco smoke (ETS) exposure after banning smoking in closed public places in other countries. Information sources were chosen based on cultural similarities between societies and by favoring sources reporting lower effect sizes to avoid overestimation. The model considered exposure reduction only among non-smokers, separately for workplaces, catering venues, and homes. For those exposed

Table 5.2 Quantification items extracted from checklist of the RAPID guidance for top-down analysis

	Key items concerning quantification
• Policy	• Identify performance and outcome indicators in the policy • List information sources to do the assessment and description
• (Wider) Determinants of health	• Consider size of population affected, severity of health effects • Consider feasibility of assessment in a quantitative way • Assess interactions between health determinants • List information sources used to make the assessment and description
• Risk factors	• Consider size of exposure change influenced by the policy, size of population affected, severity of related health outcomes • Consider feasibility of quantitative exposure assessment (availability of applicable exposure measures, numerical information on the baseline level/prevalence of exposure and on the expected change of exposure related to policy implementation)/quantitative assessment by calculating frequency (prevalence) or level (dose, concentration) of exposure • Describe exposed population and exposure pattern in different population groups (equity) • Assess exposure • Assess interaction between risk factors
• Health outcomes	• Consider strength of evidence for causality, severity (morbidity, disability, and mortality), reversibility, and frequency of occurrence in the population • Identify populations affected with special attention to susceptible subgroups (equity) • Consider availability and validity of baseline frequency data of the health condition and of dose/exposure–response functions applying dose–response coefficients or relative risk estimates • Assess change in health outcomes/quantitative assessment by calculating simple frequency measures (e.g., morbidity, hospitalization, mortality) or measures of disease burden (attributable death, potential years of life lost, and disability-adjusted life years); give preference to complex disease burden measures (e.g., disability-adjusted life years) if available and feasible • Determine cost related to health outcome if possible

to ETS in more than one location, the location with the smallest exposure reduction was applied. The outcome assessment was based on the methodology of the WHO GBD study, 2004 (WHO 2008). Age- and sex-specific prevalence rates of exposure from a population-based study and association measures from publications providing high-degree evidence were used to calculate population attributable risk fractions (PAF). Attributable death (AD) was determined using age- and sex-specific mortality rates.

To estimate the complex measure of DALY, potential YLL were calculated with age- and sex-specific Hungarian life expectancies and YLD were determined using WHO age-specific disability weights for treated cases (WHO 2008). The DisMod II software (version 1.01) provided by the WHO was used to estimate the average duration lived with a disease, as these data were not readily available. Cause- , age-,

Table 5.3 Quantification issues in selected top-down RAPID case studies

Policy	Wider determinants of health	Risk factors, other proximate factors	Health outcome	Results, comments
Tobacco policy, Hungary—Proposal for the amendment of Act No XLII of 1999 on the protection of non-smokers and on certain rules of consumption and trade of tobacco products	**Substance use** **Air quality** Built environment and land use Working environment and housing conditions Income and social status Employment and working conditions Social contacts Culture Recreation	**Active smoking** **Environmental tobacco smoke exposure** Property value Family expenses, income of the tobacco industry, government income Employment and turnover of the catering industry Exclusion of smokers Improved conditions for recreation	**Chronic respiratory diseases** **Coronary heart diseases** **Stroke** **Lung cancer** **Other smoking-related cancers** Mental diseases	Quantified annual health gain is estimated to be **1,685 attributable deaths and 21,936 DALYs** in long term. The reduction in environmental tobacco smoke exposure has a higher contribution than decreased prevalence of active smoking. The consideration of the uncertainty of input data related to, e.g., validity or limitations of extrapolation is critical for the scientifically sound assessment of health risks of policies.

(continued)

Table 5.3 (continued)

Policy	Wider determinants of health	Risk factors, other proximate factors	Health outcome	Results, comments
Housing subsidy program, Germany — North Rhine-Westphalia Housing Subsidy Programme for 2010 (*Wohnraumförderungsprogramm* 2010, circular order IV.4-250-01/10)	**Housing**	Thermal comfort Indoor air quality Noise **Environmental barriers Home safety and accidents** Social and physical quality of the housing and the immediate environment	Respiratory diseases (general symptoms, asthma, lung cancer) Mental health (depression and anxiety) **Injuries (fall, hip fracture, death due to hip fracture)**	Potentially **3,110 to 7,257 hip fractures and 622 to 1,451 deaths resulting from hip fractures** could have been avoided in the year 2009, if all homes of people aged 65 years and older in North Rhine-Westphalia were barrier-free. In case of lacking observational data, the application of a wide range for the exposure-response function based on expert judgement provides a feasible way to construct the model of assessment.

	Social and economic factors Fixed determinants Access to services	**Pandemic influenza infection** **Hospitalization due to pandemic influenza infection** **Death due to pandemic influenza infection**	Estimates for the decrease in **influenza death-related disease burden from status quo (5195 YLL65) to alternative policy 1 (13387 YLL65) and to alternative policy 2 (11535 YLL65).**
Pandemic influenza plan, Romania—Policy for preventing and limiting illness A/H1N1, Romanian Ministry of Health (order nr. 1094/10.09.2009) Policy alternative of proactive school closure Policy alternative of increasing vaccination rate	Lack of supplies and medical care Wage losses, unemployment Self-isolation lifestyle, loneliness Ageing Children under 6 months old cannot be vaccinated Elderly have priority on vaccination Education/health services/ transport Lack of education and lack of school lunch and breakfast program No access to healthcare services Internal and international travel restriction		Feasibility and effectiveness of policy implementation are important factors to be considered when assessing policy effect.

In *bold*: Elements of the causal pathway that were considered in the quantification process and sex-specific incidence, prevalence, and mortality rates, as well as age- and sex-specific population numbers and all-cause mortality rates, served as input variables for DisMod computation. The standard 3 % discount rate was used without age-weighting in the calculation of DALY. The study was able to determine the above-described measures of disease burden of both active and passive smoking for four diseases of public health importance: lung cancer, chronic obstructive respiratory diseases, coronary heart diseases, and stroke. In addition, quantitative assessment of burden of active smoking was feasible for arterial diseases and 12 additional types of cancer.

The *German* case study assessed the housing program's theoretical effect of making all homes barrier free in North Rhine-Westphalia on falls, consequent hip fracture, and death in the population aged 65 years and older. The exposure assessment estimated the number of persons aged 65 years and older living in homes with barriers in North Rhine-Westphalia, using population statistics and information from the literature. The number of falls at home, the resulted hip fractures, and the consequent deaths were calculated in the outcome assessment based on literature reports about the frequency of falls among the elderly, the proportion of falls leading to hip fracture, and the proportion of hip fractures resulting in death within one year.

The *Romanian* case study compared the effectiveness of the 2009 Romanian pandemic influenza preparedness plan on preventing pandemic influenza infection and related hospitalization and death to that of two policy alternatives based on proactive school closure and on increased vaccination rate. The baseline scenario (status quo) was determined using official national data of the AH1N1 influenza pandemic in 2009–2010 and raw data on hospitalizations collected through sentinel surveillance system. The study estimated four measures of the impact: total number of cases, hospitalizations, deaths, and years of potential life lost by the age of 65 (YLL65). The impact was analyzed for the policy of proactive school closure with the assumption of having a direct effect on virus transmission in the school age population and an indirect effect on the inter-age group transmission resulting in a drop in the number of pandemic influenza cases. Assumed reduction in infected and hospitalized cases among children and adults, as well as no effect on mortality, was used to estimate the impact of increasing vaccination rate to achieve 50 % coverage among children.

Estimation of Prevention Potentials

In contrast with the previous section, now we look at bottom-up analysis, i.e., we move "backwards" through the causal chain, starting with health effects and moving towards policies.

Again, to span the full range is not a trivial task. Just as in top-down analyses, success or failure to a large extent depends on the availability of both valid data and appropriate methods. As pointed out in Sect. "Estimation of Future Impacts",

Table 5.4 Quantification items extracted from the checklist of the RAPID guidance for bottom-up analysis

	Key items concerning quantification
• Health outcomes	• Provide available/accessible epidemiological/population health data (incidence, prevalence, hospitalization, etc.) and describe the source of data (international, national, regional, local statistics) • Consider availability and validity of baseline frequency data of the health condition and of dose/exposure–response functions applying dose–response coefficients or relative risk estimates • Consider frequency of occurrence in the population • Set objectives and define what kind of change (nature and size of it) would be desirable in occurrence of health outcome • Quantitative assessment by calculating simple frequency measures (e.g., morbidity, hospitalization, mortality) or measures of disease burden (attributable death, potential years of life lost, and disability-adjusted life years); give preference to complex disease burden measures (e.g., disability-adjusted life years) if available and feasible
• Risk factors	• Consider significance of induced health effects (size of exposure change influenced by the policy, size of population affected, severity of related health outcomes) • Consider feasibility of quantitative exposure assessment (availability of applicable exposure measures, numerical information on the baseline level/prevalence of exposure and on the expected change of exposure related to policy implementation) • Describe exposed population and exposure pattern in different population groups (equity) • Assess exposure/quantitative assessment by calculating frequency (prevalence) or level (dose, concentration) of exposure • If direct exposure measures are not available, use proxy measures • Assess interaction between risk factors
• (Wider) Determinants of health	• Consider importance of effect (size of population affected, severity of health effects, costs involved), feasibility of assessment favorably in a quantitative way • Assess interactions between health determinants
• Policy	

quantification can obscure the underlying complexities and uncertainties. Again, it is hoped that, over time, adequate evidence and robust methods will increasingly become available to support this line of analysis.

Quantification in Bottom-Up RAPID Guidance

In the RAPID guidance for bottom-up analysis, numerous quantification issues are addressed (see Chap. 4). Table 5.4 summarizes key items with regard to quantification extracted from the checklist of the RAPID guidance for bottom-up analysis.

Quantification in Bottom-Up RAPID Case Studies

Within the RAPID project, several bottom-up case studies applied various methods of quantification. For selected case studies from Spain, Germany, and Hungary, these are shown in Table 5.5.

The *Spanish* case study addressed the prospective quantification of possible reductions in road traffic fatalities (RTF) by assuming different exposure scenarios related to the use of the safety belt as a protective factor, which in turn could be promoted by the implementation of a policy (e.g., the penalty point system—PPS). In spite of the fact of the many steps undertaken across Europe to improve road safety, much still needs to be done if rising trend in RTF is to be halted or reversed (WHO 2009b). The European Road Safety Observatory (ERSO) reported that road traffic accidents during the year 2006 accounted for 0.96 % of total deaths within EU (estimations made for 19 Member States, using data from 2006), 1.10 % being the case of Spain (ERSO 2008).

The definition used in this case study for the health outcome (RTF) was the one proposed by the United Nations Economic Commission for Europe: "any person killed immediately or dying within 30 days as a result of an injury accident" (WHO 2004 p. 58).

The baseline scenario was determined using official RTF national data by subgroups for the year 2006 (prior to the implementation of PPS), obtained from the Spanish Traffic Authority's annual report (Ministerio del Interior 2006). In such reports, some inconsistent use of definitions may occur: some tables and figures provided data adjusted to the European definition for RTF (victims killed immediately or dying within 30 days of the crash), while others show direct police records presented as crash-deaths at 24 h.

The dose–response function referring to the effectiveness of the use of safety belts in preventing car occupants from being killed in a road traffic accident and the calculation method were obtained by a literature review. Two possible exposure scenarios were defined and estimated: (1) safety seat belt wearing rate registered in 2006 (pre-PPS policy implementation) for drivers of light vehicles and (2) improvement of the percentage of those wearing seat belts to the maximum possible rate (99 %). This approach excludes possible interactions with other risk factors and health determinants; therefore several assumptions needed to be defined.

From a policy risk assessment perspective, the correct characterization of exposure to different risk factors, adjusted also to specific scenarios (concrete areas and affected populations), is very important. Only in this way it will be possible to quantify a health gain if changes in the level of exposure to those risk factors could be predicted as the result of certain measures being put in place. At present this type of approach in the field of road traffic accidents are not straightforward. The European project SafetyNet addresses the difficulties in gathering information on RTF risk factors, and details the methodologies for countries to improve data collection in a uniform manner across the EU (Yannis and Papadimitriou 2005; Hakkert and Gitelman 2007).

Table 5.5 Quantification issues in selected bottom-up RAPID case studies

Case study	Health outcome	Risk factors, other proximate factors	Wider determinants of health	Policies	Results, comments
Traffic accidents, Spain	Road traffic fatalities	**Use of the safety seat belt** (protective factor)	Individual risk behavior	– Penalty Point System – Supporting education, communication, training, and public awareness	Potentially **1,500 RTF** could have been prevented among drivers of light vehicles in non-urban roads in Spain during 2006 by using properly the safety belt, assuming that the rest of risk factors remain equal Improving data collection referring to risk factors and social health determinants adjusted to specific scenarios is a critical step for optimizing policy risk assessment related to road traffic accidents
Road traffic injuries, Germany	Road traffic injuries	Age, sex; driving experience, driving style, **speeding**; physical, mental impairment, **road environment factors**	Socioeconomic factors, social attitudes Region	– Introduction of speed limits – Establishment of speed detection devices	Between **2,700 and 4,400 fatalities and serious injuries** could be avoided by implementing in NRW the speed control system. **Up to 5 lives** could be saved annually if specific speed limits are introduced in NRW Evidence-based study results on the effect of speed surveillance on RTI would improve the quantitative characterization of health impacts of various road safety policy options

(continued)

Table 5.5 (continued)

Case study	Health outcome	Risk factors, other proximate factors	Wider determinants of health	Policies	Results, comments
Chronic liver disease, Hungary	Chronic liver disease and cirrhosis	**Alcohol consumption** **Age, gender**	Substance use Socioeconomic status, education, income, employment Culture, recreation	– Regulation of the alcohol market – Addressing the availability of alcohol – Targeting illegal production and sale – Supporting the reduction of harm in drinking and the surrounding environments – Reducing drinking and driving – Supporting education, communication, training, and public awareness – Interventions for individuals with harmful alcohol consumption and alcohol dependence	**1,439 lives and over 28,500 DALYs could be saved** annually in Hungary, if all heavy drinkers reduced their alcohol consumption under 60 g/day The improvement of monitoring systems that can provide valid data on alcohol consumption and related harms as well as quantitative data on policy effect are needed in order to optimize the characterization of policy alternatives

In *bold*: Elements of the causal pathway that were considered in the quantification process

The *German* case study intends to provide policy makers with evidence-based arguments for moving forward in taking actions that would more efficiently reduce traffic accidents and their health consequences. For doing so, a quantitative predictions of road traffic injuries (RTI) being preventable is conducted regarding changes in exposure scenarios related to speeding (second most frequent crash cause outside built-up areas in Germany) as a result of the proposed implementation of two policy measures: the introduction of speed limits and the establishment of speed detection devices.

The health outcome used in this case, RTI, included RTF as described previously in the Spanish experience, plus seriously and slightly injured persons in a road traffic crash. The health data used for quantification corresponded to the RTI for the year 2009 provided by the statistics agency of North Rhine-Westphalia (IT.NRW 2010), stratified by type of road (motorways, country road, and roads in built-up areas). The quantitative dose–response functions corresponding to the effectiveness of the introduction of the two policy actions were obtained from literature reviews (WHO 2004; Wilson et al. 2009). In the case of the introduction of speed limits, the exposure scenarios considered were based on shifts to lower speed limits (i.e., from 130 to 120 km/h in motorways); the estimation of the health impacts included only fatal road traffic injuries as dose–response functions for nonfatal injuries were not available. For the effectiveness of speed control devices, the exposure scenarios proposed were implementation of systems versus no implementation, and the health impact quantification did not differentiate between various types of roads, as the evidence on the dose–response relationship was not available.

The *Hungarian* case study analyzed policy options that can reduce the disease burden of chronic liver disease and cirrhosis (ICD-10: K74) attributable to alcohol consumption. The quantitative assessment modeled the exposure change required to achieve the arbitrary target of 20 % reduction in alcohol-related cirrhosis mortality. Baseline values were determined for 2006 since data of cirrhosis morbidity and mortality as well as alcohol consumption volumes were available for that year. The large-scale meta-analysis by Rehm et al. (2010) provided relative risk values separately for morbidity and mortality by gender and exposure categories, which were determined as ranges of daily pure alcohol consumption in grams. The assessment was based on the calculation of population attributable risk fractions (PAF) that allowed for the assessment of disease burden measured in attributable death, and DALY. The quantification followed the methodology of the WHO GBD study, 2004 (WHO 2008). Potential YLL were determined using age- and sex-specific Hungarian life expectances in 2006. WHO age-specific disability weights for treated cases were applied to calculate YLD (WHO 2008). Since information on the average duration lived with cirrhosis was not readily available, these data were estimated using the DisMod II software (version 1.01) provided by the WHO. Age- and sex-specific incidence, prevalence, and mortality rates, as well as population numbers and all-cause mortality rates by sex and age groups of the total population, served as input variables for the computation. In the calculation of DALY, 3 % discount rate was applied without age-weighting.

Health Impact Quantification Tools

As indicated earlier, a suite of software tools supporting quantitative modeling has emerged. The tools incorporate mathematical models, i.e., equations describing the relationship between items of the causal web, including health determinants and health outcomes. Such models exist in both the environmental health and the general public health arena.

For input, the tools require information on the initial status of the system, and the expected changes concerning selected variables. For output, they generate estimates of changes in health. The required data input tends to be extensive.

According to Lhachimi et al. (2010), a standard tool for quantification in HIA should be able to quantify the baseline situation (population health without intervention) and then quantify changes resulting from one or more policy options.

In environmental health, current "flagship" projects—especially INTARESE[1] and HEIMTSA[2]—aim at "full-chain" modeling where the full chain is meant to start with policy options and extends all the way to health outcomes and possibly also subsequent monetization. In general public health, e.g., DYNAMO-HIA,[3] modeling tends to be limited to the route from risk (or protective) factor to health outcome.

A synoptic view of seven selected software tools for quantitative impact modeling is given in Table 5.6.

The majority of the tools were developed to be applied in the field of public health. Only HEIMTSA/INTARESE incl. ICT were established in an environmental health context. The BoD/environmental burden of disease (EBD) approach can be applied in both contexts.

This multitude of sophisticated, scientifically well-founded models and tools are developed in the scientific arena and are available for free. Some models can directly be downloaded from the Web whereas others require a simple user request (e.g., PREVENT, HEIMTSA/INTARESE for the Resource Center). The Health Forecasting Tool is hosted at the University of California in Los Angeles and models predictions of population health on request.

PREVENT and DYNAMO-HIA are stand-alone tools, which means that they do not require any other software to run. ICT can work as a stand-alone tool too, but advanced users would like to make full use of the tool and for this Analytica© is needed. ICT is part of the HEIMTSA/INTARESE toolbox, which furthermore provides a platform with an integrated set of further stand-alone modules. WHO offers spreadsheet templates and the stand-alone DISMOD software for calculation of the population BoD, expressed, e.g., in DALY.

DYNAMO-HIA and PREVENT contain integrated databases on a range of risk factors and disease, whereas all other tools are "empty-shells" which need

---

[1] Integrated Assessment of Health Risks of Environmental Stressors in Europe.

[2] Health and Environment Integrated Methodology and Toolbox for Scenario Assessment.

[3] Dynamic Modeling for Health Impact Assessment.

Table 5.6 Selected HIQ tools

Tool name	Outline	Reference/www.
• BoD/EBD	• Comprehensive and comparable assessment of mortality and loss of health due to diseases and injuries in populations. Calculates estimates of premature mortality, disability, and loss of health attributable to risk factors	http://www.who.int/healthinfo/ global_burden_disease/ http://www.who.int/ quantifying_ehimpacts/en/
• DYNAMO-HIA	• Predicts health impacts of changes in risk factor exposure on population health due to policies or interventions. The generic and dynamic model is based on scenario building and partially micro simulation	www.dynamo-hia.eu
• Health Forecasting	• Models future scenarios of lifetime health histories of a population by projecting disease and mortality rates into the future taking into account different assumptions and policy options. Developed for Californian population	www.health-forecasting.org
• ICT	• Quantifies health impacts from environmental exposures. It applies dynamic life-table modeling for calculating target population-specific mortality and morbidity impacts. Multiple scenarios can be specified and run simultaneously	http://en.opasnet.org/w/ Impact_calculation_tool
• INTARESE/ HEIMTSA	• The toolbox consists of a Guidance System (online textbook and tutorial system) and a Resource Center: an eclectic set of tools (models, datasets, risk functions) for dealing with HIA aspects in each stage in the full chain	www.integrated-assessment.eu
• Prevent	• A multiple risk factor, multiple disease dynamic population model that allows evaluation of the benefits of risk factor interventions	www.eurocadet.org; www.epigear.com

substantial input data to determine risk factors, diseases, and relationships. The HEIMTSA/INTARESE toolbox provides a platform with an integrated set of stand-alone modules which are linked to datasets. Typical input data needed for all these models include, e.g., population data for overall mortality; birth rates; incidence, prevalence, and mortality for relevant diseases by age and sex; risk factor exposure or prevalence by age and sex; and effects of interventions.

A full-chain modeling is offered by the HEIMTSA/INTARESE tool providing several models for each step of the causal pathway. The effects of the policies on health determinants can be modeled as well as the impact of changes in health determinants on health outcomes. A monetarization step may complete the full chain approach. Other models like DYNAMO-HIA and PREVENT focus on the effect of changes in risk factor exposure on health outcomes. The effect of a policy (plan, program, project) on a risk factor/health outcome is merely not part of the models, needs to be defined outside of these models, and is used as input for expected change of the risk factor exposures.

DYNAMO-HIA and HEIMTSA/INTARESE, incl. ICT, are developed specifically for investigating change, and others (e.g., BoD) by running the model under different conditions.

As each policy risk assessment or HIA is different, framing of the issues and questions of the considered policy as well as defining and characterizing the impact chains will vary as well. Considering the complexity of HIA, there is no "one-size-fits-all" software model. None of the models can be regarded as a standard HIA quantification tool applicable to every situation.

Profound knowledge of the underlying epidemiological concepts is implied, as the majority of the tools focus on epidemiological measures such as mortality, incidence, and prevalence. In order to apply the models and interpret the results correctly, good epidemiological proficiency is inevitable. For the models focusing on environmental health, users need substantiated knowledge of environmental health exposure assessment.

Efforts towards quantitative modeling of the "full chain" of causal events now have reached remarkable levels of sophistication. Cross-project debate, however, up to now is still rather limited (Fehr and Mekel 2010).

In a recent attempt to take stock of such tools, and moving the debate forward, it was found that currently, further tool development is not the overriding priority. Although several aspects (health inequalities, uncertainties) do need consideration, main current challenges refer to comparative evaluation of different tools with regard to their range of application, face validity, and end-user satisfaction. Such evaluations should be carried out in realistic conditions, where the health impact question comes from policy makers. Also challenging is the maintenance and continued availability of the toolkits, including updating their data contents. For these tools to be widely used, they should also be publicly available in a form that allows users to apply the tool without (too much) help from its developers. Developing an adequate framework for sustainability of health impact quantification toolkits is another priority for the near future (Fehr et al. 2012).

Conclusions

In risk assessment, quantification seems indispensable, and the question is not "if" but only "how" it should be applied. On the contrary, in a current debate which is fueled in part by equity considerations, the need is seen to abandon traditional dichotomous risk characterization approaches and to extend quantification.

Concerning HIA, the situation is different. Both advantages and disadvantages can be identified. In the view of many, quantitative information supports the thorough understanding of relevant phenomena and might help to reach a new and improved quality of science–policy interaction.

As Veerman et al. (2005) point out, "knowing the size of an effect helps decision makers to distinguish between the details and the main issues that need to be addressed and facilitates decision making by clarifying the trade offs that may be entailed."

According to Kemm (2013) magnitude of impact is preferably described in quantitative terms wherever possible. Trade-offs between options are easier when magnitude is precisely described, and decision-makers are more likely to be influenced when the impacts are quantified.

Quantification can be seen to serve the following purposes:

- Fullest usage of information available.
- Allowing for detailed comparisons, incl. priorities and trade-offs.
- Enabling to build, apply, and evaluate predictive models.
- Adding weight to arguments, both within and beyond the professional field.

When summary measures of population health are applied, this can help to integrate preventive and curative efforts by providing a common metric for "preventive" and "treatment" results.

Undoubtedly, however, there are also disadvantages of impact quantification, including the following: quantitative estimates incorporate numerous value- and model-based assumptions that are not always made explicit; they may give an unwarranted patina of robust science; and they may de-emphasize, or even omit, stakeholder participation (Fehr and Mekel 2013).

HIA and quantification are key tasks for public health and likely to even gain in importance. They represent some of the most demanding and potentially rewarding activities at the science–policy interface and are highly relevant for health policy-making at all levels. It is important that the public health community continues exploring and utilizing health impact quantification (Fehr et al. 2012).

References

ACS—American Chemical Society (1998). Understanding risk analysis. A short guide for health, safety, and environmental policy making. ACS and Resources for the Future: Center for Risk Management(RFF), Internet edition. http://www.rff.org/rff/publications/upload/14418_1.pdf. Accessed 2 April 2013

ATSDR/Agency for Toxic Substances and Disease Registry (2005) Public Health Assessment Guidance Manual (update). Atlanta: U.S. Department of Health and Human Services—Agency for Toxic Substances and Disease Registry

Bhatia, R., & Seto, E. (2011). Quantitative estimation in Health Impact Assessment: opportunities and challenges. *Environmental Impact Assessment Review, 31*, 301–309.

Briggs, D.J. (2008). A framework for integrated environmental health impact assessment of systemic risks. Environmental Health 7:61. doi:10.1186/1476-069X-7-61. Available from: http://www.ehjournal.net/content/7/1/61

Bronnum-Hansen, H. (2009). Quantitative health impact assessment modeling. *Scandinavian Journal of Public Health, 37*, 447–449.

Committee on Health Impact Assessment, National Research Council of the National Academies. (2011). *Improving health in the United States. The role of Health Impact Assessment.* Washington, DC: The National Academies Press.

Corvalán, C., Briggs, D., & Kjellström, T. (1996). Development of environmental health indicators. In D. Briggs, C. Corvalán, & M. Nurminen (Eds.), *Linkage methods for environment and health analysis: general guidelines. A report of the health and environment analysis for decision-making (HEADLAMP) project* (pp. 19–53). Geneva: United Nations Environment Programme, United States Environmental Protection Agency, World Health Organization.

Ministerio del Interior—Dirección general de Tráfico (2006). Anuario estadístico de accidentes. NIPO: 128-07-049-4. http://www.dgt.es/portal/es/seguridad_vial/estadistica/publicaciones/anuario_estadistico. Accessed 14 April 2013

DoH WA—Department of Health, Government of Western Australia (2006). Health Risk Assessment in Western Australia. http://www.public.health.wa.gov.au/cproot/1499/2/Health_Risk_Assessment.pdf. Accessed 2 April 2013

ERSO—European Road Safety Observatory (2008). SafetyNet—Annual statistical report 2008 based on CARE European Road Accident Database. http://ec.europa.eu/transport/wcm/road_safety/erso/safetynet/fixed/WP1/2008/SafetyNet%20Annual%20Statistical%20Report%20 2008.pdf. Accessed 14 April 2013

Ezzati, M., Lopez, A. D., Rodgers, A., & Murray, C. J. L. (Eds.). (2004). *Comparative quantification of health risks. Global and regional burden of disease attributable to selected major risk factors.* Geneva: World Health Organization.

Fehr, R., Hurley, F., Mekel, O. C., & Mackenbach, J. P. (2012). Quantitative health impact assessment: taking stock and moving forward. *Journal of Epidemiology and Community Health, 66*(12), 1088–1091.

Fehr, R., & Mekel, O. (Eds.) (2010). Quantifying the health impacts of policies—principles, methods, and models. Report of a scientific expert workshop (Düsseldorf, Germany, 16–17 March 2010). Landesinstitut für Gesundheit und Arbeit des Landes Nordrhein-Westfalen (LIGA. NRW). http://www.lzg.gc.nrw.de/_media/pdf/liga-fokus/LIGA_Fokus_11.pdf

Fehr, R., & Mekel, O. (2013). Health Impact Assessment (HIA) in Germany. In J. Kemm (Ed.), *Past achievement, current understanding, and future progress in Health Impact Assessment* (pp. 156–167). Oxford, UK: Oxford University Press. Chapter 17.

Goldstein, B. D. (2009). Toxicology and risk assessment in the analysis and management of environmental risk. Ch. 8.7. In R. Detels, R. Beaglehole, M. A. Lansang, & M. Gulliford (Eds.), *Oxford textbook of public health. The methods of public health* (Vol. 2, pp. 931–939). Oxford, UK: Oxford University Press.

Hakkert, A.S., & Gitelman, V. (Eds.) (2007). Road Safety Performance Indicators: Manual. Deliverable D3.8 of the EU FP6 project SafetyNet. http://ec.europa.eu/transport/wcm/road_safety/erso/safetynet/fixed/WP3/sn_wp3_d3p8_spi_manual.pdf. Accessed 27 December 2010

Hill, A. B. (1965). The environment and disease: association or causation? *Proceedings of the Royal Society of Medicine, 58*(5), 295–300.

IPCS. (2004). IPCS glossary of key exposure assessment terminology. In IPCS (Ed.), *IPCS risk assessment terminology. IPCS Harmonization project document no. 1.* Geneva: World Health Organization.

IPCS. (2008). Guidance document on characterizing and communicating uncertainty in exposure assessment. In IPCS (Ed.), *Uncertainty and data quality in exposure assessment. IPCS harmonization project document no 6.* Geneva: World Health Organization.

IPCS. (2010). WHO Human Health Risk Assessment Toolkit: chemical hazards. In IPCS (Ed.), *Harmonization project document no. 8.* Geneva: World Health Organization.

IT.NRW—Information und Technik Nordrhein-Westfalen (2010). Statistische Berichte. Straßenverkehrsunfälle in Nordrhein-Westfalen 2009. IT.NRW: Düsseldorf. http://www.it.nrw.de

Joffe, M., & Mindell, J. (2002). A framework for the evidence base to support Health Impact Assessment. *Journal of Epidemiology and Community Health, 56*, 132–138.

Joffe, M., & Mindell, J. (2006). Complex causal process diagrams for analyzing the health impacts of policy interventions. *American Journal of Public Health, 96*, 473–479.

Kemm, J. (2013). Quantitative assessment. Ch. 3. In J. Kemm (Ed.), *Health Impact Assessment: past achievement, current understanding, and future progress* (pp. 25–37). Oxford, UK: Oxford University Press.

Kruize, H., Hänninen, O., Breugelmans, O., Lebret, E., & Jantunen, M. J. (2003). Description and demonstration of the EXPOLIS simulation model: two examples of modeling population exposure to particulate matter. *Journal of Exposure Analysis and Environmental Epidemiology, 13*, 87–99.

Lhachimi, S. K., Nusselder, W. J., Boshuizen, H. C., & Mackenbach, J. P. (2010). Standard tool for quantification in health impact assessment a review. *American Journal of Preventive Medicine, 38*(1), 78–84.

Lioy, P. J. (2009). The science of human exposures to contaminants in the environment. Ch. 8.4. In R. Detels, R. Beaglehole, M. A. Lansang, & M. Gulliford (Eds.), *Oxford Textbook of Public Health. The methods of public health* (Vol. 2, pp. 872–893). Oxford, UK: Oxford University Press.

Lioy, P. J. (2010 August). Exposure science: a view of the past and milestones for the future. *Environmental Health Perspectives, 118*(8), 1081–1090.

McCarthy, M., & Utley, M. (2004). Quantitative approaches to HIA. Ch. 6. In J. Kemm, J. Parry, & S. Palmer (Eds.), *Health impact assessment. Concepts, theory, techniques and applications* (pp. 61–70). Oxford: Oxford University Press.

McDowell, I. (2006). *Measuring health. A guide to rating scales and questionnaires* (3rd ed.). Oxford, UK: Oxford University Press.

Mekel O, Mosbach-Schulz O, Schümann M, Okken P, Peters C, Herrmann J, et al., 2007, Evaluation of standards and models in probabilistic exposure assessment [Evaluation von Standards und Modellen zur probabilistischen Expositionsabschätzung]. WaBoLu-Hefte 02/07-05/07. Berlin, Umweltbundesamt

Mindell, J., & Barrowcliffe, R. (2005). Linking environmental effects to health impacts: a computer modelling approach for air pollution. *Journal of Epidemiology and Community Health, 59*, 1092–1098.

Mindell, J., & Joffe, M. (2005). Mathematical modelling of health impacts. *Journal of Epidemiology and Community Health, 59*(8), 617–618.

Mindell, J., Hansell, A., Morrison, D., Douglas, M., & Joffe, M. (2001). On behalf of participants in the Quantifiable HIA discussion group, what do we need for robust, quantitative impact assessment? *Journal of Public Health Medicine, 23*(3), 173–178.

Murray, C. J. L., Ezzati, M., Lopez, A. D., Rodgers, A., & Vander, H. S. (2003). Comparative quantification of health risks: conceptual framework and methodological issues. *Population Health Metrics, 1*(1), 1.

NRC—National Research Council. (2009). *Science and decisions: advancing risk assessment.* Washington, DC: The National Academies Press.

O'Connell, E., & Hurley, F. (2009). A review of the strength and weaknesses of quantitative methods used in health impact assessment. *Public Health, 123*, 306–310.

Rehm, J., Taylor, B., Mohapatra, S., Irving, H., Baliunas, D., Patra, J., et al. (2010). Alcohol as a risk factor for liver cirrhosis: a systematic review and meta-analysis. *Drug and Alcohol Review, 29*(4), 437–445.

Schütz, H., Wiedemann, P. M., Hennings, W., Mertens, J., & Clauberg, M. (2006). *Comparative risk assessment: concepts, problems and applications.* Weinheim: Wiley-VCH.

Schwartz, J., Bellinger, D., & Glass, T. (2011). Expanding the scope of environmental risk assessment to better include differential vulnerability and susceptibility. *American Journal of Public Health, 101*(Suppl 1), S88–S93. doi:10.2105/AJPH.2011.300268.

Sexton, K., Kleffman, D., & Callahan, M. (1995). An introduction to the national human exposure assessment survey and related phase I field studies. *Journal of Exposure Analysis and Environmental Epidemiology, 5*, 229–232.

US EPA—U.S. Environmental Protection Agency (2000). Risk Characterization Handbook. EPA 100-B-00-002. Office of Science Policy, Office of Research and Development, U.S. Environmental Protection Agency, Washington, DC

US EPA—U.S. Environmental Protection Agency. (2004). *Example exposure scenarios. National Center for Environmental Assessment.* Washington DC: US EPA.

Veerman, J. L., Barendregt, J. J., & Mackenbach, J. P. (2005). Quantitative Health Impact Assessment: current practice and future directions. *Journal of Epidemiology and Community Health, 59,* 361–370.

Veerman, J. L., Mackenbach, J. P., & Barendregt, J. J. (2007). Validity of predictions in Health Impact Assessment. *Journal of Epidemiology and Community Health, 61,* 362–366.

WHO. (2004). *Preventing road traffic injury: a public health perspective for Europe.* Copenhagen: World Health Organization Regional Office for Europe.

WHO. (2009a). *Global health risks: mortality and burden of disease attributable to selected major risks.* Geneva: World Health Organization.

WHO. (2009b). *Global status report on road safety: time for action.* Geneva: World Health Organization.

WHO, 2002, World health report. (2002). *Reducing risks, promoting healthy life.* Geneva: World Health Organization.

WHO—World Health Organization. (2008). *The global burden of disease: 2004 update.* Geneva: WHO.

Wilson, C., Willis, C., Hendrikz, J., & Bellamy, N. (2009). *Speed enforcement detection devices for preventing road traffic injuries (review).* The Cochrane Collaboration: The Cochrane Library.

Yannis, G., & Papadimitriou, E. (Eds.) (2005). State of the Art Report on Risk and Exposure Data. Deliverable 2.1. of the the EU FP6 project SafetyNet. http://www.dacota-project.eu/Links/erso/safetynet/fixed/WP2/Deliverable%20wp%202.1%20state%20of%20the%20art.pdf. Accessed 27 December 2010

Chapter 6
Application of RAPID Guidance on an International Policy

Gabriel Guliš, Liliana Cori, Sarah Sierig, and Odile Mekel

As higher level in terms of geo-political integration policy making goes as larger the impact of policies and consequently benefits and hazards related to policies can be. In the globalized world nations states give up their policy making roles on certain areas of policy making to higher, international or transnational level of policy making. Therefore a policy risk assessment tool should be able to assess risks related to such international or transnational policies and strategies. Previous chapters of this book described development of RAPID guidance both top-down and bottom-up methodology on level of national policies. This sub-chapter is going to discuss testing of the top-down RAPID guidance on level of a European Union (EU) policy. The EU Health Strategy 2008–2013 "Together for health" was subjected to the assessment after a negotiation process with the Executive Agency for Health and Consumers (EAHC) and the Directorate for Health and Consumer Protection (DG SANCO) of the European Commission.

The main objective of testing the developed policy risk assessment tool on a real case on international level was to identify weaknesses and missing elements which could be applicable on international level, but not necessarily relevant on national level policies. After interview with DG SANCO colleagues, the project group underwent an

G. Guliš (✉)
Unit for Health Promotion Research, University of Southern Denmark,
Niels Bohrsvej 9-10, 6700 Esbjerg, Denmark
e-mail: ggulis@health.sdu.dk

L. Cori
Institute of Clinical Physiology, National Research Council, Istituto Fisiologia Clinica
Consiglio Nazionale delle Ricerche, V.le dell'Università 11, 00185 Roma, Italy
e-mail: liliana.cori@ifc.cnr.it

S. Sierig
NRW Centre for Health (LZG.NRW), Bielefeld 33611, Germany
e-mail: sarah.sierig@gmx.de

O. Mekel
Unit Innovation in Health, NRW Centre for Health (LZG.NRW), Bielefeld 33611, Germany
e-mail: odile.mekel@lzg.gc.nrw.de

G. Guliš et al. (eds.), *Assessment of Population Health Risks of Policies*,
DOI 10.1007/978-1-4614-8597-1_6, © Springer Science+Business Media New York 2014

Table 6.1 Health outcomes mentioned in the EC Health Strategy

Health outcome	Where to find in EC health strategy
Specific diseases including genetic disorders	Objective 1
Alzheimer's	Objective 1
Injuries	Objective 2
Communicable diseases	Objective 2
Specific diseases	Objective 2

intensive discussion process to conduct the assessment. The different approaches reflected the aim to test applicability of the RAPID guidance on international level.

Implementation is always one of key factors to influence achievements of policies; in case of international policies even more. If implementation is not defined in a policy or strategy it is unlikely any change will be achieved. Lack of implementation mechanisms, tools, methods, is therefore a kind of hazard to question potential achievements of any policy. On policy level therefore more questions about implementation were added into RAPID guidance tool. It is important to describe in depth who is in charge for implementation both on international and national level; targets groups of implementers must be part of a policy in the same way as target group for action and impact. Target groups for implementation and impact are in most cases different; in case of the implementation it is mostly staff of Ministries of health, who is a target group whereas as of impact the Health strategy claims the EU citizen as a target group. Similar as implementation information upon monitoring and evaluation should be assessed on policy level within a policy risk assessment. Lack of measurable goals, lack of indicators and a monitoring system can questions achievements of a policy.

Assessment of the EC Health Strategy as Whole Document

Complex policies can be assessed as of health risks and impacts either as a whole or by specific objectives. The present assessment shows how to analyze the EC Health Strategy as a whole—by means of the RAPID tool. A main part of the RAPID methodology is the definition, inclusion and prioritization of health outcomes, risk factors and health determinants. The EC Health Strategy includes nearly all health outcomes even if only a few of them are specifically defined (see Table 6.1).

The risk factors and resources mentioned in the strategy are nearly covering all determinants of health. Especially in objective 1 "key issues" to tackle are listed which include most health relevant risk factors or determinants: "*Healthy ageing must be supported by actions to promote health and prevent disease throughout the lifespan by tackling key issues including poor nutrition, physical activity, alcohol, drugs and tobacco consumption, environmental risks, traffic accidents, and accidents in the home*" (EC 2007, p. 7).

This makes it difficult to include or exclude risk factors and health outcomes only on the basis of the Strategy. Therefore we decided to identify the most relevant health outcomes for Europe in general (share of Burden of Disease—BoD) and the current attributable fraction of BoD for risk factors mentioned in the EC strategy.

This overview is presented in following sub-chapters, using the indicators healthy life years (HLY) and disability-adjusted life year (DALY). Additionally, the Burden of Disease studies of WHO were used to identify the most important risk within EU-27. Based on this overview it is possible to examine to what extent the EC Health Strategy can contribute to reduce the differences between EU-27 countries for two main health indicators (HLY and DALY) and to exploit the full potential health gains.

Distribution of Diseases Within Europe

To assess the potential health gains of the EU Health Strategy it is important to have an overview of the distribution of diseases within Europe.

Healthy Life Years (HLY) in EU-27

The indicator Healthy Life Years (HLY) was used to compare EU-27 countries. HLY are the *"expected remaining years lived from a particular age without long-term activity limitation"*. HLY *"takes into account both mortality and ill-health, providing more information on burden of diseases in the population than life expectancy alone"* (EC, Heidi Data Tool, http://ec.europa.eu/health/indicators/indicators/index_en.htm).

Here the HLY at birth is used. For 2008 we see large differences in healthy life expectancy between the EU-27 countries (see Fig. 6.1).

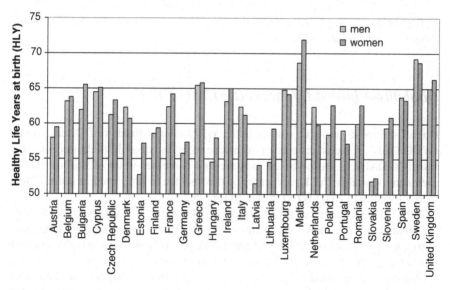

Fig. 6.1 Healthy life years at birth (HLY) in the EU-27 countries 2008 (own illustration, data adapted from the HEIDI Data Tool)

Table 6.2 Highest and lowest healthy life years (HLY) of EC-27 countries

Country	HLY — men 2008	HLY — women 2008
Sweden	69.2	–
Latvia	51.5	–
Malta	–	71.9
Slovakia	–	52.3
Difference = Potential health gain	17.7	19.6

Box 1: The disability-adjusted life year

The disability-adjusted life year (DALY) extends the concept of potential years of life lost due to premature death to include equivalent years of "healthy" life lost by virtue of being in states of poor health or disability *(3)*. One DALY can be thought of as one lost year of "healthy" life, and the burden of disease can be thought of as a measurement of the gap between current health status and an ideal situation where everyone lives into old age, free of disease and disability.

DALYs for a disease or injury cause are calculated as the sum of the years of life lost due to premature mortality (YLL) in the population and the years lost due to disability (YLD) for incident cases of the disease or injury. YLL are calculated from the number of deaths at each age multiplied by a global standard life expectancy for each age. YLD for a particular cause in a particular time period are estimated as follows:

YLD = number of incident cases in that period × average duration of the disease × weight factor

The weight factor reflects the severity of the disease on a scale from 0 (perfect health) to 1 (death). The weights used for the GBD 2004 are listed in Annex Table A6 of Mathers et al. *(11)*.

In the standard DALYs reported here and in recent *world Health Reports*, calculations of YLL and YLD used an additional 3% time discounting and non-uniform age weights that give less weight to years lived at young and older ages *(6)*. Using discounting and age weights, a death in infancy corresponds to 33 DALYs, and deaths at ages 5-20 years to around 36 DALYs.

Fig. 6.2 Definition of the DALY indicator (WHO 2008a, b)

Regarding potential maximum health gains, we compare the "best" and the "worst" countries (see Table 6.2).

Disability-Adjusted Life Years (DALY) in EU-27

One of the most extensive studies is the WHO Global Burden of Disease Study (WHO GBD). It measures burden of disease using the disability-adjusted life year (DALY). DALY is a time-based measure and combines years of life lost due to premature mortality (YLL) and years of life lost due to time lived in states of less than full health (YLD) (WHO 2008a, b) (Fig. 6.2).

WHO GBD covers more than 100 diseases (defined by ICD code). These diseases are divided into three main categories: (1) *communicable, maternal, perinatal and nutritional conditions (includes 39 defined diseases)*; (2) *non-communicable diseases (includes 57 diseases)* and (3) *injuries (includes 9 causes of injuries)*.

An initial comparison of DALY rates (DALY per 100,000 population) shows that the *non-communicable diseases* play the most important role regarding the burden

Table 6.3 DALY rates (DALY per 100,000 population by cause, WHO 2009)

EU27	DALY rate all causes	Communicable, maternal, perinatal and nutritional conditions	Non-communicable diseases	Injuries
Austria	12,069	495	10,583	990
Belgium	12,948	543	11,239	1,166
Bulgaria	18,296	943	16,044	1,308
Cyprus	12,010	833	10,275	902
Czech Republic	14,326	526	12,378	1,422
Denmark	13,447	486	11,971	990
Estonia	18,900	1,183	14,649	3,068
Finland	13,205	504	10,981	1,720
France	12,262	579	10,517	1,167
Germany	12,536	488	11,312	736
Greece	11,826	495	10,404	928
Hungary	17,941	693	15,688	1,560
Ireland	11,692	653	10,155	884
Italy	11,245	495	9,984	766
Latvia	19,615	1,150	15,341	3,125
Lithuania	18,401	1,090	13,861	3,450
Luxembourg	12,341	670	10,452	1,219
Malta	11,141	600	9,875	666
The Netherlands	11,486	578	10,294	614
Poland	14,911	699	12,454	1,759
Portugal	13,615	923	11,582	1,110
Romania	17,685	1,447	14,450	1,788
Slovakia	15,340	767	12,978	1,595
Slovenia	14,002	552	11,929	1,521
Spain	11,352	609	9,883	860
Sweden	11,478	481	10,164	833
UK	12,871	674	11,489	708
ALL average	13,961	709	11,886	1,365

of disease in Europe. In all countries of EU-27 they account for 80–90 % of the whole burden of disease in this country (Table 6.3).

Regarding possible health gains, we compare again the "best" and the "worst" countries. The "best" country, Malta has 11,141 DALY per 100,000 population for all causes. The country with the "worst" DALY rate, Latvia, has 19,615 DALY per 100,000 population for all causes. The difference between these two values is 8,474 DALY per 100,000 population (all causes) and can be interpreted as potential health gain (see Table 6.4).

To explore where the health gains can be reached concretely we need to have a closer look on specific diseases or disease categories. The three main categories of BoD-studies (*communicable, maternal, perinatal and nutritional conditions; non-communicable diseases* and *injuries* are further divided into 2–14 subcategories).

Table 6.4 EU-27 countries with highest and lowest DALY rate

EU-27 countries with highest and lowest DALY	DALY rate all causes
High Latvia	19,615
Estonia	18,900
Lithuania	18,401
Bulgaria	18,296
Hungary	17,941
Romania	17,685
Low Greece	11,826
Ireland	11,692
The Netherlands	11,486
Sweden	11,478
Spain	11,352
Italy	11,245
Malta	11,141

Table 6.5 Main non-communicable diseases subcategories which contribute as first, second or third importance to total DALY in a country

	1	2	3	Sum
Neuropsychiatric conditions	18	9	0	27
Cardiovascular diseases	9	11	7	27
Malignant neoplasms	0	7	18	25
Sense organ diseases	0	0	1	1
Unintentional injuries	0	0	1	1

Finally, per subcategory, there are 1–16 ICD-coded diseases (or causes of injuries) listed.

Within the *non-communicable diseases* three subcategories are crucial for the burden of disease in Europe:

1. Neuropsychiatric conditions.
2. Cardiovascular diseases.
3. Malignant neoplasms.

In 25 countries of EU-27 these subcategories are the first, second or third important contribution to the total DALY. Exceptional cases are Cyprus with *Sense organ diseases* and Lithuania with *Unintentional injuries*, each on the third rank (see Table 6.5).

On average (EU-27), *malignant neoplasms* account for 2,072 DALY per 100,000 population, *neuropsychiatric conditions* for 3,179 and *cardiovascular diseases* for 2,888 DALY per 100,000 population. Regarding potential health gains, we compare the "best" and the "worst" countries again: Cyprus has the lowest DALY rate for *malignant neoplasms* (971) while Hungary has the highest rate (3,044). The difference between these two values (~potential health gain) is 2,073 DALY per 100,000 population. For *neuropsychiatric conditions* the "best" country is Italy (2,546), the "worst" Finland (3,709), the difference amounts to 1,163 DALY per 100,000 population. For *cardiovascular diseases* the DALY rate of 6,924 in Bulgaria is the highest and the rate of 1,415 in France is the lowest, with a difference of 5,509 DALY (see Table 6.6).

Table 6.6 DALY rates, three major non-communicable diseases (DALY per 100,000 population by cause, WHO 2009)

EU27	Malignant neoplasms	Neuropsychiatric conditions	Cardiovascular diseases
Austria	1,882	3,211	1,828
Belgium	2,193	3,183	2,129
Bulgaria	2,162	3,166	6,924
Cyprus	971	2,591	2,258
Czech Republic	2,571	2,970	3,358
Denmark	2,350	3,199	2,093
Estonia	2,329	3,493	4,676
Finland	1,612	3,709	2,305
France	2,234	3,439	1,415
Germany	2,114	3,088	2,392
Greece	1,897	2,607	2,764
Hungary	3,044	3,645	4,193
Ireland	1,725	3,286	1,735
Italy	2,056	2,546	1,941
Latvia	2,340	3,418	5,705
Lithuania	2,175	3,455	4,319
Luxembourg	1,798	3,260	2,002
Malta	1,688	2,661	2,022
The Netherlands	2,112	3,013	1,707
Poland	2,368	3,229	3,245
Portugal	2,032	2,982	2,416
Romania	2,115	3,156	5,009
Slovakia	2,144	3,667	3,422
Slovenia	2,452	3,283	2,464
Spain	1,890	2,760	1,556
Sweden	1,680	3,387	2,004
UK	2,007	3,432	2,083
ALL average	2,072	3,179	2,888

In the 18 countries where *neuropsychiatric conditions* are the main causes of total DALY a closer look shows that *unipolar depressive disorders* lead to the most DALY within this group (see Table 6.7).

With the indicator HLY it is possible to get an overview of differences in health status between countries. The difference in HLY between the "best" (highest HLY) and the "worst" (lowest HLY) country can be interpreted as health gain potential: the highest HLY should be possible to reach for all countries; of course adequate measures are needed.

The health gain potential seems to be enormous: nearly 20 healthy life years seem to be possible.

A possible next step to assess the causes of these differences would lie in a comparison between policies and measures in "best" and "worst" countries. But it is not possible to break this indicator down into single disease or disease groups and link causal-effect-relationships for single risk factors to the healthy life expectancy.

Table 6.7 Main neuropsychiatric conditions which are the first, second or third important cause of DALY in a country

Neuropsychiatric conditions	Number of countries with rank			
	1	2	3	Sum
Unipolar depressive disorders	18	0	0	18
Alzheimer and other dementias	0	10	6	16
Alcohol use disorders	0	7	8	15
Drug use disorders	0	0	2	2
Schizophrenia	0	1	0	1
Bipolar disorder	0	0	1	1
Migraine	0	0	1	1

Table 6.8 Potential health gains based on the comparison of HLY and DALY rates between EU-27 countries

Health outcome	Potential health gain
HLY at birth for men	17.7 HLY
HLY at birth for women	19.6 HLY
All causes	8,474 DALY
Malignant neoplasms	2,073 DALY
Neuropsychiatric conditions	1,163 DALY
Cardiovascular diseases	5,509 DALY

For further assessment the indicator disability-adjusted life year (DALY) offers more detailed information.

With the DALY indicator it is possible to compare the contribution of different diseases to the total burden of disease in one country and between countries. So the DALY indicator offers more detailed information about the concrete diseases which lead to differences in healthy life expectancy.

The difference in DALY rate between the "best" (lowest DALY rate) and the "worst" (highest DALY rate) country could also be interpreted as health gain potential: the lowest DALY rate should be possible to reach for all countries, of course with adequate measures (see Table 6.8).

Major Risk Factors for Health in the EU-27 Countries

The leading risk factor in the EU-27 is tobacco (WHO 2005); it is the leading cause of the total burden of disease expressed in DALY in 16 out of 27 countries. In the remaining countries tobacco is the second or third cause of the total burden of disease (see Table 6.9).

In average tobacco accounts for 12.7 % of all DALY of a country in EU-27 (range 5.6 %—Cyprus to 20.9 %—Hungary). The prevention potential is vast, as demonstrated in the Hungarian assessment in Chap. 3.

Other leading risk factors are related to lifestyle, too. The top 5 in each country are accounting for ~50 % of all DALY.

Table 6.9 Major risk factors in EU-27 countries

Risk factor	Rank 1	Rank 2	Rank 3	Sum
	Number of countries, where the risk factor attributes to the total burden of disease on ...			
Tobacco	16	6	5	27
High blood pressure	4	10	7	21
Alcohol	7	9	4	20
High BMI	0	1	7	8
High cholesterol	0	1	4	5

Table 6.10 Strategies mentioned in the EC Health Strategy

No.	Actions	Objective
1	Measures to promote the health of older people and the workforce and actions on children's and young people's health (Commission)	1
2	*Development and delivery of actions on tobacco, nutrition, alcohol, mental health and other broader environmental and socio-economic factors affecting health* (Commission, Member States)	1
3	New Guidelines on Cancer screening and a Communication on European Action in the Field of Rare Diseases (Commission)	1
4	Follow up of the Communication on organ donation and transplantation (Commission)	1
5	Strengthen mechanisms for surveillance and response to health threats, including review of the remit of the European Centre for Disease prevention and Control (Commission)	2
6	Health aspects on adaptation to climate change (Commission)	2
7	Community framework for safe, high quality and efficient health services (Commission)	3
8	Support member states and regions in managing innovation in health systems (Commission)	3
9	Support implementation and interoperability of e-health solutions in health systems (Commission)	3

To What Extent can the EC Health Strategy Contribute to Tap the Full Potential Health Gains?

Based on this overview, we were able to examine to what extent the EC Health Strategy can contribute to reduce the differences between EU-27 countries for two main health indicators (HLY and DALY) and to tap the full potential health gains. In the first three parts of this chapter the most relevant diseases for EU-27 and the most important risk factor were identified.

In this fourth part of the chapter, the actions of the strategy to tackle diseases and risk factors are identified (see Table 6.10).

To assess the impact of these actions on health outcome we have to define how they influence health determinants, risk factors and health outcomes. A problem is that most of the actions are not concrete enough to show these connections. As an example to demonstrate how the impacts of these actions could be estimated, the second action "Development and delivery of actions on tobacco, nutrition, alcohol, mental health and other broader environmental and socioeconomic factors affecting health" was chosen.

Tobacco is the major health risk factor within the EU-27. Tackling this factor promises the largest health gain: 6–20 % of all DALY per country. It is not very probable to achieve 100 % tobacco-free environments in the EU and to tap the full prevention potential.

Conclusions

Main objective of this assessment was to test the developed policy risk assessment tool (RAPID tool or methodology) on the case of EC Health Strategy. The EC Health Strategy is a very special case for using the RAPID tool. An important aspect of the RAPID tool is to assess affected health determinants, risk factors and health outcomes, define the connections between them and prioritize. The EC Health Strategy includes nearly all health outcomes and health determinants, so it was very difficult to exclude and prioritize. Another difficulty was that the Strategy included very broad objectives, clear aims are missing, and only a few health outcomes were mentioned concretely ("specific diseases").

The approach to define important diseases and risk factors using comprehensive indicators like DALY and HLY was a very suitable extension of the RAPID tool.

We were able to show a large health gain potential for major diseases and related to major risk factors. Actions defined in the EC Health Strategy can contribute to achieve health gains but it has to be defined in what extent. In general the potential health gains regarding actions on lifestyle risk factors can be assumed as very large. A possible next step in assessment could be a comparison between policies and measures in "best" and "worst" countries to identify reasons for differences.

We have shown the enormous health gain potential by tackling specific major diseases and tackling main risk factors. But it is the wrong conclusion to neglect other diseases and risk factors. For example, the communicable diseases could lead to a huge amount of DALY if there are outbreaks. The number of DALY might be very low because of existing well implemented surveillance mechanisms. On the other hand a low DALY rate or a small amount of DALY is not necessarily a product of a good prevention or treatment policy. For some diseases underreporting might be a cause of a low DALY rate.

Assessment of EC Health Strategy by Specific Objectives

Four specific, single issue assessments were conducted on three objectives of the EC Health strategy:

- Two related to "Strengthen mechanisms for surveillance and response to health threats, including review of the remit of the European Centre for Disease prevention and Control"—case of meningococcal meningitis and influence pandemic preparedness.
- One on "Support Member States and Regions in managing innovation in health systems"—cardiovascular disease mortality and morbidity.
- One on "Development and delivery of actions on tobacco, nutrition, alcohol, mental health and other broader environmental and socioeconomic factors affecting health"—tobacco policy.

In all four cases a national policy or programme was clearly linked to the EC Health strategy; the Slovenian public health policy, Romanian influenza preparedness plan, Polish invasive cardiology program and the Hungarian anti-tobacco legislation were identified as national counterparts of the EC health strategy. This confirms the finding from interviews with DG SANCO representatives on need to include different levels of policies into main policy step while conducting policy risk assessment of an international policy.

To integrate all the characteristics of the discussion developed previously, be more specific and facilitate the understanding of argumentation on the need of inclusion of different policy levels the following scheme presents all policy levels, target groups (European Commission and Member States), actions for the two target groups and specific influenza pandemic countermeasures.

The first policy level is the EC Health Strategy followed by its second objective "Protecting citizens from health threats" from the two target group perspective (second policy level). For each of these two, using official documents actions related to the Health Strategy Objective and specific pandemic influenza countermeasures and health outcomes (third and fourth policy level) were identified.

The first policy level identified in the Health Strategy targets the European Commission in order to display the goals to be achieved by member states in respect of health care.

The second level of policy drifts from the European Commission to Member States. An important aspect characterizing this level consists in the fact that is bipolar, catching simultaneously the European institutional level as well as member states health institutions.

The third policy level is identified as the specific actions for each of the two actors of the second level.

The fourth policy level is the ultimate level of implementing health services and is drifting from the ones above it. It also represents the translation into practice of all the rules and principles regarding the health protection system and related to both member states and European Commission apparatuses. European Commission's actions of applying a mechanism of surveillance in order to prevent health threats imply in the fourth level of health policy a decreased prevalence of influenza pandemics. It is natural that the measures taken in order to diminish the prevalence of health threats at macro level to be universally available for all member states so as to action equally and apply the same steps in reducing the widespread of influenza pandemics. Analyzing the facts from this perspective, we can identify two objectives to focus on to European level: travel and trade restrictions and general personal hygiene.

Travel and trade restrictions are welcomed in case of influenza pandemics because they represent the heart of social and business activities nowadays, and the main measures which should be taken in case of outbreak consists of travel advice so as to offer information about the risks people are exposed to, entry screening to identify and control the infected people, borders closure to stop the widespread of the virus and ultimately international travel restrictions so as to block it to become a global issue.

Promoting general personal hygiene is also a feasible action, which can be put in practice by all the citizens of Europe. Some of the measures identified in the scheme are part of the natural course of personal daily hygiene, consisting in hand washing so as to protect the human body from ingesting bacteria and respiratory hygiene. Other measures are focusing on protecting the citizens in case of pandemics, advising them to wear masks in order to prevent the contact with the virus and self-isolation so as to protect other people from getting the virus.

These are the measures proposed by Health Strategy document which may be applied in case of pandemic influenza break out, insisting on the one hand on prevention and providing protection for European citizens, and on the other hand on establishing the measures should be taken in such situation to action immediately and cease the illness.

The other aspect of the fourth policy level regarding member states is focusing on the implementation of the measure but at a national level. The main goal identified is to change the incidence of pandemic influenza. The same pattern as in Romanian top-down case study, inscribing in the scheme the two measures proposed at the national level, namely, school closure and vaccination was followed. Adopting these two steps may have a great impact on the ordinary course of the society, but they are mandatory to prevent, control and cease a case of pandemic influenza at national level.

School closure may constitute a limitation for continuing the usual social life, firstly causing social distancing and quarantine. Even though the magnitude of such action could paralyze the entire social order, it is increasingly important to appeal to isolation and quarantine so as to separate from the healthy people and avoid infesting them. Workplace closure is also a manner for preventing the extent of disease, moreover avoiding personal contact could decrease the percentage of infected people. Another measure taken on national level, which may have a great contribution in stopping pandemics, may reside in cancelling the public events.

Starting a vaccination campaign could be the most preventive achievement in order to assure and shelter population's health. Furthermore, surveillance for prisons and elderly homes, prophylaxis and animal and bird surveillance for thwarting the transmission of the virus from animals to human beings should be included.

The four health policy levels are functioning after top-down mechanism; policy content is translated into practice on the one hand, at member states level by vaccination campaign and school closure and on the other hand at European level by promoting general personal hygiene notions and by asserting travel and trade restrictions.

The main objective of the detailed explanation of the scheme delivered below lies in the attempt to offer a justification for strengthening the role and the implication of the European Commission in managing situations involving pandemics (Together for Health: A Strategic Approach for the EU 2008–2013, 2007).

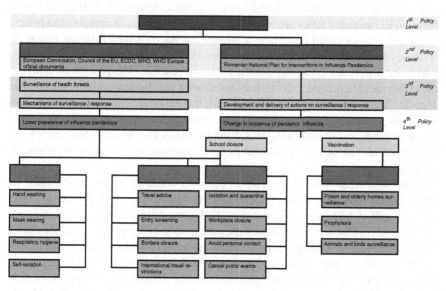

From Policy to Level of Determinants of Health is Crucial

The determinants were selected upon literature review and discussion process.

Determinants of health are influencing each other so the top down model is rather a circle or loop model. Therefore one policy with just one positive impact on one determinant is likely to launch a chain reaction on few determinants and the other way around. The assessment of surveillance of meningococcal meningitis illustrated well the "circle or loop mechanism."

Strengthened surveillance mechanisms and response to health threads would have positive impact on socio-economic status, which is one of the most important socio-economic determinant and that influences public health. Socio-economic determinants of health (for example housing conditions) have strong impact on the environmental determinant of health (for example indoor environment). Poor and less affluent population groups tend to be more often affected by inadequate housing conditions and higher environmental burden in their residential environments. Social status and low income is strongly associated with increased exposure to environmental risks in the private home or related to residential location. Living and housing conditions are the basis of many factors influencing easier transmission of meningococcal. Epidemiological findings suggest strong associations between housing conditions and health effects. Social status has impact on the behavioural and personal determinants of health. It is known that smoking and excessive drinking is more common among less affluent people.

This process must be considered while doing policy risk assessment and has been included into RAPID guidance tool.

Another important issue to consider for assessment of policies on international level could be the differences regarding the economic development. The differences between EU member states are involving different pathways of applying the policy. These differences could contribute at improving interrelations between European countries so as to maintain permanent communication and regulate the implementation process in order to equally put the policy in practice. The process of applying the policy could encounter difficulties because of the dissimilarities regarding the Member States healthcare systems and also, the national economical contribution due to the variance of state budget income. Availability and accessibility of appropriate methods and mechanisms does differ by health care systems and needs to be considered also as part of assessment as the cardiologic treatment methods assessment has shown.

Time is another important factor to consider while doing risk assessment of international (and any) policies. Depending on type of the health effect the time period needs to take in account not only the known latency period (onset of exposure to onset of disease) but also the time period form development of a policy to its full implementation. Changes in determinants of health and consequently risk factors occur only after a policy is fully implemented delaying so the onset of exposure. It is rather rare that short term effects could be seen in the immediate period of time (1–2 weeks) from applying the policy because the urgent character demanded by its content and, most often long term effects could be observed at institutional level after a longer period of time (1 year). Time period is extremely relevant in cases like the tobacco policy for example.

In the study, the health impact of the tobacco tax policy was evaluated applying integrated quantitative impact assessment. The full impact structure of the hypothesized policy action of increasing price of tobacco products by 10 % was mapped. Influenced health determinants, risk factors and health outcomes were identified and prioritized so as to select one causal chain of high importance for detailed quantitative assessment. In this process, the guidance provided by the methodological tool developed in a previous phase of the RAPID project was used and found to be applicable for the task.

The selected impact chain included substance use as determinant, active smoking as risk factor and lung cancer as health outcome. Quantitative exposure and outcome assessment was found feasible for the selected causal pathway. The study used –0.5 and –0.34 price elasticity that is 5 and 3.4 % reduction in tobacco use induced by

10 % price increase among males and females, respectively. The calculated measure was attributable death determined for the baseline and the projected scenario after the price increase. The difference, perceived as the health gain of the policy measure, was calculated to be 12,326 lives (7,668 among males and 4,658 among females) that can be saved annually as a result of increasing tobacco prices by 10 % in all member states of the European Union.

The health consequences of tobacco smoking pose a high burden on the European population, especially in older age groups, since smoking-related diseases of public health importance are typically chronic conditions that need long lag phase for development. Therefore, the importance of tackling the issue of smoking becomes more and more evident in an aging population. The inclusion of smoking into the First objective "Fostering good health in an aging Europe" of the EU Health Strategy, as a factor to be dealt with, is supported by the finding of this study. The selected tobacco policy proved to be effective measure providing example for how to manage the public health problem caused by smoking in the European population in the future.

In the study, quantitative assessment was integrated in the policy health impact assessment process in a structured way and proved to be feasible for four health outcomes that are diseases of high public health priority. Full chain approach and prioritization on each level of the impact chain proved to be essential for systematic quantification and the followed guidance provided valuable help in this process. Some difficulties were noted in the consistent rigid separation of health determinants and risk factors that can be hardly discussed in an isolated way in some cases. It has also been pointed out that those who intend to use the guidance with limited previous practice in health impact assessment may find the methodological instructions (How to do) insufficient. In spite of the noted shortcomings of the applied tool, the demonstrated methodology offers a practicable example for using quantitative assessment integrated in the health impact assessment of policies carried out on EU level.

Discussion of the Risk Assessment Process

The RAPID guidance proved to be a useful tool to assess potential risks related to EC Health strategy. The guidance allowed identifying major hazards and outlining possible impacts (in selected cases lead to quantification of impact). It seems to be obvious that a full chain policy risk assessment using the RAPID guidance needs to combine these approaches; the policy level could be described by risk assessment approach, yet quantification of risks need more work. For practice even identification of hazards, which might question success of policy in terms of its impact, is a positive phenomenon. The remaining three levels, determinants of health, risk factors and health effect, could be assessed by more impact assessment methodology.

References

EC—Commission of the European Communities. (2007). *White paper. Together for health: A strategic approach for the EU 2008–2013.* Brussels: Commission of the European Communities.

WHO. (2005). *European Health Report. Public health action for healthier children and populations.* Copenhagen, Denmark: World Health Organization.

WHO. (2008a). *The global burden of disease: 2004 update.* WHO Library Cataloguing-in-Publication Data. http://www.who.int/healthinfo/global_burden_disease/2004_report_update/en/index.html

WHO. (2008b). *WHO statistical information system (WHOSIS)—Indicator definitions and metadata—Indicator definitions and metadata—Indicator definitions and metadata, 2008.* Retrieved November 16, 11, from http://www.who.int/whosis/indicators/compendium/2008/1hat/en/

WHO. (2009). Health statistics and health information systems. Disease and injury country estimates. Death and DALY estimates for 2004 by cause for WHO Member States. Table: "Persons, all ages". http://www.who.int/healthinfo/global_burden_disease/estimates_country/en/index.html

Chapter 7
Use of Policy Risk Assessment Results in Political Decision Making

Liliana Cori, Gabriel Guliš, Joanna Kobza, Ágnes Molnár, and Jana Kollárová

Introduction

The RAPID project established, during the first period, a thematic network of risk assessment experts, including relevant partners in the ten countries involved, the "Risk assessor database". RAPID partners selected relevant policies (for top-down approach) and health outcomes (for bottom-up approach), as a starting point to develop and practise RAPID full-chain methodology.

The project devoted a specific activity, a single work package, to the dissemination and discussion of the methodology developed during the first 2 years of the project.

National workshops were planned in each country to facilitate integrated knowledge translation activity, using a participatory approach to increase potential knowledge-users awareness on the RAPID project, and to engage them in using the RAPID guidance.

L. Cori (✉)
Institute of Clinical Physiology, National Research Council, Istituto Fisiologia Clinica
Consiglio Nazionale delle Ricerche, V.le dell'Università 11, 00185 Roma, Italy
e-mail: liliana.cori@ifc.cnr.it

G. Guliš
University of Southern Denmark, Niels Bohrsvej 9-10, 6700 Esbjerg, Denmark
e-mail: ggulis@health.sdu.dk

J. Kobza
Medical University of Silesia, 18 Medykow Street, 40-752 Katowice, Poland
e-mail: koga1@poczta.onet.pl

Á. Molnár
Centre for Research on Inner City Health, Li Ka Shing Knowledge Institute,
St. Michaels's Hospital, 209 Victoria St., Rm. 3-26.22, Toronto, ON M5B 1C6 Canada
e-mail: MolnarAg@smh.ca

J. Kollárová
Regional Public Health Authority, Ipelska 1, 04011 Kosice, Slovakia
e-mail: kollarova@ruvzke.sk

G. Guliš et al. (eds.), *Assessment of Population Health Risks of Policies*,
DOI 10.1007/978-1-4614-8597-1_7, © Springer Science+Business Media New York 2014

Workshops were conceived to present case studies and the RAPID guidance to a targeted audience, to discuss and collect further insights, and integrate different perspectives in the final version of the policy evaluation methodology.

However, national workshops also actively contributed to develop evidence based methodological guidance and increase its quality and relevance for potential users by bridging know–do gap between researchers and stakeholders; by involving decision makers and potential users in the knowledge creation process; by facilitating diverse stakeholder participation from governmental, academic and private sectors, carefully identified by national RAPID surveys as having direct expertise in the field of risk assessment. The cultural and administrative differences existing in the countries involved in RAPID guarantee the inclusion of a wide range of perspectives.

Results of the national workshops helped to identify barriers and solutions for using the guidance, for adapting necessary changes to it and for communicating results to other potential users.

One-year time to organize workshops was planned, facilitating the discussion of needs and requirements of partner organizations. This chapter describes the process and content of national workshops.

The differences existing in legislation and competence in each country explain the variability to be expected in national workshops organization and implementation. One of the distinctions is in the legal context of the countries involved in RAPID, referred to the existence of a binding legislation about Health Impact Assessment, HIA. In fact, where legislation exists, there is a more generalized knowledge of the issue of assessment, as well as a higher background level of expertise in the country.

Notwithstanding the differences in scientific and political contexts, the discussion around risk assessment has been grown up during the last years, and several methods and tools have been developed and presented, with particular reference to the evaluation of specific projects or technologies. In the ten countries promoting RAPID project, there was a general interest by the experts included in the data base, particularly to identify a methodology to analyze policies.

Methods: Organization of the Workshops

When the RAPID dissemination and implementation work package started its activities, the discussion among partners was carried out via email, conference calls and during meetings, in particular the European Public Health Association (EUPHA) annual conferences. The discussion was intense and focused around the need of fine-tuning methodologies, through an appropriate exchange of experiences and knowledge.

A 2-day RAPID seminar was held in Pisa, Italy, in January 2011. The objective was to have a comprehensive discussion among partner organizations:

- To discuss the obstacles met during the case studies development
- To plan together the national workshops and explain workshop implementation process and
- To practise together the workshop methodology

The national workshops target group was composed by: public health experts working in risk assessment area; environmental health experts; policy makers; local level politicians; administrators at national, regional and municipal level; university lecturers and researchers; private consultants in the field of risk assessment.

It has been agreed that the Metaplan technique is going to be used as workshop conduct method. The Metaplan technique (Copyright by Thomas Schnelle GmbH; www.metaplan.com), also called the "card technique", consists in a brainstorming process with different steps, allowing people to collect ideas, suggestions or to take decisions. In the case of Pisa meeting, it was adapted with minor changes by the developer, based on her professional and personal experience (L'Astorina, 2011). The formalized procedure is easy: it needs a skilled coordinator that is crucial to guide and monitor the process. The participants answer to a starting question individually, writing on cards, attached to a pin board. A discussion and sharing of ideas helps to build clusters of answers by topics, a process also called "framing". Another discussion round helps to assess the weight of topics as priorities. A written report illustrates results to be further discussed, to draw conclusions at the end of the process. By using this method, participants can express their ideas anonymously, without pressure to disclose thoughts or evaluations of specific experiences. It encourages active involvement among the participants even in case of different levels of hierarchy. The crucial roles for workshop organization are: one coordinator and one facilitator. One or more members of the RAPID national team can support them, and the additional presence of an international representative can be attractive for the audience.

The production of a common set of materials was proposed and accepted. The dissemination and information format included: a general presentation of RAPID Project; a presentation of RAPID risk assessment method; a four pages/slides presentation for each of the cases (ten top-down, eight bottom-up); a slide presentations in English, to be translated if necessary; a draft press release format.

Finally, to drive the collection of conclusions and recommendations, an evaluation and outcome format was proposed, including: a description of workshop organization (people contacted, instruments, participation); a copy of dissemination documents used, article published, press releases, etc.; a detailed workshop report; a collection of proposals and recommendation produced as a result.

Preparatory Survey

A preparatory questionnaire to identify common issues to be covered was completed by RAPID partner organizations, before the meeting, and the Pisa seminar completed the first phase, developing a format for national workshops. A synthesis of questionnaire results offers an outline of the topics discussed to prepare RAPID workshops.

The first issue emerged in relation to the *differences in national contexts* already mentioned. The two central topics, *legislation regarding HIA* and *competence*, present variability and change both in administrative levels and in field of competence.

In Germany, for example, the HIA situation is notoriously "sensitive". A first book completely dedicated to HIA was published in 1997 (Kobusch, Fehr, & Serwe, 1997), the first national workshop was held in 2002, and the efforts to establish HIA started earlier than in many other European countries. Even if the implementation of HIA was limited, a scientific competence exists in the country, especially in Universities. HIA practice facilitated a discussion among experts, and the scientific community currently uses different approaches. There are reservations from various actors, pointing at specific issues like tackling the lack of time and resources, the existence of already well-established methodologies for impact evaluation, or the lack of reliability of results.

In Italy, the experience in HIA practice is more recent but is experiencing a phase of intense development, especially applied to plans and policies impacting the environment. Epidemiologists and public health officials operating in research bodies (National Research Council), Universities (Hygiene and Public Health Departments), the National Health Service, Regional Public Health and Prevention Services and Environment Protection Agencies, developed the first experiences of HIA in early 2000s (Bianchi & Cori, 2013; Figueras & McKee, 2012). The core reason for introducing this practice was the weak or absent inclusion of the assessment of health impacts in Environmental Impact Assessment (EIA), and Strategic Environmental Assessment (SEA), even if it is required. In many critical circumstances, like building of new or industrial plants, when the awareness of an existing environmental problem emerges or when cases of unexpected diseases emerge in a limited area, citizens complain and require information. HIA have been frequently the best answer, as it is directly linked to the people well being, and provides answers about the health status of the community. The debate around its potential uses is interesting and includes several disciplinary areas; it is quite polarized, from a negative position stating that HIA is proposed to block activities and innovation to strong supporters, maintaining that HIA is an essential tool for public health protection. A lively debate is going on in Italy related to health condition of population living in high-risk areas: part of the debate regards the opportunity to implement binding instruments for health impact evaluation such as HIA.

In Spain, the recent introduction of HIA in national legislation provides the opportunity to spread information, train specialists and administrators, enhance expertise and support active citizenship.

Another important question is *the significant difference between EU countries as regards to the administrative structure, competences, decision making process and legislative procedures.*

Most EU Member States have some basic political and administrative structures for the delivery of public services at national, regional and local levels common, but they differ and depend on how responsibility is divided among levels. The most important parameters for assessing the different institutional models for decision making process including health goals across the European Union include effectiveness, efficiency, responsiveness, sustainability, integration and financing (Figueras and McKee, 2012). Decentralized governmental structures may be more responsive to the expectations and needs of the local communities. Local decision makers are often better informed; regional strategies may be more effective in balancing inequities in resources and coordinating activities in communities than national interventions. On the other hand a centralized function has more potential to take a strategic and whole of government approach and to respond to main health risks and challenges.

The national level is responsible for the framework and guidance for national policies. In many countries like Spain, Poland, Italy and Germany, health priorities differ across regions, as a consequence the importance of regional level decision making is increased. Authority is needed at the local level where it is necessary to coordinate action efficiently. Local level is often defined as operational because at this level is the most direct access to the population in implementation process of policies.

Over past years, some EU Member States adopted several intersectoral policies but the capacity to implement them is still weak, local governments and municipalities have no formal structures to support intersectoral working. Responsibility for health risks and consequences of political decisions is almost divided among departments and decision makers with unclear lines of communication. Experts recommendations, if only appear, although often evidence-based, are also implemented very selectively. Decision making process represents a complex process with formal and informal influences. There is also a lack of good documented research on the complex mechanisms of decision making process in most EU states. Analyzing the decision making processes across Europe it is important to raise some conceptual backgrounds. In some countries the national role is relatively limited compared to the responsibilities and autonomy of the regions.

Germany for instance reflects the decentralized responsibility for public services delivery and population health status. The federal role in decisive process is limited and the Lander have almost complete autonomy. The Lander are subdivided into administrative regions, district presidents are appointed by the land president. The smallest administrative units are the municipalities. The Land level is most relevant to decision making process.

In Denmark, the county/municipal level has considerably political autonomy and the national level coordinates national programmes, develops national policies and monitors their implementation.

In Slovakia, public health and risk assessment are related mostly to environmental and occupational issues, done either by regional and district based public health authorities or by private occupational health assessment institutions. The second are dealing naturally with occupational hazards only. HIA and health related impact assessment is mandatory; the regional public health authority on one hand gives license those who wants to do it, and on other hand evaluates the reports produced.

HIA procedure is not presently binding in Italy, neither at national nor at regional level, with the exception of limited provisions that will be described. The Italian National Health Service, NHS, applying a universalistic model, has the responsibility for public health prevention, cure and rehabilitation for the general population. In this domain, there is a potential interest in adopting HIA as a formalized process for evaluating programmes and policies. The organization and functioning of the prevention, cure and rehabilitation services is assigned to regional health systems administered by Regional Governments. Although HIA could represents a useful method and a tool to evaluate programmes, policies and projects of regional and local interest, up to now only in few Regions significant applications were done Moreover, even if the amount of economic resources is planned at national level and it is distributed to each Region on the basis of homogeneous criteria (number of inhabitants, population-age structure), the regionalization of the health system (i.e. devolution of responsibility for management and decision making) is producing wide differences among regions, both in prevention and in health care service, depending on cultural, economic and political factors (Costa et al., 2011). In this context, it's easily comprehensible that HIA has been up to now differently considered and used (Bianchi & Cori, 2013). Even the definition of Health Impact Assessment is controversial, because it is sometime used for studies concerning the evaluation of past exposures or facts, omitting two HIA distinguished features, recently properly defined by Kemm (2013): "HIA has two essential features: It seeks to predict the future consequences for health of possible decisions. It seeks to inform decision making" (Kemm, 2013, p. 3) and "One confusing aspect of some of the early literature on HIA is the use of the terms 'prospective', 'concurrent' and 'retrospective'. If HIA is concerned with prediction then clearly it is prospective and the term 'prospective HIA' in tautologous, while the terms 'concurrent HIA' and 'retrospective HIA' make no sense. Those activities that were called retrospective HIA should more accurately be called evaluation and those that were described as a concurrent HIA should be described as monitoring" (Kemm, 2013, p. 4). This misuse of concepts generates confusion both in decision makers and citizens, which are often highly interested in understanding and participating in the fulfilment of HIA studies. The circulation of information around RAPID development and guidance production was used as a further opportunity to build knowledge and training around those topics.

The example of Poland clearly shows the complexity of risk assessment implementation.

In Poland there is a three-level administrative division with the following units: voivodeship, poviats and municipalities. Each of the administrative level has its own authorities, which are divided into decision making and executive. Implementation of law on all three authority levels is similar. The decision making body, i.e. municipality, city, poviat council, the voivodeship parliament promulgates, within its competences and in accordance with the delegation resulting from primary acts, normative acts, as well as legal acts, which do not contain binding legislation. These acts are published in the form of resolutions, which undergo control of suitable voivodes in terms of their coherence with primary law-acts. The executive authority, i.e. administrator, mayor, city mayor, poviat board, voivodeship board, executes resolutions of the decision making authority by a detailed specification of the manner of their execution in the form of orders. The majority of local government units hold binding strategic documents: development and sector strategies, action, plans and the majority of them are drawn up mandatorily. This results from acts, part of them for the purpose of participating in aid programmes, or they are created because of a specific need of a given unit. The resolution-passing initiative in local government units belongs generally to those authorities as well as their commissions, clubs and members as well as executive authorities. The authors of bills of decision making authorities are most often executive authorities. The order-passing initiative is the sole competence of executive offices and most often it also undergoes a procedure of verifying the coherence with binding law, in this case, also with local law. The process of implementing policy health risks assessment methods in local government units should be discussed on several levels: strategic management concerning long-term strategies and programmes, current establishment of law, including: by the decision making authority (resolutions) and by the executive authority (orders) and finally by current administration (issuing administrative decisions).

In the practical experience, HIA knowledge and implementation is more and more linked to the activity of international research groups that should contribute to strengthen the methodology as well as the effectiveness of the instrument.

Workshops Experience

The *methodology for workshop organization* was another issue emerged in preparation of the RAPID national workshops, strictly linked to each national context.

Three different *programme formats* were distributed, for a two days or one day workshop. National partners had to decide about the main focus of the workshop, and, consequently, to choose the best organization setting. A format for *dissemination and information* provides a presentation of RAPID project and instruments; the explanation of top-down and bottom-up methodologies for risk assessment, as well as one or two case studies; the participants are required to present their experience, with a limited discussion session. The presentation of RAPID can be also articulated giving an international and national background about risk assessment and HIA implementation. A format for *proposal and discussion* provides short presentations, done by the organizers and the participants sharing their professional experience and presenting one of the case study developed by RAPID partners; a discussion around critical points, obstacles and perspectives focused on the case examined; recommendations can be drawn as a conclusion, aimed at improving the process and supporting the best use of the RAPID guidance. A format for *practicing the methodology* includes presentations of the RAPID top-down or bottom-up methodology, and the application on a case-study, one of the cases developed within RAPID project, or a new one identified by workshop participants; focusing around possible practical developments, obstacles and improvements; recommendations could be drawn in this case to improve the methodology and its application to perform policy evaluation.

Considering the different situation in the countries involved, in addition to a dissemination function, both around HIA thinking and RAPID thinking, a collection of information will be even more crucial, on the current European HIA landscape and by country. This perspective was proposed and included in the format for national workshops.

An *interactive discussion session* was proposed, to be organized as a group exercise, discussion rounds or a proper working session, where people can share experience and competence, to be carefully adapted to the specific situation. The proposal of Metaplan technique, to be practiced during the meeting in Pisa, was identified for this reason. The RAPID team directly experienced a time saving procedure, a method to discuss and work together, which makes participants feel deeply involved in the group process with a common objective. During the meeting in Pisa, the Metaplan question, "when I think of risk in my life I think of ...", was particularly stimulating for the group. Apparently simple and well known, it gave the possibility to open a broad discussion involving several professional and personal aspects.

As for the *participants*, the involvement of national health sector and academia in national workshops was established, as well as an accurate selection of the reference people to invite in the discussion, with the differences due to the local situation and the network built around RAPID project. To raise the attention around national RAPID workshops and attract participants, each partner will choose the suitable information channels, using the experts' database and mailing list, relationship with professional associations and other sources, as well as press releases, articles, specific instruments to be identified and produced.

The issue of *language* is central and different in each country, to allow an open discussion within the workshop, and to decide about the participation of RAPID team members. As we will see, most of the seminars were hold in national languages.

The preferences expressed by partners during the preparation phase composed a complex picture, to be integrated and combined.

One of the main differences is the level of knowledge and implementation of risk assessment by researchers and scholars, the demand for evaluation by public bodies and private organizations in each country. The risk assessment of policies is an innovative field of application, but there might be a positive ground for acceptance or a negative prejudice, specifically by public officials. The network of experts and officials is also different in the ten countries involved in RAPID project.

During the seminar held in Pisa the choice among different approaches was focused around the three proposed formats: dissemination and information, proposal and discussion and practice of the methodology. Each of them was translated in timing and content organization.

As a deliverable of each national workshop it was established to produce a document describing: the organization (people contacted, instruments, participation); copy of the dissemination documents used, article published or press releases, if any; a short report on workshop development; a collection of recommendation produced as a result of national workshops.

Finally, the practice of Metaplan technique during the Pisa seminar was useful to understand its potential use in national workshops, the added value of introducing participation methodologies within group discussions. It was also a positive and collaborative relationship-building exercise for the RAPID group.

A synthesis of the whole experience of national workshop implementation is presented in the following Table 7.1.

Table 7.1 Review of workshops

Partner country	Date	Agenda	RAPID tool and method	Participants
Italy	16-12-11	Wide picture + RAPID + case study	Top-down Metaplan	13
Denmark	19-01-12	RAPID + EU case study	Top-down Metaplan	12
Spain	3-11-11	RAPID + case studies	Top-down	14
Hungary	25-10-11	Wide picture + RAPID + case studies	Top-down Metaplan	14
Germany	19-10-11	Wide picture + RAPID + case studies	Top-down	13
Poland	5-11-11	RAPID + case studies	Top-down and bottom-up	9
Slovak Republic	20-10-11	Wide picture + RAPID + case studies	Top-down	30
Slovenia	6/7-12-11	Wide picture + RAPID + case studies	Top-down and bottom-up	46
Romania	20-01-12	RAPID + case studies	Top-down	16
Lithuania	19-01-12	WAPID + case studies	Top-down and bottom-up	30

It is possible to observe here: the differences in the agenda, the issues covered, the explanation of the whole methodology or part of it, the presentation of one or more case-studies and the use of Metaplan technique; the time-spam, only one country held a 2-day workshop; the number of participants.

A total of 197 experts were involved in ten countries. The participants to the workshops were primarily contacted from the list of risk assessors that had been composed in a previous phase of the project. However, policy makers from the local, regional and national levels were also invited to reach a broader audience and increase diversity of participants. Their willingness to participate reflected the interest in evidence based policy-making and policy risk assessment, and the need for training. The involvement of policy makers was a critical area: the countries where decision makers participated in the seminar were Hungary and Poland. In other countries like Italy, Spain, Germany and Denmark, the participation was mainly from risk assessment experts, public health practitioners, lecturers and students as well as public administrators, whose competence is relevant for policy implementation. Participants represented various expert areas linked to risk assessment and environmental impact assessment, such as health policy, health promotion, epidemiology, environmental health, occupational health and radiation health. Diverse professional backgrounds of the participants reflected that multiple sectors are the multiplicity of potential stakeholders. Few representatives participated from NGOs and from the private sector. Finally, this participation reflected the already mentioned historical, legal and scientific status of risk assessment and HIA in different countries: whether HIA is mandatory or not; which component and levels of government are responsible for impact assessment, what is the role of private sector, what technical and practical capacities are available (e.g. competency frameworks, guidelines, expertise) highly influence the awareness and the interest of stakeholders.

During the RAPID workshops, the rationale of the project and selected top-down and/or bottom-up RAPID case studies were presented. The discussion around RAPID guidance produced the suggestions presented in the next paragraph, and included in the last revision of RAPID guidance methodology.

The results of workshops, including the evaluation by participants, were summarized quantitatively, and analyzed qualitatively. A wide range of contextual issues in relation to risk assessment practice in participant countries emerged, to be used to understand how to use RAPID products, the object of the next paragraph.

In general, the RAPID workshop findings showed the differences in policy health risks assessment and HIA implementation reflecting the already mentioned wide diversity in decision making process among project partner states, consistent with constitutional arrangements of the countries, which affect legislative procedures, formal mechanisms, governance, financing and provision of public services. The workshop findings reflect the complex decision making process and competences and different tradition in policy health risk approach also because of the broad national priorities in public health policy of the different countries, they in certain sense illustrate how public health objectives are implemented and in some cases evaluated across Europe. As we already noted above, over past years intersectoral policies have been implemented in many States, but the capacity to support them is still weak. The promotion of formal mechanisms to prioritize political activities and interventions would be beneficial, with the objective of connecting more strictly health objectives, population health status and the available resources, and to strengthen local and regional capacities through good governance, monitoring and surveillance.

How to Use the RAPID Products

The main results and suggestions emerged from national workshops are described in the following pages. Most of the recommendations directly related to the RAPID guidance tool were accepted and included in the last version. Further elements are also added here as a support for the users, for example regarding communication and public participation.

The major discussion points and participants opinions focused on terminology, specific concept such as health determinants and risk factors, structure of the tool, different contexts of policy and risk assessment, consultation process and communication strategies.

The *terminology* was one of the first discussion points, both in the workshops done in national languages and in English. One of the main reasons is that several participants brought together different knowledge and background in risk assessment practice. The definitions of "risk assessment", "impact assessment" and "policy evaluation" had to be clarified in order to enable further discussion around specific features and potential uses of the RAPID guidance. Differences between lay and professional knowledge generated questions around the meaning of terms such as "scope of policy", "strength of evidence", "transparency" which impeded to understand checklist tasks. As noted by participants an initial chapter or a glossary of terms would be desirable in the final guidance. Participants were lacking precise the definition of "health outcome" in order to make it easier to evaluate. One suggestion was to change the wording "tool" in "guidance" in the title of the RAPID document.

Referred to this topic, the RAPID working group suggests that an ad hoc glossary presented in national languages can be a useful supporting tool when a multidisciplinary group is beginning the activity of policy evaluation; the discussion and clarification of terms is an initial task that can be highly productive for relation building as well as definition of boundaries and scope of the work to be developed.

The *distinction between health determinants and risk factors* is one of the operative difficulties that clearly appear when a policy evaluation is needed.

There were even conflicts among different areas of expertise when discussing how to define and identify "determinants" and "risk factors". As implied by some participants these terms, in fact, could be merged and determinants can be considered as clusters of risk factors, or maintained separated. The relation to health effects is more apparent in some cases, yet caution is needed to avoid over-simplification. Some experts underlined that during practical use of the guide, problems concerning separation between health determinants and risk factors can emerge because of the close interactions between them. A lack of solid and clear differentiation between "determinants" and "risk factors" is challenging for terminology and translation as well, therefore an operative discussion and a clarification seemed necessary. In order to reach a scientifically sound agreement on the debate around "determinants of health" as well as to support the analysis of possible interactions among health determinants, a list of determinants were recommended to be compiled, based on the updated model of the WHO Commission on Social Determinants of Health (CSDH, 2008). Definition of "socio-economic" exposure was debated as well as a lack of focus on the protector was noted in the model.

In relation with the *structure of the RAPID guidance* several points were underlined during national workshops. In terms of quantification, participants agreed in the feasibility of quantifying impacts from risk factors to health effects (sufficient literature was thought to be available in most cases), but they noted difficulties in relation to the strain from determinants of health towards risk factors. Interactions between risk factors were considered to be too complex and their full investigation as impossible. In order to enhance the use of the guidance participants recommended incorporating a descriptive summary from guidelines on how to use the best scientific evidence, as well as to provide brief summary of quantitative tools available.

The RAPID guidance was positively considered by participants in general, judged as an applicable and useful tool, with specificities like in Spain, where mandatory HIA is being finally adopted, and training is needed. They deliberated both approaches (bottom-up and top-down) as necessary and valuable as a starting point. If the user has prioritized which strain is going to be analyzed, the duality might be eliminated. It is important to harmonize both approaches in order to avoid confusion.

The first step—analysis of the policy—seemed to be of crucial importance for the participants; the "translation" of policy contents into health determinants was deemed to be one of the most difficult steps. Top-down tool was referred by some participants as being easier to implement, and as a useful tool at regional, municipal and local level, rather than on national level; those differences should be reflected in the guidance as well. In general, the top-down approach was better accepted to fit in a prospective HIA. The bottom-up approach is more complex to identify as directly applicable for decision making, but very useful for the evaluation and planning of several connected policies as well as putting health issues on agenda of all sectors. More information on the links to HIA as broader framework of assessment was noted as desirable to include.

Specific suggestion were formulated regarding the *aim and target users* of the guide that can be more clearly defined, making special emphasis on the appraisal phase of policy level HIA. Someone ask for a more detailed technical description of each steps, providing examples, as well as a guideline on how the final report should be presented considering the different stakeholders (policy makers, general public, etc.), acknowledged as a possible addition to the guide. It was suggested to provide a description on how to bridge the information gathered in the scoping and screening phases, with the characterization of the impact itself in the appraisal phase.

The *definition of target population* should be broadened, different population subgroups, should be described according to social class, gender and other axis of inequalities. *Latency* of policy impacts should also be taken into consideration. Concern was raised about the possibility that *quantification approaches*, although very important, might hide relevant health determinants and risk factors that modulate the final results of the impact of a policy on health. Participants agreed on the importance of the quantification process in providing more robust HIA outputs for policy makers. However, in many fields the scientific evidence available does not allow currently to move forward in this direction. It would be very useful to provide some information on how to proceed when the quantification is not possible (instructions on how to conduct qualitative assessment in a systematic way, description of sources of information, databases).

Cautions were raised by participants when discussing the comprehensiveness of the assessment. They agreed in *the limitations* of the risk assessment process, as not all the negative and positive health impacts can be assessed. The need for recommendations on how to *prioritize factors* (e.g. how many should be analyzed) was articulated by participants, along with the importance of strengthening analytic focus on *socio-economic determinants* and *vulnerable populations*.

All these issues require further practice based research. The developed RAPID guidance needs to be applied on different policies under different societal and policy making contexts and experience should be gathered and evaluated.

Regarding the context of risk assessment implementation and use, the decision makers participating in workshops mainly focused on differences and contradictions sometimes existing among national, regional or local strategies. Conflict of interests, political culture and economic influences were noted as the most important contextual factors that influence implementation and use of the guidance. As noted by a participant, models of health determinants (e.g. Dahlgreen & Whitehead model, Lalonde model) are not taken into consideration during decision making process in health departments of the municipalities. Even health department employees often lack basic knowledge concerning those aspects. It can be challenging for them to identify and describe health determinants and risk factors or to undertake a literature review. Existing local level procedures at the local level may hamper the application of health risk assessments as well.

As regards to professional communities, there is still an issue of poor knowledge about the difference between HIA, SEA and policy risk assessment, such questions should always be discussed at the beginning of any workshop. In some cases problems arise *in using quantification methods/tools* because of the limited expertise available in health risk assessment, lack of data, *difficulty in reaching consensus among specialists, interaction with politicians.* Although there is a theoretical possibility of using expertise in the decision making process there are *administrative obstacles* concerning indication of expert or institution, which would be preferred to support the policy making process. Participants agreed in the importance of institutionalizing health impact assessment by mandatory legislation across Europe, in which process the European Union could take a leading role along with HIA experts and research community.

The *consultation process* is a topic of interest. The participation of policy makers and citizens in the policy risk assessment was identified as an essential element throughout the whole process in order to ensure the acceptance and application of recommendations. However, a "real" participation of the civil society was visualized as a complex issue not easy to accomplish due to political conflicts. Participants suggested incorporating recommendations on how to overcome those barriers in the final guidance. Participants recommended extending the consultation around the guidance and its validation by the wider involvement of health and public policy makers, national public health agencies, non-health sectors, academic institutes, NGOs.

Closely linked, there is the issue of the different dissemination and communication strategies. The participants, as main barriers to promote RAPID guidance noted the limited knowledge regarding social determinants of health as well as low awareness on the use of impact assessment. Suggestions to overcome these challenges were focusing on the availability of detailed information on the RAPID case studies and guidance via Internet, and through publications, roundtables, workshops and conference presentations.

Use of sector-specific *communication strategies* as well as direct communication with relevant ministries, institutions, local health authorities and NGOs were recommended. Tailored dissemination of the results to risk assessors and impact assessment experts through professional societies and mailing lists were noted as of high importance.

Referred to this topic, the RAPID working group suggests RAPID guidance users to dedicate a specific attention to communication and participation, to understand if participation is necessary and its scope. Crucial elements to understand are, for example: is the policy controversial? Is there a risk connected to its implementation? It is to consider that the involvement of stakeholders implies a methodological and ethical commitment to transparency and protection of people (privacy, health, culture). In the recent period, several activities have been devoted to the relationship between scientific production and policy making. It is a controversial relation, and a specific attention is needed when those spheres of competencies and interests are closely connected. A first possible exercise, that is defining roles and competencies of stakeholders, is crucial. A second step can be the draft of a "context analysis", simply describing the situation, the expectations of each actor, the foreseen objectives, in order to share and agree about future development. Before starting the activities of risk assessment, it is possible in this way to discuss and understand many issues that can have an influence on the analysis and on future developments. Each actor can be further supported, for example the ERA ENVHEALTH network has developed a checklist for researcher, to facilitate the research results transfer to decision making (www.era-envhealth.eu).

References

Bianchi, F., & Cori, L. (2013). HIA in Italy. In J. Kemm (Ed.), *HIA – Past achievements, current understanding and future progress*. London: Oxford University Press.

Costa, G., Paci, E., & Ricciardi, W. (Eds.). (2011). United Italy, 150 years later: has Equity in Health and Health Care improved?. *Epidemiol Prev*, 35(5–6) suppl. 2, 1–136.

CSDH (WHO Commission on Social Determinants of Health). (2008). Closing the gap in a generation: Health equity through action on the social determinants of health. *Final report of the commission on Social Determinants of Health*. Geneva: World Health Organization.

Figueras, J., & McKee, M. (Eds.). (2012). *Health systems, health, wealth and societal well-being*. Maidenhead: Open University Press, MacGraw-Hill Education.

Kemm, J. (2013). *HIA – Past achievements, current understanding and future progress*. London: Oxford University Press.

Kobusch, A.-B., Fehr, R., & Serwe, H.-J. (Eds.). (1997). *Gesundheitsverträglichkeitsprüfung*. Baden-Baden: Grundlagen - Konzepte - Praxiserfahrungen. Nomos Verlagsgesellschaft.

L'Astorina, A. (2011). *Pisa meeting metaplan report*. Pisa: CNR Report.

Index

A

Ádám, B., 37–121, 131–191, 199–229
U.S. Agency for Toxic Substances and Disease
    Registry (ATSDR), 19

B

Barton, H., 185
Bhatia, R., 26, 27
Bianchi, F., 1–10
Boehlert, G.W., 51
Boldo, F., 66
Bolivar, J., 131–191
Bottom-up policy risk assessment
  asthma, Slovakia
    epidemiological approaches and
      designs, 155
    health determinants, 153–154
    health outcome, 152–153
    local environment plans, 156
    policy impact, 154–155
    prevalence data, 155
    risk factors, 153–154
  COPD, Slovenia
    health determinants, 148–150
    health outcome, 147–148
    policy impact, 150–151
    risk factors, 148–150
  cost-benefit analysis, 132
  factors, 131–132
  HIA method, 133
  life expectancy, Poland
    alcohol consumption, 182
    health determinants and risk factors,
      177–180
    health outcome, 176–177

    health promotion programs, 180–181
    National Health Fund, 181–182
    physical activity, 182
    smoking, 182
  liver cirrhosis, Slovak and Hungarian
    experience, 156, 158
    alcohol policy interventions, 163–166
    excessive alcohol consumption, 156,
      158–160
    health outcome description, 157
    Hepatitis B and C, 160–161
    horizontal interactions, 163
    inherited liver diseases, 162
    non-alcoholic fatty liver disease, 161
    non-alcoholic steatohepatitis, 161
    policy interventions, 156
    quantitative assessment, 162–163
    tobacco use and high blood
      pressure, 156
    toxic substances, 161–162
  methodological guidelines, 186–187
    checklist, 188–191
    cross-cutting issues, 187–188
    health determinants, 185–186
    health outcomes, 183–184
    risk factors, 184–185
  osteoporosis, Denmark
    health outcome, 168–170
    policy impacts, 175
    prevalance, 168
    risk factor and health determinants,
      170–175
  quantification approach, 133
  RAPID guidance, 133
  road traffic fatalities in Spain
    data collection, 139

Bottom-up policy risk assessment (*cont.*)
    direct and indirect costs, 134
    health determinants, 136–137
    health outcome, 134–136
    National Strategic Plan on Road Safety
      2005–2008, 138
    Penalty Point Driving License
      System, 138
    quantitative approach, 139
    risk factors, 136–137
    RTF reduction, 138–139
   road traffic injuries in German
    dose–response relationship, 146
    health determinants, 140–142
    health outcomes, 140
    injury reduction, 143
    limitations, methodological studies,
      146–147
    motorists, 139
    policy impacts, 142
    risk factors, 140–142
    speed cameras, 146
    speed control, 145–146
    speed enforcement detection
      devices, 142–143
    speed limits, 142–144
Brand, D.A., 69
Brower, M., 51, 52

C
Chereches, R., 37–121
Cocarta, D.M., 52
Coffman, S., 78, 79
Cole, B.L., 26, 27
Coles, R.W., 51, 52
Cori, L., 233–247, 249–262
Corrao, G., 161

D
Danish energy policy 2008–2020
    fossil fuels, 50
    GHG emission reduction, 49
    health and risk factor
      determinants, 51–52
    health impact assessment, 50
    health outcomes, 52–55
    initiatives, 50
Davenport, C., 26
Dincer, I., 51, 52
Disability-Adjusted Life Years (DALY)
    BoD-study, 237
    health outcome, 240

    non-communicable diseases, 238
    population rate, 237
Dynamic Modeling for Health
    Impact Assessment (DYNAMO-
    HIA), 226, 227

E
EC Health strategy assessment
    DALY (*see* Disability-Adjusted Life Years
      (DALY))
    health determinants, 245–247
    HLY, 235–236
    objectives, 243–245
    potential health gain, 241–242
    RAPID guidance tool, 234–235
    risk factors, 240–241
Environmental impact assessment (EIA),
    26–27
Epidemiological health risk assessment
    approach, 23–24

F
Fehr, R., 37–121, 131–191, 199–229
Fletcher, W.J., 22
Framework convention on tobacco control
    (FCTC), 42

G
Gandini, S., 46
Gekas, V., 52
Geremek, M., 1–10, 131–191
Grant, M., 185
Gras, M.E., 136
Grass, S.W., 51, 52
Greenhalgh, R., 52
Greenland, S., 23
Grohmann, J., 131–191
Guliš, G., 1–10, 37–121, 233–247, 249–262

H
Halliburton, S.S., 84
Harris, E., 26, 28
Harris-Roxas, B., 26, 28
Health and Environment Integrated
    Methodology and Toolbox for
    Scenario Assessment (HEIMTSA),
    226, 227
Health impact assessment (HIA), 25
    categorization and forms
      criteria, 25

participatory approach, 26
procedural approach, 26–27
quantitative/analytic approach, 26
outputs, 28–29
procedure
    assessment of impacts, 29
    monitoring and evaluation, 28
    reporting to decision-makers, 28
    scoping, 28
    screening, 28
Health in all policies (HiAP), 4–5
Healthy Life Years (HLY), 235–236
Healthy public policy, 4
    behavioral risks, 13
    design and implementation, 14
    European Union, 15
    health determinants, 14
    health impact assessment (*see* Health
        impact assessment (HIA))
    health services, 13
    public health evolution, 13
    risk assessment (*see* Risk assessment)
Higgins, C., 132
Hungarian anti-smoking policy
    health and risk factor determinants, 46
        air quality, 44
        built environment and land use, 45
        economic impact, 44–45
        housing and working conditions, 45
        social contacts and recreation, 45
        tobacco smoking, 43–44
    health outcomes, 49
        active smoking, 46–47
        passive smoking, 47–48
    policy description, 41–43
    political decision-makers, 41

I
Icks, A., 60
Impact assessment (IA), 8–9. *See also* Health
    impact assessment (HIA)
Influenza Preparedness Plan of Romania
    data, 99
    health and risk factor determinants
        community infection control, 101
        general personal hygiene, 101
        horizontal interactions, 104
        pandemic influenza vaccination rate,
            103
        proactive school closure, 102–103
        public and private school systems,
            101–102
        quantification-related assessment, 104

racial/ethnic minority groups, 103–104
        social distancing and quarantining, 101
        travel and trade restrictions, 101
    health outcomes, 105–107
    policy description
        AH1N1 virus, 99–100
        case study, 99
        day care and school settings, 100–101
        ECDC reports and WHO guidelines, 99
        vaccination, 100
Integrated Assessment of Health Risks of
    Environmental Stressors in Europe
    (INTARESE), 226, 227

J
Jaakkola, J.K., 52
Jaakkola, M.S., 52
Jenkins, B.M., 51, 52
Joffe, M., 26, 136

K
Kallayova, D., 131–191
Kemm, J., 9, 26, 229, 254
Kingdon, J.D., 7
Kobza, J., 1–10, 37–121, 131–191, 249–262
Kollárová, J., 1–10, 37–121, 131–191,
    249–262
Kowalska, M., 66
Kræmer, S.R.J., 131–191
Kvakova, M., 131–191

L
Lalonde, M., 14, 37
Lhachimi, S.K., 226
Linzalone, N., 37–121
Lithuanian National Road Safety Program
    health determinants
        behavioral determinants, 82–83
        biological determinants, 82
        environmental determinants, 83
        socioeconomic factors, 83
    health outcomes, 84–85
    policy description, 80–82
    road traffic injuries, 80
Lock, K., 154
Lunevicius, R., 83

M
Mahoney, M., 26
Majdan, M., 37–121

Maldonado, G., 23
Martin-Olmedo, P., 13–32, 131–191, 199–229
McKee, M., 154
Mekel, O., 13–32, 37–121, 131–191, 199–229,
  233–247
Metcalfe, O., 132
Mindell, J.S., 26, 132
Mochungong, P., 37–121
Molnár, A., 1–10, 37–121, 131–191, 249–262
Murray, C.J., 23

N
National Environmental Policy Act (NEPA),
  16
North Rhine-Westphalia Housing Subsidy
    Program 2010
  health and risk factor determinants
    endogenous/personal risk factors,
      58–59
    exposure assessment, 59
    housing, 58
  health outcomes
    fall-related injuries, 59–60
    poor housing conditions, 59
    quantification-related assessment,
      60–61
  policy description
    Germany and NRW, 56–57
    policy selection, 56
    WoFP objectives, 57–58

O
Otorepec, P., 37–121, 131–191

P
Pastuszka, J.S, 37–121
Policy evaluation, 30–31
Political decision making
  models
    normative models, 6
    positive models, 6–7
    rational model, 5
  RAPID (*see* RAPID national workshops)
Potential impact fraction (PIF), 23
Public health
  decision making process and policy, 3
  definition, 1
  European perspective, 2
  functions, 2
  health threats and epidemics, 2
  operations, 3–4

policy making models
  normative models, 6
  positive models, 6–7
  rational model, 5

Q
Quantitative approach, health risk assessment
  causal attribution, health potentials,
    203–204
  causal web/web, 202–203
  exposure and risk assessment
    characterization, 212–214
    chemical hazards, 205
    CRA approach, 205
    environmental health paradigm, 206
    exposure/dose–response curves,
      211–212
    hazard identification, 207
    ingestion exposure, 207–208
    inhalation and dermal exposure,
      207–208
    measurements, 209–211
    potential exposure pathways, 208
    US EPA, 205
  health determinants and risk factors,
    201–202
  health impact tools, 226–228
  individual health and disease, 200
  population health, 200–201
  top-down RAPID Guidance, 215–220

R
Rahman, M.H., 83
Ramos, P., 84
RAPID national workshops
  discussion and participants opinions
    administrative obstacles, 261
    aim and target users, 260
    communication strategies, 261
    consultation process, 261
    health determinants and risk factors, 259
    political culture and economic
      influences, 260–261
    quantification process, 260
    RAPID guidance structure, 259–260
    risk assessment limitations, 260
    stakeholders, 262
    terminology, 258–259
  national workshops, 249–250
  organization
    Denmark, 253
    European Union, 252–253

evaluation and outcome format, 251
Germany, 252
health experts, 251
HIA procedure, 253–254
Italy, 252
Metaplan technique, 251
objectives, 250
Poland, 254–255
preparatory survey, 251–252
Slovakia, 253
Spain, 252–253
workshops experience
contextual issues, 258
dissemination and information, 256
interactive discussion session, 256
language issue, 256
participants, 256
policy health risk approach, 258
policy makers, 257–258
programme formats, 255
review, 257
Rehm, J., 162, 225
Risk assessment, 7–8
dose–response assessment, 17
Environmental Protection Agency, 16–17
exposure assessment, 17–18
hazard identification, 17
hazardous agent, 15–16
independency, 18
National Environmental Policy Act, 16
National Research Council (NRC), 17
NRC's Science and decisions, 24–25
outputs
probabilistic approach, 22–23
qualitative risk assessments outputs, 22
quantitative risk assessments outputs, 22
physical environment, 16
policies and strategies
ATSDR, 19
food safety, 19–21
International Programme on Chemical
Safety (IPCS), 19
risk management, 20–21
risk profile, 21
risk characterization, 18
scientific judgments and policy options, 18
terminology and approach, 16
Road traffic fatalities (RTF) in Spain
data collection, 139
direct and indirect costs, 134
health determinants, 136–137
health outcome, 134–136
National Strategic Plan on Road Safety
2005–2008, 138

Penalty Point Driving License System, 138
quantitative approach, 139
risk factors, 136–137
RTF reduction, 138–139
Road traffic injuries (RTI), German
dose–response relationship, 146
health determinants, 140–142
health outcomes, 140
injury reduction, 143
limitations, methodological studies,
146–147
motorists, 139
policy measures, 142
risk factors, 140–142
speed cameras, 146
speed control, 145–146
speed enforcement detection devices,
142–143
speed limits, 142–144
Road Traffic Legislation in Slovakia
health determinants
behavioral determinants, 76
environmental determinants, 75–76
socioeconomic determinants, 75
health outcomes, 77–79
policy description, 74–75
risk factors, 76–77
Rosen, M.A., 51

S
Schoenhagen, P., 84
Schwartz, J., 213
Seifert, H., 52
Seto, E., 26, 27
Sierig, S., 37–121, 233–247
Slovak National Action Plan on alcohol
problems
health determinants
behavioral determinants, 69
health care, 71
social class, 71
health outcomes, 72–73
interventions, 70
policy description, 68–69
risk factors, 71–72
state health policy, 68
Slovenian National strategy on wine
production
health determinants
behavioral and personal determinants,
88
environmental determinants, 87
exposed groups, 89

Slovenian National strategy on wine
    production (*cont.*)
  horizontal interactions, 89
  socioeconomic determinants, 87–88
  health outcomes, 89–91
  policy description, 86–87
Speight, J.G., 51, 52

T
Taylor, I., 51
Taylor, J., 52
Thompson, D.C., 78
Top-down policy risk assessment
  checklist for, 118–121
  Danish energy policy 2008–2020
    fossil fuels, 50
    GHG emission reduction, 49
    health and risk factors
        determinants, 51–52
    health impact assessment, 50
    health outcomes, 52–55
    initiatives, 50
  guidance
    cross-level issues, 116–118
    health determinants, 111–113
    health outcomes, 115–116
    horizontal interrelations, 117
    latency of effects, 118
    policy, 108–111
    quantitative assessment, 116–117
    risk factors, 113–114
    transparency, 117
    uncertainty, 117–118
  Hungarian anti-smoking policy
    health and risk factors determinants,
        44–46
    health outcomes, 46–49
    policy description, 41–43
    political decision-makers, 41
  Influenza Preparedness Plan of Romania
    AH1N1 virus, 99–100
    case study, 99
    data, 99
    day care and school settings, 100–101
    ECDC reports and WHO
        guidelines, 99
    health and risk factors determinants,
        101–104
    health outcomes, 105–107
    vaccination, 100
  Lithuanian National Road
        Safety Program

  behavioral determinants, 82–83
  biological determinants, 82
  environmental determinants, 83
  health outcomes, 84–85
  policy description, 80–82
  road traffic injuries, 80
  socioeconomic factors, 83
North Rhine-Westphalia Housing Subsidy
      Program 2010
  health and risk factor determinants,
      58–59
  health outcomes, 59–61
  policy description, 56–58
particulate matter standards in Poland
  exposure-effect relationships, 62–63
  health determinants, 64–65
  health outcomes, 65–66
  policy description, 63–64
  risk factors, 65
  total suspended particles, 62
radioprotection policy, Italy
  context and aims, 92–93
  CT scans, 92
  ethical issues, 98
  health and risk factor determinants,
      94–97
  health outcomes, 97
  imaging techniques, 91–92
  policy description, 93–94
Road Traffic Legislation in Slovakia
  behavioral determinants, 76
  environmental determinants, 75–76
  health outcomes, 77–79
  policy description, 74–75
  risk factors, 76–77
  socioeconomic determinants, 75
Slovak National Action Plan on alcohol
      problems
  behavioral determinants, 69
  health care, 71
  health outcomes, 72–73
  interventions, 70
  policy description, 68–69
  risk factors, 71–72
  social class, 71
  state health policy, 68
Slovenian National Strategy on wine
      production
  behavioral and personal
      determinants, 88
  environmental determinants, 87
  exposed groups, 89
  health outcomes, 89–91

    horizontal interactions, 89
    policy description, 86–87
    socioeconomic determinants, 87–88
Tsoutsos, T., 51, 52

V
Veerman, J.L., 26, 27, 214, 215, 229

W
Wcisło, E., 66
Werham, A., 26

Z
Zejda, J.E., 66
Zurlyte, I., 1–10, 37–121

Printed in the United States
By Bookmasters